HEPATOCELLULAR CARCINOMA - FUTURE OUTLOOK

Edited by **Ahmed O. Kaseb**

Hepatocellular Carcinoma - Future Outlook
http://dx.doi.org/10.5772/50274
Edited by Ahmed O. Kaseb

Contributors

Dengfu Yao, Rafik Ghobrial, Emad Asham, Howard Monsour, Hojjat Ahmadzadehfar, Amir Sabet, Hans Jürgen Biersack, Bruno C. Odisio, Ravi Murthy, Ana Martinelli, Andraza Texeira, Zhou Yuan, Biswajit Mukherjee, Toshitsugu Nakamura, Francisco J. Vizoso, Noemi Eiro, Koichi Matsuzaki, Miki Murata, Alessandro Uzzau, Maria Laura Pertoldeo, Giorgio Soardo, Claudio Avellini, Vittorio Cherchi, Serena Bertozzi, Yasunobu Matsuda, Daniela Cesselli, Francesca Morassi, Valerio Barghini, Debora Donnini, Ahmed Kaseb, Laura M. Kulik

Published by InTech
Janeza Trdine 9, 51000 Rijeka, Croatia

Publishing Process Manager Sandra Bakic
Technical Editor InTech DTP team
Cover InTech Design team

Additional hard copies can be obtained from orders@intechopen.com

Hepatocellular Carcinoma - Future Outlook, Edited by Ahmed O. Kaseb
p. cm.
ISBN 978-953-51-1202-0

For EU product safety concerns:
IN TECH d.o.o., Prolaz Marije Krucifikse Kozulić 3, 51000 Rijeka, Croatia,
info@intechopen.com or visit our website at intechopen.com.

Meet the editor

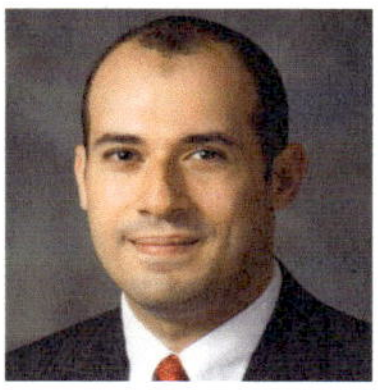

Dr. Ahmed Kaseb is an Associate Professor and program director of Hepatocellular Carcinoma (HCC) at The University of Texas MD Anderson Cancer Center, Houston, Texas, USA. Dr. Kaseb received his medical degree from Cairo University, and worked at University of Michigan, and Wayne State University and Henry Ford Hospital, in Detroit, Michigan. Dr. Kaseb has contributed greatly to the understanding of HCC interdisciplinary therapies and molecular staging, and received funding for several projects and clinical trials. Dr. Kaseb serves as an Editor and reviewer for several international journals, and has received several national and international awards throughout his career. Dr. Kaseb has authored and co-authored over 50 papers and book chapters.

Contents

Preface IX

Chapter 1 **Role of Alleles and Genotypes of Polymorphisms of IL-18 (-607 C/A; and -137 C/G), IFN-γ (+874 A/T) and TNF-α (-238 A/G and -308 A/G) and HLA-G Genes in the Susceptibility of Hepatocellular Carcinoma 1**
Andreza Correa Teixeira, Ana de Lourdes Candolo Martinelli and Eduardo Antonio Donadi

Chapter 2 **Liver Transplantation for Hepatocellular Carcinoma 21**
Emad H. Asham, Howard Mansour and Mark Ghobrial

Chapter 3 **Radioembolization for the Treatment of Unresectable Hepatocellular Carcinoma 41**
Hojjat Ahmadzadehfar, Amir Sabet and Hans Jürgen Biersack

Chapter 4 **Image-Guided Therapies for Hepatocellular Carcinoma in Hepatocelluar Carcinoma — Future Outlook 63**
Bruno C. Odisio, Ravi Murthy and Michael J. Wallace

Chapter 5 **Neoadjuvant Chemotherapy for Hepatocellular Carcinoma 81**
Xin-yu Huang, Qi Zheng and Zhou Yuan

Chapter 6 **Targets and Approaches to Control Hepatocellular Carcinoma in Future 97**
Mukherjee Biswajit, Hossain Chowdhury Mobaswar , Bhattacharya Sanchari and Shampa Ghosh

Chapter 7 **Early Chronic Inflammation and Subsequent Somatic Mutations Shift Phospho-Smad3 Signaling from Tumor-Suppression to Fibro-Carcinogenesis in Human Chronic Liver Diseases 113**
Miki Murata, Katsunori Yoshida and Koichi Matsuzaki

Chapter 8 **Surgical Treatment Strategies and Prognosis of Hepatocellular Carcinoma 143**
Alessandro Uzzau, Maria Laura Pertoldeo, Vittorio Cherchi, Serena Bertozzi, Claudio Avellini and Giorgio Soardo

Chapter 9 **Conditions that Predispose to the Development of HCC: The Role of Tumor Associated Fibroblasts and of microRNA 173**
C. Avellini, D. Cesselli, A.P. Beltrami, M. Orsaria, S. Marzinotto, F. Morassi and S. Uzzau

Chapter 10 **Signs and Symptoms 197**
Valerio Barghini, Debora Donnini, Alessandro Uzzau and Giorgio Soardo

Chapter 11 **Sorafenib in the Continuum of Care for Hepatocellular Carcinoma: Challenges in Defining Optimal Practice 217**
Ahmed O. Kaseb and Laura M. Kulik

Chapter 12 **Sorafenib-Inhibited Signaling: Emerging Evidence of RAF-Independent Pathways as Potential Therapeutic Targets in Hepatocellular Carcinoma 239**
Yasunobu Matsuda, Toshifumi Wakai, Masayuki Kubota, Mami Osawa and Shun Fujimaki

Chapter 13 **Insulin-Like Growth Factor-II: Molecular-Targeted Therapy for Hepatocellular Carcinoma 255**
Min Yao, Li Wang, Meijuan Yan, Xiaodi Yan and Dengfu Yao

Chapter 14 **Simultaneous Changes in Expression of Bile Canalicular CD10 and Sinusoidal CD105 (Endoglin) in Chronic Hepatitis and Liver Cirrhosis 281**
Toshitsugu Nakamura

Chapter 15 **Hepatocellular Carcinoma, Steroid Hormones and Metalloproteases 295**
Noemí Eiró, Belen Fernandez-Garcia, Antonio Altadill, Luis O. González and Francisco J. Vizoso

Preface

Liver cancer is the fifth most frequently diagnosed cancer in men worldwide, and is the second leading cause of cancer-related death. Hepatocellular carcinoma (HCC) is the most common type of primary liver cancers, and has unique age, sex, and geographic distributions that are most likely determined by specific etiologic factors. HCC is potentially curable by surgical resection and liver transplantation. However, the majority of patients present with unresectable, advanced-stage disease, which is most commonly accompanied by severe background liver disease. Therefore, management of HCC is complicated by its highly variable biologic behavior and the frequent coexistence of underlying liver disease in affected patients. Hence, the care of patients with HCC has long been based upon a multidisciplinary approach, which involves experts from multiple specialties collaborating from the earliest stages of treatment planning to ensure personalizing the treatment for each individual patient. Thus, our book will describe not just diagnosis and treatment of HCC, but also the entire range of existing and evolving interdisciplinary surgical, local and systemic therapies for this complex disease.

Furthermore, the demonstration of improved patient outcome in clinical trials of targeted agents in this very challenging malignancy has generated renewed enthusiasm in the field which led to a wide expansion of clinical research efforts in all aspects of HCC management. However, clinical development of targeted therapy in HCC suffers from several handicaps including lack of effective ways of choosing patients who are likely to respond, and monitoring biologic activity as measured by plasma and tissue biomarkers or imaging-based biomarkers to assess tumor response. Therefore, we have chosen to present some relevant literature reviews and research studies related to recent research advances in HCC.

We are very grateful for the dedication and work of all authors in putting together this interdisciplinary collection of the clinical and research knowledge on the management of HCC, and for their steadfast efforts in bringing this book to life.

We believe that this description of HCC multidisciplinary care will be a valuable resource for physicians and researchers from multiple specialties and in different practice settings and an example for other multidisciplinary endeavors.

Dr. Ahmed O. Kaseb
Assistant Professor, Department of Gastrointestinal (GI) Medical Oncology,
Division of Cancer Medicine, The University of Texas,
Anderson Cancer Center, Houston, USA

Chapter 1

Role of Alleles and Genotypes of Polymorphisms of IL-18 (-607 C/A; and -137 C/G), IFN-γ (+874 A/T) and TNF-α (-238 A/G and -308 A/G) and HLA-G Genes in the Susceptibility of Hepatocellular Carcinoma

Andreza Correa Teixeira,
Ana de Lourdes Candolo Martinelli and
Eduardo Antonio Donadi

Additional information is available at the end of the chapter

http://dx.doi.org/10.5772/56350

1. Introduction

Hepatocellular carcinoma (HCC) is a primary malignant tumor of the liver which represents a serious public health problem in the world, corresponding to the fifth more frequent malignant neoplasia among men, the eighth among women, and the third cause of cancer death in the world [1,2]. Seventy to ninety percent of HCC cases occur in patients with cirrhosis or with chronic liver disease, with cell injury followed by regeneration mediated by the immune response playing an important role in hepatocarcinogenesis [3].

In Brazil, a national survey to update HCC epidemiology and clinical profile of patients with HCC (29 centers, with 1,405 patients diagnosed with HCC from 2004 to 2009) showed that the median age at diagnosis was 59 years (1–92 years old; 78% male) and 98% of the patients had cirrhosis (1279/1308), with the hepatitis C virus being the main etiology (54%), followed by hepatitis B virus (16%) and alcohol (14%). In Southeastern and Southern Brazil, hepatitis C virus accounted for over 55% of cases. In the Northeast and North, hepatitis C virus accounted for less than 50%, and hepatitis B virus accounted for 22–25% of cases [4]. In Ribeirão Preto, Southeastern Brazil, the clinical characteristics of 130 patients with HCC attended at the University Hospital of the Faculty of Medicine of Ribeirao Preto, University of São Paulo (HCFMRP-USP) was revised. The mean (± SD) age at the time of HCC diagnosis was 55.6±11.2 years, with 81.5% of them being males. Cirrhosis was present in 89.2% of cases, with 53.4% of the patients being ChildPugh A; chronic hepatitis B or C without cirrhosis was detected in 3.2%, nonalcoholic steatohepatitis (NASH) in 3.8%, and a normal liver in 3.8% [5].

The human major histocompatibility complex (MHC) represents a set of genes responsible for coding histocompatibility molecules. It is a high density region [3.6 Mb DNA) located on the short arm of chromosome 6, region 6p21.3, which contains more than 200 genes grouped into three classes denoted class I, II and III. Class I genes (classic or class Ia) code for the classic histocompatibility molecules HLA-A, B and C; class II genes code for the histocompatibility molecules HLA-DR, DQ and DP, and class III genes, although included in the MHC, do not code for histocompatibility molecules. Among class I genes, there are also those denoted non-classic or class Ib, which code for the non-classic histocompatibility molecules HLA-E, F and G [6].

HLA-G is a class I non-classic HLA gene consisting of eight exons and seven introns with a stop codon in exon 6 (exon 7 is always absent from mature mRNA and, due to the stop codon in exon 6, exon 8 is not translated), a 5' promoter region and a 3' untranslated region (3'UTR) [7,8]. The characteristics of *HLA-G* are: low polymorphism, alternative splicing in the primary transcript that codes for seven protein isoforms, limited distribution in normal tissues, and immunsuppressive properties [9]. Of the seven proteins coded by the *HLA-G* gene, four are linked to the membrane (HLA-G1 to HLA-G4) and three are soluble (HLA-G5 to HLA-G7). The HLA-G1 and HLA-G5 proteins are the main isoforms described in healthy issues such as trophoblast, thymus, cornea, and erythroid and endothelial precursors. On the other hand, the expression of *HLA-G* can be induced in pathological situations such as autoimmune and inflammatory diseases, viral infections, cancer, and transplantation. *HLA-G* exerts inhibitory activity by binding to inhibitory receptors denoted immunoglobulin-like transcript (ILT)-2 and ILT-4, which are expressed by lymphoid and myeloid cells and by myeloid cells only, respectively, and killer immunoglobulin-like (KIR)2DL4 receptor, present only in natural killer cells [9].

Thus far, 47 alleles have been attributed to the *HLA-G* gene, which code for 15 distinct functional proteins with all isoforms (*HLA-G**01:01, *01:02, *01:03, *01:04, *01:06, *01:07, *01:08, *01:09, *01:10, *01:11, *01:12, *01:14, *01:15, *01:16, and *01:17) and truncated (G*01:05N allele) or no proteins at all (G*01:13N allele). Polymorphic sites are observed in the coding and non-coding regions. The promoter and 3′UTR regions of *HLA-G* are highly polymorphic, with the variations in the 3′UTR being associated with the levels of *HLA-G* expression. Two main polymorphic sites were identified in the 3′UTR: a 14bp insertion/deletion, in which the insertion has been associated with reduced levels of HLA-G, and the presence of guanine at position +3142, which increases the affinity of specific microRNAs for *HLA-G* mRNA, reducing the expression of HLA-G [8,10].

The expression of *HLA-G* is frequently detected in malignant tumors of various origins and in some situations has been significantly correlated with tumor size, degree of invasion, metastasis, clinical stages of the disease, and mortality [11,12]. Regarding HCC, few studies evaluating the role of alleles and genotypes of *HLA-G* polymorphism are available in the literature, and evolve different population. Jiang et al, studying a Chinese population showed that the heterozygote and the 14bp II homozygote confer a lower risk of HCC compared with

14bp DD, and that the associations were stronger in the hepatitis B-positive than the hepatitis B-negative population [13] Zhang et al, examining fifteen single-nucleotide polymorphisms (SNPs) in the non-classical class I alleles, found that the SNPs rs17875380, rs41557518, rs114465251, and rs115492845 were associated with susceptibility to chronic hepatitis B infection or HCC, and HLA-F*01:04, HLA-G*01:05N, and HLA-E*01:01 were associated with hepatitis B or hepatitis B with HCC [14].

In general, the inflammatory response mediated by the immune system is beneficial to the host; however, when tissue homeostasis is chronically affected the interactions between innate and adaptive immune responses may be deregulated, culminating with chronic inflammation, excessive tissue remodeling, loss of tissue architecture, apoptosis/necrosis and oxidative stress which, under certain circumstances, may increase the risk of tumor development [15]. The cytokines are responsible for the regulation of growth differentiation and activation of immune cells. The ability to produce cytokines by an individual is influenced by genetic components that have been attributed to molecular mechanisms, including variations in the transcription, translation and secretion pathways [16].

2. Problem statement

Over the last years, regarding HCC, few studies evaluating the role of alleles and genotypes of *HLA-G* polymorphism are available in the literature, and included diverse patient populations. Moreover, previous studies have concentrated on cytokine promoters, encouraged by the identification of a series of SNPs [17]. However, the relation of these polymorphisms with susceptibility to HCC or disease severity has not been clarified.

Application area

Immune response and carcinogenesis

Research course

Alleles and genotypes of cytokines polymorphisms and 14bp of HLA-G gene in HCC patients.

3. Method and patients

We evaluated, in a Brazilian cohort, the association of alleles and genotypes of the 14bp insertion/deletion polymorphism of the *HLA-G* gene, and alleles and genotypes of polymorphisms of genes *IL-18* (-607 C/A; rs1946518 and -137 C/G; rs187238), *IFN-γ* (+874 A/T; rs62559044) and *TNF-α* (-238 A/G; rs361525 and -308 A/G; rs1800629) with susceptibility to HCC and with the type of tumor presentation (infiltrative diffuse, multinodular and uninodular), with nodule size (>10 cm, 5-10 cm and <5 cm), with the Milan criteria (fulfills or does not fulfill), the evaluation of metastasis (present or absent), and the histological classification of the tumor (Edmondson-Steiner Classification) [18,19, 20,21].

This was a retrospective cross-sectional study conducted on 109 patients (89 men) with mean age 55.8±11.4 years for the 14bp insertion/deletion polymorphism of the *HLA-G* gene, and 112 consecutive patients [Mean (±SD) age was 55.6±11.2 years, and 81.5% were males] for the polymorphisms of genes *IL-18* (-607 C/A; rs1946518 and -137 C/G; rs187238), *IFN-γ* (+874 A/T; rs62559044) and *TNF-α* (-238 A/G; rs361525 and -308 A/G; rs1800629) followed up from 2001 to 2009 at the Focal Hepatic Injuries Outpatient Clinic of the Faculty of Medicine of Ribeirão Preto, University of São Paulo (HCFMRP-USP). The study was approved by the Research Ethics Committee of HCFMRP-USP. Individuals of both genders who fulfilled the following criteria were included in the study: a) diagnosis of HCC defined by the Barcelona 2000 criteria [22] for the diagnoses performed up to 2006 and according to the recommendations of the American Association for the Study of Liver Disease (AASLD) [23] for the diagnoses performed since 2007; b) with DNA stored in the Biological Sample Bank of the Laboratory of Gastroenterology, Department of Internal Medicine. Exclusion criteria were patients with focal hepatic injuries other than HCC according to the Barcelona 2000 criteria and the recommendations of the AASLD and patients with other concomitant neoplasias.

The evaluation of the severity of HCC was based on: a) tumor presentation (uninodular, multinodular or diffuse infiltrative); b) nodule size (<5 cm, 5-10 cm or >10 cm); c) Milan criteria (fulfills or does not fulfill); d) metastasis (present or absent); e) histological classification according to Edmondson & Steiner, 1954 (grades I, II, III or IV) [24].

A total of 202 healthy individuals (56 females and 146 males) with a mean age (±SD) of 33.3±8.3 years and from the same geographic region as the patients studied were used as controls for the evaluation of the frequency of 14bp, *IL-18, IFN-γ* and *TNF-α* alleles and genotypes.

For the determination of the 14bp insertion/deletion, IL-18 (-607 C/A; rs1946518 and -137 C/G; rs187238), IFN-γ (+874 A/T; rs62559044) and TNF-α (-238 A/G; rs361525 and -308 A/G; rs1800629) genotypes, we first extracted genomic DNA from peripheral leukocytes by the salting out technique [25]. The HLA-G 14bp insertion/deletion genotypes at exon 8 of the HLA-G locus was analyzed as described: 200ng of genomic DNA were amplified in a 25mL reaction mixture containing 0.20mM dNTP (Invitrogen, Carlsbad, CA), 0.2mM of each primer, 0.5U Taq DNA polymerase (Invitrogen, Carlsbad, CA), 1.5mM MgCl2 and a 1x PCR buffer (0.2M Tris–HCl, pH 8.5; 0.5M KCl). After an initial denaturation step at 94°C for 5 minutes, samples were submitted to 30 additional cycles at 94°C for 45 seconds, 56°C for 45 seconds and 72°C for 1 minute, with a final extension cycle at 72°C for 7 minutes with 5′-TGTGAAA-CAGCTGCCCTGTG-3′ as the forward primer and 5′-AAGGAATGCAGTTCAGCATGA-3′ as the reverse primer [26,27]. After DNA amplification by PCR, the reaction products were submitted to 10% polyacrylamide gel electrophoresis under non-denaturing conditions followed by silver impregnation. The presence of 345 bp fragments corresponded to the deletion allele, while the 359 bp fragment corresponded to the 14bp insertion allele.

The alleles and genotypes of *IL-18* (-607 C/A; rs1946518 and -137 C/G; rs187238), *IFN-γ* (+874 A/T; rs62559044) and *TNF-α* (-238 A/G; rs361525 and -308 A/G; rs1800629) polymorphisms were analyzed by the polymerase chain reaction using allele-specific primers (PCR-SSP) (Table 1). For SNP *IL-18* −607, a generic reverse primer 5′-TAACCTCATTCAGG

SNP	Primer	Sequence (5'-3')
IL-18 -607 C/A	*IL-18* 607.2	TAACCTCATTCAGGACTTCC
	IL-18 607C	GTTGCAGAAAGTGTAAAAATTATTAC
	IL-18 607A	GTTGCAGAAAGTGTAAAAATTATTAA
	HGBA.S	CGGTATTTGGAGGTCAGCAC
	HGBA.A	CCCACCACCAAGACCTACTT
IL-18 -137 C/G	*IL-18* 137.2	AGGAGGGCAAAATGCACTGG
	IL-18 137C	CCCCAACTTTTACGGAAGAAAAC
	IL-18 137G	CCCCAACTTTTACGGAAGAAAAG
	HGBA.S	CGGTATTTGGAGGTCAGCAC
	HGBA.A	CCCACCACCAAGACCTACTT
IFN-γ +874 A/T	*IFN-γ* 874 *IFN-γ* 874 T *IFN-γ* 874 A	TCAACAAAGCTGATACTCCA TTCTTACAACACAAAATCAAATCT TTCTTACAACACAAAATCAAATCA
	GH 1	GCCTTCCCAACCATTCCCTTA
	GH 2	TCACGGATTTCTGTTGTGTTTC
TNF-α -238 A/G	TNF 238 UP	AGGCAATAGGTTTTGAGGGCCAT
	TNFAS238G	CCCCATCCTCCCTGCTCC
	TNFAS238A	TCCCCATCCTCCCTGCTCT
	HGBA.S	CGGTATTTGGAGGTCAGCAC
	HGBA.A	CCCACCACCAAGACCTACTT
TNF-α -308 A/G	TNFAA 308.2	CAGCGGAAAACTTCCTTGGT
	TNFAS 308G	ATAGGTTTTGAGGGGCATGG
	TNFAS 308A	ATAGGTTTTGAGGGGCATGA
	HGBA.S	CGGTATTTGGAGGTCAGCAC
	HGBA.A	CCCACCACCAAGACCTACTT

IL-18: interleukin-18; *IFN-γ*: interferon-gamma; *TNF-α:* tumor necrosis factor-alpha; HGBA.S and HGBA.A: human hemoglobin; GH1 and GH2: human growth hormone.

Table 1. Primers for the detection of single nucleotide polymorphisms (SNPs) of genes IL-18 (-607 C/A and -137 C/G), IFN-γ (+874 A/T) and TNF-α (-238 A/G and -308 A/G).

ACTTCC-3′ and two allele-specific forward primers (5′-GT TGCAGAAAGTGTAAAAAT-TATTAC-3′ and 5′-GTTGCAG AAAGTGTAAAAATTATTAA-3′) were used to amplify a 196-bp product. For SNP *IL-18* −137, a common reverse primer 5′-AGGAGGGCAAAATG-CACTGG-3′ and two allele-specific forward primers (5′-CCCCAACTTTTACGGAAG AAAAG-3′ and 5′-CCCCAACTTTTACGGAAGAAAAC-3′) were used to amplify a 261-

bp product. An internal positive amplification control was performed using the primers 5′-CG GTATTTGGAGGTCAGCAC-3′ and 5′-CCCACCACCAAGA CCTACTT-3′, which are specific for the human hemoglobin genes. The reactions were performed in a final volume of 10μL containing 200ng of genomic DNA, 3pmol of each primer (the generic one and a specific one), 2pmol of each control primer, 0.25mM dNTP (Pharmacia Biotech, Paris, France), 1.5mM MgCl2, 0.75U of Taq DNA poly- merase (Invitrogen, Carlsbad, CA), and 1× PCR buffer (0.2 M Tris – HCl, pH 8.5, 0.5 M KCl). The cyclingconditions were 3min at 94°C, followed by seven cycles of 20s at 94°C, 40s at 64°C for *IL18* -607 or 60s at 68°C for *IL18* -137 and 40s at 72°C and 25 cycles of 20s at 94°C, 40s at 57°C for *IL18* -607 or 20s at 62°C for *IL18* -137 and 40s at 72°C, and final stage of 5min at 72°C [9]. For the *TNF-α* (-238 and -308) and *IFN-γ* +874 specific amplification, the primers were identical to those previously described [28,29]. All amplification products were visualized using 10% non-denaturing polyacrylamide gel electrophoresis (PAGE) followed by silver staining.

For statistical analysis, the allele and genotype frequencies were calculated by the direct count method in all groups. Adherence of genotypic proportions to Hardy-Weinberg expectations was determined by the exact test of Guo and Thompson [30] using the GENEPOP software v. 4.0.10. The presence of a significant association between polymorphisms of the same gene was evaluated by a likelihood ratio test of probability of linkage disequilibrium using the ARLEQUIN software, v. 3.1 [31]. If a positive association was detected, but the gameteic phase was unknown, the PHASE (v. 2 package) [32] and EM algorithms [33] were used to reconstruct the TNF or IL haplotypes. Allele, genotype and haplotype frequencies were compared by the two-tailed Fisher exact test using the GraphPad InStat 3.06 software, which was also used to estimate the odds ratio (OR) and its 95% confidence interval (95%CI). The level of significance was set at $P<0.05$.

4. Results

Cirrhosis was observed in 89% of the patients, and major underlying causes included: hepatitis C (35%), alcohol plus hepatitis C (25%), alcohol (18%), hepatitis B (9%), alcohol plus hepatitis B (4%), alcohol plus hepatitis C plus hepatitis B (1%), hereditary hemochromatosis (1%), non-alcoholic steatohepatitis (1%), autoimmune hepatitis (1%) and cryptogenic cirrhosis (5%). Four percent of the patients had no underlying liver disease, 4% non-alcoholic steatohepatitis and 3% chronic hepatitis without cirrhosis (two hepatitis B and one hepatitis C). Fifty-four percent (59/109) of the patients met the Milan criteria for liver transplantation [34]. Metastasis search was performed in 88% of cases (17% had metastasis and 93% did not). Tumors <5cm, 5-10cm and >10 cm were found in 57%, 18% and 8% respectively. Diffuse infiltrative HCC totaled 15% of the cases. Histological evaluation of HCC was performed in 39% (42/109) of subjects with 62% presenting Edmondson-Steiner I or II and 38% III or IV.

4.1. 14bp insertion/deletion polymorphism

Genotype frequencies of patient and control groups were in accordance to Hardy-Weinberg Equilibrium. The 14bp*D allele was more frequent in cases of HCC than in controls (0.6514 vs. 0.5619; *P*=0.0326), conferring an OR=1.46 (95%CI=1.04-2.05). Evaluation of genotype frequency (genotypes 14pb DD, DI and II) did not show significant difference between the groups studied (*P*=0.0871; OR=1.54; 95%CI=0.96-2.48; *P*=0.7182; OR=0.89; 95%CI=0.56-1.44; and *P*=0.1343; OR=0.60; 95%CI=0.32-1.12, respectively). However, the 14bp DD genotype was marginally more frequent among individuals with HCC than among controls, with 10.3% difference (0.4495 vs. 0.3465, respectively) (*P*=0.0871; OR=1.54; 95%CI=0.96-2.48). Patients were stratified according to the characteristics of HCC (type of tumor presentation, nodule size, Milan criteria, presence of metastasis and Edmondson-Steiner classification), and no significant differences were detected between groups regarding the 14bp insertion/deletion allele frequencies (14bp*D and 14bp*I alleles) or genotype frequencies (14bp DD, DI and II genotypes). Table 2 shows the frequency of the 14bp insertion/deletion polymorphism and Table 3 shows the results of the statistical analyses.

Samples	14bp alleles		14bp genotypes		
I	D	II	DI	DD	
Groups	n(frequency)	n(frequency)	n(frequency)	n(frequency)	n(frequency)
Control	177 [0.4381]	227 [0.5619]	45 [0.2228]	87 [0.4307]	70 [0.3465]
HCC	76 [0.3486]	142 [0.6514]	16 [0.1468]	44 [0.4037]	49 [0.4495]
Tumor presentation					
Diffuse	7 [0.2500]	21 [0.7500]	1 [0.0714]	5 [0.3571]	8 [0.5714]
Multinodular	14 [0.3684]	24 [0.6316]	13 [0.1579]	9 [0.4211]	6 [0.4211]
Uninodular	55 [0.3667]	95 [0.6333]	12 [0.1600]	31 [0.4133]	32 [0.4767]
Nodule size					
>10cm	6 [0.3333]	12 [0.6667]	1 [0.1111]	4 [0.4444]	4 [0.4444]
5-10cm	11 [0.2750]	29 [0.7250]	1 [0.0500]	9 [0.4500]	10 [0.5000]
<5cm	51 [0.4113]	73 [0.5887]	13 [0.2097]	25 [0.4032]	24 [0.3871]
Metastasis					
Present	4 [0.2857]	10 [0.7143]	0 [0.0000]	4 [0.5714]	3 [0.4286]
Absent	63 [0.3539]	115 [0.6461]	13 [0.1461]	37 [0.4157]	39 [0 4382]
Milan criteria					
Yes	46 [0.3898]	72 [0.6102]	11 [0.1864]	24 [0.4068]	24 [0 4068]
No	30 [0.3000]	70 [0.7000]	5 [0.1000]	20 [0.4000]	25 [0 5000]
Edmondson					
I-II	24 [0.4615]	28 [0.5385]	5 [0.1923]	14 [0.5385]	7 [0.2692]
III-IV	16 [0.5000]	16 [0.5000]	4 [0.2500]	8 [0.5000]	4 [0.2500]

HLA-G: *Human Leukocyte Antigen-G*; bp: base pairs; HCC: hepatocellular carcinoma; I: insertion; D:deletion

Table 2. Distribution of the *HLA-G* 14bp insertion/deletion allele and genotype frequencies.

Comparisons	14bp alleles		14bp genotypes		
I	D	II	DI	DD	
Groups					
HCC *vs.* control	0.0326	0.0326[a]	0.1343	0.7182	0.0871[b]
Tumor presentation					
Diffuse *vs.* multinodular	0.4238	0.4238	0.6197	1,0000	0.4905
Diffuse *vs.* uninodular	0.2839	0.2839	0.6830	0.7738	0.3863
Multinodular *vs.* uninodular	1.0000	1.0000	1.0000	1.0000	1.0000
Nodule size					
>10 cm *vs.* 5-10 cm	0.7577	0.7577	0.5320	1.0000	1.0000
>10 cm *vs.* <5 cm	0.6132	0.6132	0.6769	1.0000	0.7318
5-10 cm *vs.* <5 cm	0.1372	0.1372	0.1698	0.7963	0.4382
Milan criteria					
Yes *vs.* no	0.1995	0.1995	0.2794	1.0000	0.3421
Metastasis					
Present *vs.* Absent	0.7739	0.7739	0.5883	0.4556	1.0000
Edmondson-Steiner					
I-II *vs.* III-IV	0.8232	0.8232	0.7109	1.0000	1.0000

HLA-G: Human Leukocyte Antigen-G; bp: base pairs; HCC: hepatocellular carcinoma; I: insertion; D:deletion

[a] Odds ratio= 1.46 [95% confidence interval: 1.04-2.05]

[b] Odds ratio= 1.54 [95% confidence interval: 0.96-2.48]

Table 3. Probability values obtained by means of two-tailed Fisher exact test in the comparisons of HLA-G 14bp insertion/deletion allele and genotype frequencies between different groups.

4.2. IL-18 (-607 C/A; rs1946518 and -137 C/G; rs187238), IFN-γ (+874 A/T; rs62559044) and TNF-α (-238 A/G; rs361525 and -308 A/G; rs1800629) polymorphism

The genotypification of the polymorphisms of the genes *IL-18* (-607 C/A and -137 C/G), *IFN-γ* (+874 A/T) and *TNF-α* (-238 A/G and -308 A/G) was performed in 112 patients with HCC and in 202 healthy controls. The genotype distribution of the two groups adhered to the theoretical proportions of Hardy-Weinberg equilibrium. Significant associations were detected between HCC and the following alleles (Table 4): *IL-18* -607*A (*P*=0.0235; OR=1.48; 95%CI=1.06-2.08); *TNF-α* -238*A (*P*=0.0025; OR=2.12; 95%CI=1.32-3.40), and *TNF-α* -308*A (*P*=0.0351; OR=1.82; 95%CI=1.07-3.08). When the genotypes were evaluated (Table 5), the following associations with HCC were detected: *IL-18* -607 AA (*P*=0.0048; OR=3.03; 95%CI=1.40-6.55); *TNF-α* -238 GA (*P*=0.0011; OR=2.44; 95%CI=1.45-4.12); and *TNF-α* -308 GA (*P*=0.0031; OR=2.51; 95%CI=1.39-4.51). Alleles and genotypes from *IL-18* -137G/C and *IFNγ* +874T/A were not associated with susceptibility to HCC. The inference of haplotypes was performed for the polymorphisms of *IL-18* and *TNF-α*. Haplotypes -607A/-137G IL-18 and TNF-α -308G/-238A -308A/-238G were more frequent in patients with HCC compared with the control group (P = 0.0180, OR = 1.69, 95% CI 1.10 to 2.59, P = 0.0036, OR = 2.06, 95% CI 1,28-3.31 and P = 0.0480, OR = 1.75; 95% CI = 1.03 to 2.97, respectively). On the other hand, TNF-α -308G/-238G haplotype was more frequent in the group of healthy subjects (P = 0.0001, OR = 0.46, 95% CI 0.32 to 0.68), providing protection against HCC.

SNP			**Allele frequency**			
	allele	HCC n (frequency)	Control n (frequency)	P	OR	95%CI
IL-18 -137C/G	C	62 [0.2768]	120 [0.2970]	0.6464	0.90	0.63-1.30
	G	162 [0.7232]	284 [0.7030]	0.6464	1.10	0.77-1.59
IL-18 -607A/C	A	92 [0.4107]	129 [0.3193]	0.0235	1.48	1.06-2.08
	C	132 [0.5893]	275 [0.6807]	0.0235	0.67	0.48-0.94
IFN-γ +874A/T	A	130 [0.5856]	240 [0.5941]	0.8652	0.96	0.69-1.35
	T	92 [0.4144]	164 [0.4059]	0.8652	1.03	0.74-1.44
TNF-α -238A/G	A	41 [0.1847]	39 [0.0965]	0.0025	2.12	1.32-3.40
	G	181 [0.8153]	365 [0.9035]	0.0025	0.47	0.29-0.76
TNF-α -308A/G	A	30 [0.1351]	32 [0.0792]	0.0351	1.82	1.07-3.08
	G	192 [0.8649]	372 [0.9208]	0.0351	0.55	0.32-0.93

Table 4. Distribution of the allele frequencies of polymorphisms of the *IL-18* (-607 C/A and -137 C/G), *IFN-γ* (–874 A/T), and *TNF-α* (-238 A/G e -308 A/G) genes among patients with hepatocellular carcinoma (HCC) and healthy controls.

When the -607C/A SNP of *IL-18* was evaluated in terms of the different presentations of the HCC, the frequencies of the -607*C and -607*A alleles between individuals with multinodular and uninodular HCC, showed that the -607*C allele confers significant susceptibility to multinodular lesions (*P*=0.0289; OR=2.4; 95%CI = 1.09-5.28). Evaluation of the genotype frequency in SNP -607C/A of *IL-18* revealed that genotype 607CC was significantly more frequent in cases of multinodular HCC compared to uninodular tumors (*P*=0.0284; OR=3.5; 95%CI=1.24-9.86). On the other hand, genotype +874AT was found to be more frequent among patients with infiltrative diffuse HCC compared to uninodular HCC (*P*=0.0443; OR=3.6; 95%CI=1.04-12.47), thus conferring greater susceptibility to the diffuse tumor.

SNP	Genotype frequency					
	genotype	HCC n (frequency)	Control n (frequency)	P	OR	95%CI
IL-18 -137C/G	CG	48 [0.4286]	84 [0.4185]	0.9051	1.05	0.66-1.68
	CC	7 [0.0625]	18 [0.0891]	0.5157	0.68	0.27-0.68
	GG	57 [0.5089]	100 [0.4950]	0.9063	1.06	0.67-1.68
IL-18 -607A/C	CA	56 [0.5000]	105 [0.5198]	0.8138	0.92	0.58-1.47
	AA	18 [0.1607]	12 [0.0594]	0.0048	3.03	1.40-6.55
	CC	38 [0.3393]	85 [0.4208]	0.1845	0.71	0.44-1.14
IFN-γ +874A/T	AT	50 [0.4505]	82 [0.4059]	0.4741	1.20	0.75-1.91
	AA	40 [0.3604]	79 [0.3911]	0.6276	0.88	0.54-1.42
	TT	21 [0.1892]	41 [0.2030]	0.8823	0.92	0.91-1.65
TNF-α -238A/G	GA	41 [0.3694]	39 [0.1931]	0.0011	2.44	1.45-4.12
	AA	0 [0.0000]	0 [0.0000]	1.0000	1.81	0.03-92.15
	GG	70 [0.6306]	163 [0.8069]	0.0011	0.40	0.24-0.69
TNF-α -308A/G	GA	30 [0.2703]	26 [0.1287]	0.0031	2.51	1.39-4.51
	AA	0 [0.0000]	3 [0.0149]	0.5548	0.25	0.01-4.99
	GG	81 [0.7297]	173 [0.8564]	0.0098	0.45	0.25-0.80

Table 5. Distribution of the genotype frequencies of polymorphisms of the *IL-18* (-607 C/A and -137 C/G), *IFN-γ* (+874 A/T), and *TNF-α* (-238 A/G and -308 A/G) genes among patients with hepatocellular carcinoma (HCC) and healthy controls.

No significant differences in the allele or genotype frequencies of SNPs of *IL-18, IFN-γ* and *TNF-α* were detected between the various tumor sizes, although the *TNF-α* -238*A allele was slightly more frequent in tumors larger than 10cm compared to tumors smaller than 5cm (*P*=0.0889; OR=2.82; 95%CI: 0.94-8.41). Similarly, genotype *TNF-α* -238AG indicated a marginally greater susceptibility to tumors >10cm (*P*=0.0565; OR=4.63; 95%CI=1.05-20.48) than to tumors < 5 cm, whereas genotype *TNF-α* -238GG conferred marginal protection against large lesions (>10 cm vs. <5cm) (*P*=0.0565; OR=0.22; 95%CI=0.05-0.95).

Evaluation of SNP -607C/A of *IL-18* revealed no significant difference in allele and genotype frequencies between patients with HCC with or without metastasis. In contrast, evaluation of SNP -137C/G of *IL-18* revealed that the -137*C allele was more frequent among individuals with metastasis than among individuals with no meatastasis (*P*=0.0240; OR=4.00; 95%CI=1.32-12.14). The frequencies of genotypes -137CC, CG or GG did not differ significantly between patients with and without metastasis, although genotype -137CC tended to confer greater susceptibility to metastasis (*P*=0.0564; OR=8.80; 95%CI=1.29-60.13) and genotype -137GG presented marginal protection against secondary lesions (*P*=0.0548; OR=0.14;

95%CI=0.02-1.21). Regarding genes *IFN-γ* and *TNF-α*, the allele and genotype frequencies did not differ significantly between the groups with and without metastasis.

The 14bp*D allele in gene *HLA-G* was more frequent in cases of HCC compared to control, with the 14bp DD genotype tending to be more frequent among individuals with HCC. The alleles and genotypes of the 14bp insertion/deletion polymorphism of the *HLA-G* were not associated with disease severity.

Chen et al., in a study of 150 individuals of the Chinese Han population, showed that genotypes of the 14bp insertion/deletion polymorphism of *HLA-G* were significantly associated with the expression of soluble HLA-G in plasma in this population [35]. These authors detected a dramatically lower expression of soluble HLA-G in plasma in the presence of the 14 bp I/I genotype than in the presence of the 14 bp I/D (P = 0.004) or D/D (P = 0.003) genotypes. No significant difference in plasma expression of soluble HLA-G was detected between 14 bp I/D and D/D genotypes.

Many mechanisms of tumor escape have been proposed in the literature, some of them local and others systemic. Particularly important among them is the expression of immunomodulatory molecules in the tumoral microbiota, as well as the expression of soluble suppressive factors by the tumoral cells. HLA-G represents one of these immunomodulatory molecules, playing an important role in the mechanisms of immunotolerance by the inhibition of the activity of NK cells, cytotoxic T lymphocytes and antigen-presenting cells [9,36].

The 14bp insertion/deletion polymorphism in exon 8 of *HLA-G* (3′UTR of the transcript) has been associated with the magnitude of protein production through the modulation of the stability of HLA-G mRNA, although the mechanisms involved still need to be elucidated. It has been demonstrated that the *HLA-G* allele containing the insertion polymorphism may suffer an additional splicing stage, so that 92 bp are removed from the primary mRNA. Thus, smaller *HLA-G* transcripts, without the 92 bp, are more stable than the complete mRNA forms. The alternative splicing may also be related to the presence of other polymorphisms in linkage disequilibrium with the 14bp insertion [8,10]. Overall, HLA-G expression may be modulated by many actors including transcription factors (influenced by the 5′ polymorphisms of the promoter region) and the rate of mRNA degradation or translation, highly influenced by polymorphisms observed at 3′UTR [8]. Ferguson et al. recently reported that the risk for invasive cancer of the uterine cervix in a Canadian population was significantly higher in the presence of 14 bp I/I genotype (OR=2.17, 95% CI: 1.10-4.27, P=0.020) as well as homozygous genotypes HLA-G*01:01:02 (OR=3.52, 95% CI: 1.43-8.61, P=0.006) and *01:06 (OR=19.1, 95% CI: 2.29-159, P=0.005) [12]. Similarly, Chen et al. studying the relationship between HLA-G gene polymorphism and the susceptibility of esophageal cancer in Kazakh and Han nationality in Xinjiang, found that the risk of developing esophageal cancer was significantly increased in individuals with 14 bp I/I genotype compared with 14 bp D/D genotype (OR=2.69, 95% CI: 1.30-5.55, P=0.04) in Kazakh population [11].

The tumoral microbiota or even the cells that underwent mutation per se can induce the expression of HLA-G. Studies have demonstrated the expression of HLA-G in various malignant tumors, although with variations in the percentage of lesions expressing the molecule. In studies involving renal cell carcinoma [37], endometrial adenocarcinoma [38] and gastric cancer [39], at least 30% of the tumors exhibited HLA-G expression.

Regarding hepatic diseases, Souto et al., in a study of 74 liver biopsies of individuals with chronic HBV infection and 10 specimens obtained from previously healthy cadaver liver donors, demonstrated that 77% of the samples of chronic HBV hepatitis presented HLA-G expression in the hepatocytes, as opposed to none of the controls [40]. These authors detected a case of HCC, in which HLA-G expression was not detected in the tumor cells but was detected in adjacent non-tumoral hepatic tissue.

Lin et al. evaluated by immunohistochemistry the expression of HLA-G in 219 HCC and adjacent nontumoral tissue samples. The expression of HLA-G was observed in 50.2% of HCC samples vs. 0% of normal corresponding adjacent tissue. Evaluation of HCC stages showed that HLA-G expression was detected in 37.8%, 41.9% and 71.4% of cases in stages I, II and III, respectively. The data reported by these authors revealed that the expression of HLA-G was strongly correlated with advanced HCC stage and that soluble HLA-G was significantly more elevated in the plasma of patients with HCC compared to healthy controls [41]. Similarly, Cai et al. studied the expression of HLA-G by immunohistochemistry in 173 HCC specimens and observed that HLA-G expression was associated with the prognosis of HCC, especially in the early stages of the disease, with higher HLA-G expression being independently associated with shorter overall survival and greater tumor recurrence after surgical resection [42].

Recently, a study involving 267 patients divided as anti-HBs positive healthy individuals (n=50), chronic HBV carriers (n=45), active hepatitis B (n=46), liver cirrhosis (n=46) and early-stage HCC patients (n=80) showed that serum concentrations of soluble human leukocyte antigen-G (sHLA-G) were significantly higher in the active hepatitis B and HCC groups compared to the other groups ($P<0.05$). Moreover, the concentrations of sHLA-G were higher in the patients with HCC than in those with liver cirrhosis or active hepatitis B, suggesting that serum sHLA-G concentrations may be associated with the different phases of hepatitis B infection. They did not find any association between sHLA-G concentrations and HCC stage, number of tumors, pathologic grade and presence of vascular invasion [43]. Another study, examining fifteen SNPs in the non-classical class I alleles, found that the SNPs rs17875380, rs41557518, rs114465251, and rs115492845 were associated with susceptibility to chronic hepatitis B infection or HCC, and HLA-F*01:04, HLA-G*01:05N, and HLA-E*01:01 were associated with hepatitis B or hepatitis B with HCC, concluding that these polymorphisms may play an important role in immune surveillance of hepatitis B and HCC, possibly leading to immune responses to virus or cancer cells [14].

It has been demonstrated that, in addition to genetic factors, the microbiota, for example, strees inducers, hypoxia and cytokines (interferons, IL-10, TNF-α), influences the expression of HLA-G, so that more studies are needed for a better understanding of the interaction of molecules derived from the tumor and from host factors [9].

In summary, the present findings show that the deletion allele of the *HLA-G* 14bp insertion/deletion polymorphism was more frequent among patients with tumors than among healthy individuals, a fact that may confer greater susceptibility to HCC.

A higher frequency of the *IL-18* -607*A allele and -607AA genotype was found among HCC patients compared to healthy individuals in the present study. Mi et al. analyzed a pool of studies on the association between polymorphisms of the *IL-18* gene and the risk of cancer (cancer of renal cells, of the ovary and breast, nasopharyngeal an cervical cancer, cancer of the esophagus, prostate, lung and stomach, and colorectal cancer) involving approximately 2137 cases and 3117 controls for the -607C/A variant, and 2372 cases and 3476 controls for the -137G/C polymorphism, and they observed that the -607*A and -137*C alleles were associated with an increased global risk of cancer compared to patients with the wild allele. Analysis of the different ethnic groups showed that these polymorphisms were associated with an increased risk of cancer in Asians but not in Europeans or Africans [44]. Regarding the evaluation of SNP -137C/G, in the present study no significant differences in allele or genotype frequencies were detected between patients with HCC and healthy individuals. However, the *IL18* -137G/-607A haplotype was more frequent among individuals with HCC than among control. These results suggest that, even though no association was detected between SNP -137G/C and HCC, the interaction between the two polymorphisms may have been involved in the susceptibility to HCC. Regarding the polymorphism of the *IFN-γ* gene (+874 A/T), no significant difference in allele or genotype frequencies were observed between patients with HCC and healthy controls. Migita et al. studied 236 Japanese patients with chronic HBV infection who were divided into two groups: with (n=48) and without (n=188) HCC, for the evaluation of the association of polymorphisms of the *TNF-α*, *IFN-γ*, *TGF-β1*, *IL-6* and *IL-10* genes with the risk of HCC. When evaluating the SNP +874 of *IFN-γ*, the authors did not detect a statistically significant difference between the two groups, as also observed in the present study [45].

We observed that alleles *TNF-α* -238*A and -308*A confer significant susceptibility to HCC, and that genotypes *TNF-α* -238GA and -308GA and haplotypes *TNF-α* -238A/-308G and -238G/-308A are also more frequent among patients with HCC compared to control. Also in agreement with these results, Akkiz et al. when analyzing 110 patients with HCC and 110 healthy controls from the Turkish population, observed that patients with HCC had a higher frequency of genotype *TNF-α* -308GA and a lower frequency of genotype *TNF-α* -308GG compared to control and after logistic regression, genotype -308GA was found to be associated with risk of HCC. In addition, individuals with the -308*A allele (genotypes -308AA and -308GA) had a 4.75-fold higher chance to develop HCC compared to individuals with the GG genotype [46]. Similarly, Jung et al., studying 227 Korean patients with HCC and 365 controls, detected a higher frequency of allele -238*A among patients with HCC than among healthy controls [47]. On the other hand, Yang et al., did not find statistical difference in *TNF-α* -308G/A alleles or genotypes frequencies between Chinese HCC patients (n=772) and healthy controls (n=852), but they observed that *TNF-α* -863AA genotype may increase the risk of HCC compared with the wild-type *TNF-α* CC [48].

The expression of *TNF-α* is regulated both at the transcriptional and post-transcriptional level and polymorphisms in the promoter region of *TNF-α* have been related to the production of this cytokine [22]. Greater TNF-α production up to five-fold the basal level and induction of mRNA expression have been associated with the *TNF-α* -308*A allele, with elevated serum TNF levels being observed even in heterozygous patients [49]. Many mechanisms of the cancerigenous activity of TNF-α have been suggested, such as induction of pro-malignant chemokines, metalloproteinases, cell adhesion molecules, angiogenic mediators, reactive oxygen intermediates and inflammatory enzymes. Increased TNF-α levels are correlated with hepatic inflammation, fibrosis and tissue damage [46].

Studies evaluating the association of polymorphisms of *IL-18* with the severity of cancer have been reported. Saenz-Lopez et al. investigated whether the presence of SNPs -137G/C and -607A/C of *IL-18* were associated with size, grade, and TNM Classification of 158 patients with renal cell carcinoma. These authors observed that genotype -607CC was significantly associated with larger tumor size (P=0.001), grade (P=0.030), and T (P=0.001) and M (P=0.012) stage, while genotype -137GG was correlated with larger tumor size (P=0.036), grade (P=0.017), and stage T (P=0.026) [50]. Another authors, studing the association of SNPs -607A/C and -137G/C of *IL-18* with histology of colorectal and gastric cancer (moderately differentiated or undifferentiated vs. well differentiated), noticed that no difference in genotype frequency was detected, although the combination of genotypes -607AA/-137GC was more frequent among patients with less differentiated tumors [51].

Literature evidence has demonstrated that IL-18 is a pleiotropic cytokine that enhances the Th1 or Th2 immune response according to the medium and to genetics. In the presence of IL-12, IL-18 induces IFN-γ secretion by NK and T cells, activating the Th1 response, important for defense against tumor cells. On the other hand, IL-18 can increase tumor growth via increased stimulation of VEGF and of the immune response, and also stimulate solid tumor metastasis [52]. A possible explanation for this fact is the increased Th1 response in the early stages of the cancer which, however, is replaced with Th2 as tumor malignancy worsens with tumor development. Thus, as the tumor develops, *IL-18* polymorphisms, which induce great IL-18 production, may contribute to the promotion of more advanced tumors due to the activation of angiogenesis, differentiation of tumor cells and regulation of stimulators of cell proliferation [53]. To corroborate these data, Tangkijvanich et al., in a study of 70 patients with HCC and 10 healthy controls, observed that serum IL-18 levels were significantly correlated with the presence of vascular invasion and of more advanced tumors according to the Okuda classification. In addition, the survival of patients with high serum levels of IL-18 was worse. Multivariate analysis showed that serum IL-18 levels proved to be a significant and independent prognostic factor regarding survival [54].

Regarding the +874 A/T polymorphism of the *IFN-γ* gene, study involving 100 patients with chronic HCV infection and different degrees of disease severity (chronic hepatitis, n=42; cirrhosis + HCC, n=58) and 103 healthy controls detected that the TT and AT genotypes were significantly more frequent among patients with cirrhosis and HCC. These genotypes were associated with a 2.5 higher risk of progression to more severe forms of hepatic disease. In addition, the +874*T allele was approximately twice more frequent among patients in an advanced stage of hepatitis C than among patients with chronic hepatitis, although multivariable analysis did not show that the +874*T allele was an independent predictive factor of severity [55].

5. Conclusions

Our results suggest that the 14bp-deletion allele in *HLA-G* gene is associated with HCC susceptibility in a Brazilian population, and that the alleles *IL-18* -607*A and *TNF-α* (-238*A and -308*A) may confer susceptibility to HCC, whereas IL-18 -607*C and -137*C alleles may confer susceptibility to multinodular and diffuse HCC, respectively. Furthermore, deletion/deletion genotype was marginally associated with greater risk of HCC. More studies in different populations are needed to confirm these findings.

Author details

Andreza Correa Teixeira[1,2*], Ana de Lourdes Candolo Martinelli[1] and Eduardo Antonio Donadi[1]

*Address all correspondence to: andrezacteixeira@gmail.com

1 Department of Internal Medicine, Faculty of Medicine of Ribeirão Preto – University of São Paulo, Ribeirão Preto, São Paulo, Brazil

2 Department of Surgery and Anatomy, Faculty of Medicine of Ribeirão Preto – University of São Paulo, Ribeirão Preto, São Paulo, Brazil

References

[1] Bosch, F. X, Ribes, J, Díaz, M, & Cléries, R. Primary liver cancer: worldwide incidence and trends. Gastroenterology (2004). Supplement 1.

[2] Jemal, A, Siegel, R, Ward, E, Hao, Y, Xu, J, & Thun, M. J. Cancer statistics, 2009. CA: a cancer journal for clinicians (2009).

[3] Rockey, D. C, & Friedman, S. L. Hepatic fibrosis and cirrhosis. In: Boyer TD, Wright TL, Manns MP. Hepatology. Philadelphia: Elselvier, (2006).

[4] Carrilho, F. J, Kikuchi, L, Branco, F, Goncalves, C. S, & De Mattos, A. A. Brazilian HCC Study Group. Clinical and epidemiological aspects of hepatocellular carcinoma in Brazil. Clinics (2010). , 65(12), 1285-1290.

[5] Teixeira, A. C, & Mente, E. D. Cantao CAB, Sankarankutty AK, Souza FF, Motta TC, Monsignore L, Elias-Junior J, Muglia VF, Abud DG, Peria FM, Zucoloto S, Castro-Silva O, Martinelli ALC Clinical Characteristics of 130 Patients With Hepatocellular Carcinoma Followed at a Tertiary Hospital From Brazil. World Journal of Oncology (2012). , 3(4), 165-172.

[6] Abbas, A. K, Lichtman, A. H, & Pillai, S. The major histocompatibility complex. In: ______. Cellular and Molecular Immunology. Philadelphia: Elsevier; (2007). , 97-112.

[7] Castelli, E. C, & Mendes-junior, C. T. Deghaide NHS, de Albuquerque RS, Muniz YCN, Simoes RT, et al. The genetic structure of 3′untranslated region of the HLA-G gene: polymorphisms and haplotypes. Genes and Immunity (2010).

[8] Donadi, E. A, Castelli, E. C, Amaiz-villena, A, Roger, M, Rey, D, & Moreau, P. Implications of the polymorphism of HLA-G on its function, regulation, evolution and disease association. Cellular and Molecular Life Sciences (2011).

[9] Carosella, E. D, & Moreau, P. LeMaoult J, Rouas-Freiss N. HLA-G: from biology to clinical benefits. Trends in immunology (2008).

[10] Menier, C, Rouas-freiss, N, & Favier, B. LeMaoult J, Moreau P, Carosella ED. Recent advances on the non-classical major histocompatibility complex class I HLA-G molecule. Tissue Antigens (2010).

[11] Chen, Y, Gao, X. J, Deng, Y. C, & Zhang, H. X. Relationship between HLA-G gene polymorphism and the susceptibility of esophageal cancer in Kazakh and Han nationality in Xinjiang. Biomarkers (2012).

[12] Ferguson, R, Ramanakumar, A. V, Koushik, A, Coutlée, F, & Franco, E. Roger M; Biomarkers of Cervical Cancer Risk Study Team. Human leukocyte antigen G polymorphism is associated with an increased risk of invasive cancer of the uterine cervix. International Journal of Cancer (2012). E, 312-9.

[13] Jiang, Y, Chen, S, Jia, S, Zhu, Z, Gao, X, Dong, D, & Gao, Y. Association of HLA-G 3′ UTR bp insertion/deletion polymorphism with hepatocellular carcinoma susceptibility in a Chinese population. DNA Cell Biology (2011). , 14.

[14] Zhang, J, Pan, L, Chen, L, Feng, X, Zhou, L, & Zheng, S. Non-classical MHC-I genes in chronic hepatitis B and hepatocellular carcinoma. Immunogenetics (2012).

[15] Budhu, a. Wang xw. The role of cytokines in hepatocellular carcinoma. J Leukoc Biol (2006). , 80, 1197-213.

[16] Bidwell, J, Keen, L, Gallagher, G, Kimberly, R, Huizinga, T, Mcdermott, M. F, Oksenberg, J, Mcnicholl, J, Pociot, F, Hardt, C, & Alfonso, D. S. Cytokine gene polymorphism in human disease: on-line databases. Genes Immun (2001). , 2, 61-70.

[17] Bayley, J. P, Ottenhoff, T. H, & Verweij, C. L. Is there a future for TNF promoter polymorphisms? Genes Immun (2004). , 5, 315-29.

[18] Teixeira, A. C, Mendes-júnior, C. T, & Souza, F. F. Cantão CAB, Ferreira SC, Deghaide NHS, Castelli EC, Mente ED, Sankarankutty AK, Zucoloto S, Elias Jr J, Muglia V, Castro-Silva O, Donadi EA, Martinelli AC. Alleles and Genotypes of IL-18 and TNF-α Promoter Polymorphisms are Associated with Higher Risk of Hepatocellular Carcinoma (HCC) in Brazilian Population. J Hepatol. (2010). Suppl1): S236.

[19] Teixeira, A. C, Castelli, E, Souza, F, Cantão, C, Ferreira, S, Mendes-júnior, C, Deghaide, N, Mente, E, Sankarankutty, A, Zucoloto, S, Ramalho, L, Crispim, J, Castro-e-silva, O, & Donadi, E. Martinelli ALC. The 14BP-Deletion Polymorphism in HLA-G Gene Confers Susceptibility to the Development of Hepatocellular Carcinoma (HCC) in Brazilian Population. J Hepatol. (2010). Suppl1): S236.

[20] Teixeira, A. C, Mendes-junior, C. T, Souza, F. F, & Marano, L. A. Deghaide NHS, Ferreira SC, Mente ED, Sankarankutty AK, Elias-Junior J, Castro-Silva O, Donadi EA, Martinelli ALC. The 14bp-deletion allele in the HLA-G gene confers susceptibility to the development of hepatocellular carcinoma (HCC) in the Brazilian population. Tissue Antigens. 2013 Mar 18. doi: 10.1111/tan.12097. [Epub ahead of print]

[21] Teixeira, A. C, Mendes-junior, C. T, & Marano, L. A. Deghaide NHS, Secaf M, Elias-Junior J, Muglia V, Donadi EA, Martinelli ALC. Alleles and genotypes of polymorphisms of IL-18, TNF-α and IFN-γ are associated with a higher risk and severity of hepatocellular carcinoma (HCC) in Brazil Human Immunology (accepted for publication).

[22] Bruix, J, Sherman, M, Llovet, J. M, Beaugrand, M, Lencioni, R, Burroughs, A. K, et al. Clinical Management of Hepatocellular Carcinoma. Conclusions of the Barcelona-2000 EASL Conference. Journal of hepatology (2001).

[23] Bruix, J, & Sherman, M. AASLD Practice Guideline. Management of hepatocellular carcinoma. Hepatology (2005).

[24] Edmondson, H. A, & Steiner, P. E. Primary carcinoma of the liver: a study of 100 cases among 48900 necropsies. Cancer (1954).

[25] Miller, A. S. A simple salting out procedure for extracting DNA for human nucleated cells. Nucleic acids research (1988).

[26] Bermingham, J, Jenkins, D, Mccarthy, T, & Brien, O. M. Genetic analysis of insulin-like growth factor II and HLA-G in pre-eclampsia. Biochemical Society Transactions. (2000).

[27] Castelli, E. C, & Mendes-junior, C. T. Viana de Camargo JL, Donadi EA. HLA-G polymorphism and transitional cell carcinoma of the bladder in a Brazilian population. Tissue antigens (2008).

[28] MarshHP; Haldar, NA; Bunce, M; Marshall, SE; le Monier, K; Winsey, SL; Christodoulos, K; Cranston, D; Welsh, KI; Harris, AL. Polymorphisms in tumour necrosis factor (TNF) are associated with risk of bladder cancer and grade of tumour at presentation. Br J Cancer (2003)., 89(6), 1096-101.

[29] PravicaV; Perrey, C; Stevens, A; Lee, J-H; Hutchinson, IV. A single nucleotide polymorphism in the first intron of the human IFN-gamma gene: absolute correlation with a polymorphic CA microsatellite marker of high IFN-gamma production. Human Immunol (2000)., 61(9), 863-66.

[30] Guo, S. W, & Thompson, E. A. Performing the exact test of Hardy-Weinberg proportion for multiple alleles. Biometrics (1992).

[31] ExcoffierL; Laval, G; Schneider, S. Arlequin ver. 3.0: an integrated software package for population genetics data analysis. Evolutionary bioinformatics online (2005). , 1, 47-50.

[32] Stephens, M, Smith, N. J, & Donnelly, P. A new statistical method for haplotype reconstruction from population data. American journal human genetics (2001). , 68(4), 978-89.

[33] Excoffier, L, & Slatkin, M. Maximum-likelihood estimation of molecular haplotype frequencies in a diploid population. Mol Biol Evol (1995). , 12, 921-927.

[34] Mazzaferro, V, Regalia, E, Doci, R, Andreola, S, Pulvirenti, A, Bozzetti, F, Montalto, F, Ammatuna, M, Morabito, A, & Gennari, L. Liver Transplantation for the Treatment of Small Hepatocellular Carcinomas in Patients with Cirrhosis. N Engl J Med (1996). , 334, 693-700.

[35] Chen, X. Y, Yan, W. H, Lin, A, Xu, H. H, Zhang, J. G, & Wang, X. X. The 14 bp deletion polymorphisms in HLA-G gene play an important role in the expression of soluble HLA-G in plasma. Tissue antigens (2008).

[36] Yie, S. M, & Hu, Z. Human Leukocyte Antigen-G (HLA-G) as a marker for diagnosis, prognosis and tumor immune escape in human malignancies. Histology and histopathology (2011).

[37] Seliger, B, & Schlaf, G. Structure, expression and function of HLA-G in renal cell carcinoma. Seminars in cancer biology (2007).

[38] Barrier, B. F, Kendall, B. S, Sharpe-timms, K. L, & Kost, E. R. Characterization of human leukocyte antigen-G (HLA-G) expression in endometrial adenocarcinoma. Gynecologic oncology (2006).

[39] Yie, S. M, Yang, H, Ye, S. R, Li, K, Dong, D. D, & Lin, X. M. Expression of human leukocyte antigen G (HLA-G) correlates with poor prognosis in gastric carcinoma. Annals of surgical oncology (2007).

[40] Souto, F. J, Crispim, J. C, & Ferreira, S. C. da Silva AS, Bassi CL, Soares CP, et al. Liver HLA-G expression is associated with multiple clinical and histopathological forms of chronic hepatitis B virus infection. Journal of viral hepatitis (2011).

[41] Lin, A, Chen, H. X, Zhu, C. C, Zhang, X, Xu, H. H, Zhang, J. G, et al. Aberrant human leucocyte antigen-G expression and its clinical relevance in hepatocellular carcinoma. Journal of cellular and molecular medicine (2010).

[42] Cai, M. Y, Xu, Y. F, Qiu, S. J, Ju, M. J, Gao, Q, Li, Y. W, et al. Human leukocyte antigen-G protein expression is an unfavorable prognostic predictor of hepatocellular carcinoma following curative resection. Clinical cancer research (2009).

[43] Park, Y, Park, Y, Lim, H. S, Kim, Y. S, Hong, D. J, & Kim, H. S. Soluble human leukocyte antigen-G expression in hepatitis B virus infection and hepatocellular carcinoma.Tissue Antigens (2012).

[44] Mi, Y. Y, Yu, Q. Q, Yu, M. L, Xu, B, Zhang, L. F, Cheng, W, Zhang, W, Hua, L. X, & Feng, N. H. Review and pooled analysis of studies on-607(C/A) and-137(G/C) polymorphisms in IL-18 and cancer risk. Med Oncol. (2011)., 28(4), 1107-15.

[45] Migita, K, Miyazoe, S, Maeda, Y, Daikoku, M, Abiru, S, Ueki, T, Yano, K, Nagaoka, S, Matsumoto, T, Nakao, K, Hamasaki, K, Yatsuhashi, H, Ishibashi, H, & Eguchi, K. Cytokine gene polymorphisms in Japanese patients with hepatitis B virus infection--association between TGF-beta1 polymorphisms and hepatocellular carcinoma. J Hepatol (2005)., 42, 505-10.

[46] Akkiz, H, Bayram, S, Bekar, A, Ozdil, B, Akgöllü, E, Sümbül, A. T, Demiryürek, H, Doran, F. G, & Tnf-alpha, A. polymorphism is associated with an increased risk of hepatocellular carcinoma in the Turkish population: case-control study. Cancer Epidemiol (2009)., 33, 261-4.

[47] Jung, K. W, Ha, E, Yu, G. I, Kim, S. J, Chung, W. J, Jang, B. K, Lee, J. J, Shin, D. H, & Hwang, J. S. TNFalpha promoter polymorphism is a risk factor for susceptibility in hepatocellular carcinoma in Korean population. Clin Chim Acta (2009)., 407, 16-9.

[48] Yang, Y, Qiu, X. Q, Yu, H. P, Zeng, X. Y, & Bei, C. H. TNF-α-863 polymorphisms and the risk of hepatocellular carcinoma. Exp Ther Med. (2012)., 3(3), 513-518.

[49] Abraham, L. J, & Kroeger, K. M. Impact of the-308 TNF promoter polymorphism on the transcriptional regulation of the TNF gene: relevance to disease. J Leukoc Biol (1999)., 66, 562-6.

[50] Sáenz-lópez, P, Carretero, R, Vazquez, F, Martin, J, Sánchez, E, Tallada, M, Garrido, F, Cózar, J. M, & Ruiz-cabello, F. Impact of interleukin-18 polymorphisms-607 and-137 on clinical characteristics of renal cell carcinoma patients. Human Immunol (2010)., 309-313.

[51] Haghshenas, M. R, Hosseini, S. V, Mahmoudi, M, Saberi-firozi, M, Farjadian, S, Ghaderi, A, & Serum, I. L. level and IL-18 promoter gene polymorphism in Iranian patients with gastrointestinal cancers. J Gastroenterol Hepatol (2009)., 26(6), 1119-22.

[52] Nakanishi, K, Yoshimoto, T, Tsutsui, H, & Okamura, H. Interleukin-18 is a unique cytokine that stimulates both Th1 and Th2 responses depending on its cytokine milieu. Cytokine Growth Factor Rev (2001)., 12(1), 53-72.

[53] Mojtahedi, Z, & Interleukin, I. L. may enhance Th1 response in early cancer but aggravate malignant disease in its later stages. Med Hypotheses (2005)., 65(5), 995-6.

[54] Tangkijvanich P; Thong-NgamD.; Machachai, V.; Theamboonlers, A.; Poovorawan, Y. Role of serum interleukin-18 as a prognostic factor in patients with hepatocellular carcinoma. World J Gastroenterol (2007)., 13(32), 4345-9.

[55] Bouzgarrou, N, Hassen, E, Farhat, K, Bahri, O, Gabbouj, S, & Maamouri, N. Ben Mami, N.; Saffar, H.; Trabelsi, A.; Triki, H.; Chouchane, L. Combined analysis of interferon-gamma and interleukin-10 gene polymorphisms and chronic hepatitis C severity. Human Immunol (2009). , 70(4), 230-6.

Chapter 2

Liver Transplantation for Hepatocellular Carcinoma

Emad H. Asham, Howard Mansour and
Mark Ghobrial

Additional information is available at the end of the chapter

http://dx.doi.org/10.5772/55374

1. Introduction

The incidence of hepatocellular carcinoma (HCC) has increased exponentially. Liver cancer, primarily HCC, has become the third cause of death from cancer worldwide and the ninth cause of cancer deaths in the U.S.A. According to the center for disease control and prevention statistics, the annual incidence of HCC has increased significantly to an average of 3.0 per 100,000 persons. The annual percentage change in incidence (APC) is 3.5% and the highest APC was found in age group 50-59 years [1]. These statistics should be tampered with caution as only biopsy proven HCC, histology code 8170 and 8175, were counted. This definitely underestimates the scope of the disease.

2. Risk factors

While HCC may arise in healthy livers, the majority of cases develop in a back ground of chronic liver disease i.e. cirrhosis which makes management even more challenging. Viral hepatitis, both B (HBV) and C (HCV), cause 78% of primary liver cancer worldwide [1]. Other risk factors include alcoholic liver disease [2], fatty liver disease (FLD) and non-alcoholic steatohepatitis (NASH) [3, 4], hemochromatosis [5], primary biliary cirrhosis [6] and primary sclerosing cholangitis [7]. Moreover, liver adenoma carries a 10% risk for malignant transformation [8]. Tobacco smoking increases the incidence of HCC [9]. Fungi *Aspergillus flavus* present in poorly stored grains produce Aflatoxin, an environmental hazard for HCC [10]. Hepatic venous occlusive disease has been implicated in HCC development in anecdotal case reports [11].

3. Who is eligible?

Orthotropic Liver transplantation (OLT) offers the *prima facie* cure for both HCC and liver cirrhosis. Historically, while orthotropic liver transplantation (OLT) was at its infancy, courageous attempts by Dr. Thomas Starzl and colleagues to offer OLT as a cure for HCC were complicated by early recurrence [12]. As experience with OLT grew, researchers explored HCC benchmarks that would guarantee comparable survival in tumor and non-tumor patients. These efforts lead Mazzafero et al to Milan criteria. In HCC confined to the liver without macrovascular invasion single tumor ≤ 5cm or up to three tumors each ≤ 3 cm had a five year survival of 75% and a disease free survival of 83% [13]. Milan criteria results for OLT were reproducible and ushered a new dawn for HCC patients. This success led to pushing the size limits even further and University of California San Francisco (UCSF) criteria were introduced. Such criteria include single tumor ≤ 6.5 cm or up to three tumors the maximum diameter of which ≤ 4.5 cm or the total diameter ≤8cm. The one- and five -year survivals were 90% and 75% respectively [14].

It is intriguing that both criteria gained wide acceptance by the transplant community when they focused on number and size of HCC lesions and ignored biological signature of the tumor at a molecular level. To fuel the argument even more, according to data from Euro Transplant, current imaging modalities when compared with explanted liver pathology were found to underestimate by 10.4% or overestimate by 36.2% tumor size [15].

University of Toronto liver group took matters even further. They developed a protocol biopsy for tumors up to 10cm in diameter and excluded poorly differentiated ones. Ablative therapies were employed intensively to downstage/control the tumor while waiting for liver transplantation. Patient survival was similar for those with HCC within Milan criteria compared to patients beyond such criteria [16].

Mazzafero et al recently reevaluated Milan criteria to find if they are restrictive to patients with more tumor burden who may achieve similar outcomes. A multicenter data base was established. A retrospective analysis came up with the up-to-seven (Up-to-7) criteria; with 7 being the sum of the size and number of tumors for any given hepatocellular carcinoma [17]. OLT listing criteria are summarized in table 1.

Criteria	UNOS	TNM	Definition
UNOS/ TNM	I	T1	1 nodule ≤ 1.9 cm
	II	T2	1 nodule, 2 to 5 cm, or 2 to 3 nodules, all≤ 3 cm
	III	T3	1 nodule > 5 cm or 2 to 3 nodules, 1 > 3 cm
	IV	T4a	≥4 nodules, any size; no gross vascular invasion
		T4b	Any T with gross vascular invasion
		N1,M1	Metastases
Milan			1 nodule ≤ 5cm or up to three nodules each ≤ 3cm
UCSF			1 nodule ≤ 6.5 cm or up to 3 nodules, all ≤ 4.5 cm; total diameter ≤ 8 cm
Up-to-7			Diameter of the largest nodule (cm) + number of nodules ≤ 7

Table 1. Current criteria employed in liver allocation for HCC patients.

4. Patient evaluation for OLT

Thorough history and physical examination by transplant surgeons and hepatologists are the corner stone in assessment for OLT candidacy. Thereafter, patients undergo stringent testing literally from head to toe.

4.1. Blood tests

An extensive laboratory tests are essential for patients' evaluation. 1. Blood type and antibody screen, panel of reactive antibody (PRA). 2. Full hepatitis profile, to include serum HCV-RNA titers, HCV genotype, HBV-DNA, HBV-E antigen and antibody. 3. Full autoimmune markers to include iron and copper studies, immune protein electropheresis. 4. Cancer markers, i.e. alpha fetoprotein (AFP), CEA, PSA (prostate specific antigen) for males and CA 19-9. Another diagnostic HCC marker has been recently introduced is descarboxyprothrombin (DCP) also known as Prothrombin Induced by Vitamin K absence II (PIVKA II) [18]. 5. Complete blood count (CBC), complete metabolic panel (CMP) to include magnesium and phosphate. 6. Coagulation studies, i.e., PT/INR, fibrinogen levels and 7. Cytomegalovirus (CMV) status, varicella titers, cryptococcal antibodies

4.2. Endoscopy

Esophago-gastro-duodenoscopy (EGD); to screen for esophageal/gastric varices, to identify the extent of portal hypertensive gastropathy (PHG). This is important for bleeding risk stratification while the patient is on the waiting list. Usually the esophageal varices are ligated with rubber bands endoscopically.

Colonoscopy: All patients with cirrhosis older than age 35, or younger patients with higher risk with history of colitis or family history of early colon cancer, undergo screening colonoscopy with prostatic digital exam being performed in men at the same time. Polyps are identified and endoscopically removed. Patients with precancerous polyps and with history of colitis will require further screening colonoscopies every few years following OLT.

Endoscopic retrograde cholangio-pancreatography (ERCP): may be required in certain cases at the discretion of the transplant surgeons e.g. tumors at the porta hepatis or involving the confluence of the bile ducts.

4.3. Imaging

Ultrasound of liver for HCC surveillance and to determine vessels patency by Doppler studies

Liver protocol 4- phase dynamic contrast computerized tomography (CT) of abdomen and pelvis with oral and intravenous contrast is pivotal for HCC patients. Liver and spleen volumes are computed, and the spinal bone density is detected during the procedure. Number, largest diameter and location as well as macrovascular invasion are well documented to stratify the tumor within transplant candidacy criteria. HCC has a characteristic pattern on 4-phase CT scan. During the arterial phase it appears enhanced by taking up the i.v. contrast and in the following portal phase and delayed venous phase it appears hypointense the so called "wash out" [19].

In addition, CT of lungs and brain as well as nuclear bone scan are obtained to look for potential metastatic disease. Any extra hepatic disease precludes the patient from candidacy for OLT.

Magnetic resonance scan (MRI): may be required if the CT scan is not conclusive to further delineate the diagnostic patterns of HCC. During gadolinium contrast dynamic MRI, on T1 weighted images the tumor appears hypointense, isointense or hyperintense. On T2 weighted images HCC appears hyperintense on the arterial hepatic phase [20].

4.4. Cardiac assessment

In Cirrhotic patients, cardiomyopathy can compound the situation [21, 22]. All patients get base line echocardiogram. Further testing such as cardiolyte cardiac stress testing and coronary angiogram is at the discretion of the transplant cardiologist.

4.5. Pulmonary assessment

Chest roentgenogram (X R) is the base line test. Pulmonary function tests and ABG are ordered as indicated e.g. ex-smokers, pulmonary hypertension (HTN) and hepatopulmonary syndrome. Pulmonary HTN requires right sided heart catheterization and pressure measurement. Hepatopulmonary syndrome is evaluated by bubble echocardiogram.

Sinus XR, panorex XR of teeth may be required according to history and physical examination. Any sinus infection or dental caries has to be treated prior to transplantation.

4.6. Vaccinations

Prior to OLT, candidates should receive the following vaccines guided by their history of previous vaccination 1.Hep A and B vaccination, if there is no evidence of prior immunity indicated by antibody titers. 2. Pneunomax (pneumonia vaccine needs to be repeated every five years). 3. Flu vaccination once a year. 4. PPD skin test for TB screening is also applied.

Also, Mammogram / Pap smear for women as appropriate for age are part of the pre transplant evaluation tests.

4.7. Biopsy

The role of liver biopsy is contentious. The most dreaded complications are hemorrhage and tumor seeding rate of 2%-3%. HCC recurrence rates were found to be higher in patients who underwent liver transplant and had tumors >3cm, alpha feto protein >200ng/l and underwent biopsy [23]. Liver biopsy is not routinely required for patients' evaluation as long as the imaging characteristics are diagnostic [24]. Correlation with serum alpha feto protein levels can shed more light. In rare cases; lesion image guided biopsy is required for definitive diagnosis. Liver biopsy can be done via trans jugular approach in coagulopathic patients. Hepatic venous pressure gradient (HVPG) can be measured at the same time HVPG objectively assess the degree of portal hypertension [25]. As future research unfolds molecular signatures and proteomics profiling of HCC; the role of pre transplant biopsy in liver transplant candidacy for HCC patients will gain grounds. On a molecular level, proliferating indices, tumor promoter genes, tissue invasion and metastases markers, angiogenic markers, growth factors and genetic biomarkers and micro RNA have been implicated in diagnosis and prognostication of HCC patients [26].

Barcelona clinic scheme for management of HCC offers a practical staging and treatment strategy for HCC patients (Figure 1)

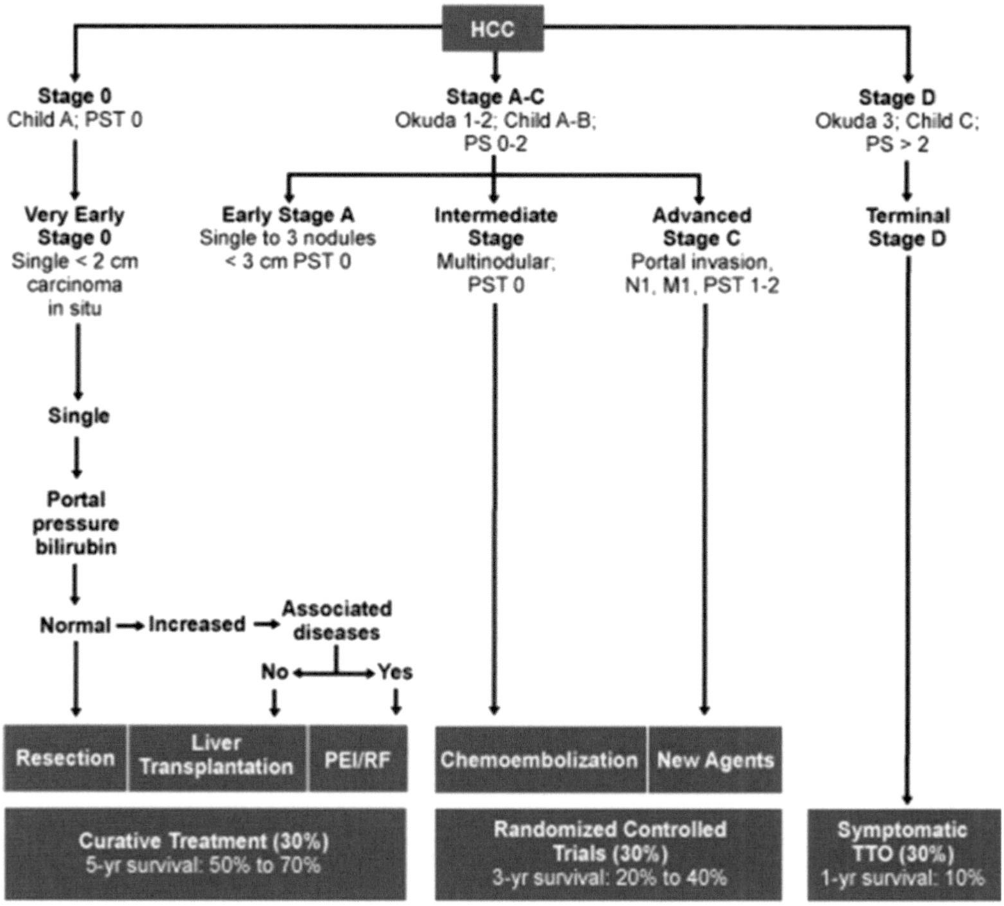

PEI, percutaneous ethanol injection; PS performance status; PST, performance status test; RF, radiofrequency; TTO, time trade off.

Figure 1. Bracelona Clinic Scheme from Llovet et al [27]

5. Diagnostic dilemmas

Often times, diagnosis of HCC is not that straight forward. Currently used markers such as serum alpha feto protein and PIVKA II as well as imaging study can be equivocal. The lesion may be too small to characterize with current imaging modalities. Also, hyperplastic or macroregenrative nodules in cirrhotic livers can be difficult to distinguish from HCC. The guide lines of the American Association for the Study of the liver disease (AASLD) recommends repeat ultrasound for lesions < 1cm at three month [28].

Positron emission tomography (PET) scan using F-18 fluoro-2-deoxy-D-glucose (FDG) has a limited role in HCC diagnosis because of low sensitivity of 50%-55% [29].

Mixed tumors HCC/intrahepatic cholangiocarcinoma may have unconventional enhancement patterns on CT and MRI scans. Usually, they are diagnosed on the explanted liver histopathology and carry worse survival than HCC [30, 31].

Even more, some small HCC are hypovascular and only diagnosed by biopsy or at the explant pathological examination [32]

6. Care of HCC patients while on the waiting list:

6.1. Surveillance

Patients on the transplant waiting list with risk factors for HCC should be screened for HCC. Once screening is positive they should join a surveillance protocol. For those who have HCC enhanced follow up is required to monitor tumor development and treat as appropriate. Liver ultrasound (US) and serum alpha feto protein at six months interval is the gold standard according to AASLD are the main stay for surveillance. US reported sensitivity is between 65%- 80% and specificity is greater than 90% [33]. Nodular cirrhotic livers, small tumors and obese patients impose a challenge for US. In such cases contrast enhanced dynamic CT or MRI is invaluable for lesion characterization.

6.2. The concept of down staging and bridging therapy

Only 5% of HCC patients evaluated for OLT are amenable for transplant [34]. This led to adoption of techniques to control tumor size. The rapidly evolving loco-regional therapies have served well HCC patients by; (i) down staging the tumor to acceptable, within criteria, size and number, (ii) disease control, while the patient is awaiting deceased donor OLT, so called "bridging therapy" i.e. bridge to transplantation and (iii) and improving post OLT survival with particular reference to tumor recurrence [35, 36]. Treatment has to be "tailored" for each patient according to their Child-Pugh score, tumor burden and location and available expertise and resources. T2 patients who are predicted to wait more than six months on the list benefit from tumor therapy [35].Loco regional therapies include percutaneous alcohol injection (PEI), thermal ablation such as radio frequency ablation (RFA) and microwave, chemotherapy delivered directly to the tumor tissue i.e. transarterial chemoembolization (TACE), radiotherapy delivered in various ways such as transarterial Yttrium- 90, three dimentional conformal radiotherapy and proton beam radiotherapy. In a prospective study including forty eight patients, Graziadei et al reported tumor control and survival using TACE for HCC patients while on the waiting list for OLT. The intention to treat 5- year survival was 93% and patients 5 year survival was 93%. Tumor recurred in one patient only, 2.4% rate [37]. Different modalities of radiotherapy are usually reserved for advanced HCC beyond transplant candidacy.

RFA as a bridge to transplantation was studied in a series of 52 patients with 87 HCC nodules. Mean tumor diameter was 2.5 cm (range 0.4-5.07). Radiographic local tumor control was achieved in 74 out of 87 tumors. In the 41 patients who received OLT; complete tumor necrosis was found on explant pathology in 46 out of 70 lesions (65.7%) [38].

Combining two modalities can have a synergistic effect, ameliorate complications of each and reduce the number of sessions to achieve tumor necrosis in patients with well compensated liver functions.

Combination of RFA and PEI has increased the efficacy of RFA to produce coagulative necrosis of HCC [39]. Another study employed TACE and laparoscopic RFA each as a single modality or in combination for down staging a series of sixty one patients who had tumors exceeding T2 stage i.e. a single lesion 2–5 cm or up to three lesions <3 cm. Tumor down staging was achieved in 70.5% of patients and thirty five patients (57.4%) became candidates for OLT. The explanted liver histology showed complete tumor necrosis in thirteen patients and down staging to T2 in seventeen patients [40].

Irreversible Electroporation (IRE or Nano knife): This is an emerging technology that is still undergoing clinical trials yet promising. Short pulses of high voltage current through electrodes inserted into the target tissue produces Nano size pores in the cell membrane that leads to cell death. It has been validated in animal models [41] and limited number of patients with variable inoperable tumors [42]. No intense heat is produced which makes it applicable for tumors near major vessels, bile ducts and porta hepatis.

Molecular targeted therapies have emerged as an effective treatment for a variety of tumors. Sorafineb is an oral multikinase inhibitor that blocks tumor cell proliferation by targeting raf/MEK/ERK signaling. It also has antiangiogenic properties by targeting the vascular endothelial growth factor receprtor-2/-3 and platelet derived growth factor beta tyrosine kinases [43]. Using the Markov model for decision making analysis [44], assuming that therapy starts on the day of listing Sorafineb was found to be cost effective as compared to no therapy [45]. This theoretical model does not take into account side effects of sorafineb particularly its antiangiogenic effect in proximity to major surgery as liver transplant. Clinical trials are awaited to examine if sorafineb improves out comes and reduce post-transplant recurrence.

6.3. Liver resection as bridge to transplantation

In view of organ shortage and unpredictable waiting list time for deceased organs donors, liver resection may be a rational option for patients with favorable lesions and well compensated livers. However, only a small percentage, 10%-15%, of HCC is resectable at time of presentation due to advanced cirrhosis, extensive burden of the neoplasm or patients cardiopulmonary status [46]. This rate of recetability is higher in Asian centers. One explanation is the higher prevalence of HBV than HCV in Asia. In the natural history and hepatocarcinogensis of HBV, HCC can develop in earlier stages of the disease than HCV. In a review of 271 patients who are candidate for OLT, 98 of whom treated by liver resection multivariate analysis showed that liver resection as a first line of treatment was a negative independent factor for disease free survival as compared to primary OLT. Only 20% of the 98 patients who were suitable for transplant but treated by resection received OLT later 17% for tumor recurrence and 3% for liver decompensation [47].

In another series of 107 patients who underwent OLLT for HCC; 88 patients were within Milan criteria. Of those 88 patients, 70 underwent primary OLT and 18 patients had liver resection first before "salvage" transplantation. The mean time between liver resection and listing was 20 months (range 1-84). Indication for salvage transplant was tumor recurrence in 11 patients, liver decompensation in 4 patients and high risk for recurrence in 3 patients. Three- year survival (82 versus 82%) and five year survival (59%versus 61 %) were comparable in the two groups [48].

It seems that the role of liver resection is limited to a highly selected group of HCC patients with single small well differentiated lesion, no vascular invasion and well compensated cirrhosis without portal hypertension. Therapeutic options has to be individualized taking into consideration tumor biology, organ availability, patient preference, center practice and regional rules for organ allocation.

7. Organ allocation

Shortage of deceased organ donors led to the development of organ allocation schemes to ensure that such scarce resource is allocated to those patients who need it the most regarding justice in distribution of organs amongst different patients groups. Model for end stage liver disease (MELD) score is adopted by United Network for Organ sharing to prioritize patients on the waiting list. MELD was originally developed to predict mortality for patients with portal hypertension undergoing transjugular intrahepatic porto-systemic shunts (TIPS). MELD mathematical equation is 0.957 x log (serum creatinine, mg/dl+ 0.378 x log (serum bilirubin, mg/dl + 1.120 log (INR) + 0.643 [49]. Patients who have T2 (2-5 cm) HCC tumors within Milan criteria gain 22 exceptional MELD points. If the patient with stable disease is still waiting for OLT for three month the exceptional points are increased to 25 [50]. These exceptional points led to an exponential increase in the number of registered HCC patients for OLT [51].

8. Living liver donors

One of the major challenges facing the liver transplant community is donor organ shortage especially in Asia where deceased organ donation is limited. High mortality while on the transplant waiting list compounds the challenge. Living donor liver transplant (LDLT) programs have emerged as one of the solutions to bridge the gap between the overwhelming demand and the limited supply. Live donation offers many advantages to the recipients; it eliminates waiting time on the list, offers the convenience of scheduling the operation at an opportune time and optimal short cold ischemia time. Nevertheless, it subjects healthy donors to a major operation with possible 1% mortality and significant morbidity [52]. Healthy volunteers for donation undergo scrutinizing tests to validate their candidacy for liver donation including psychological evaluations. In a large number of living donor volunteers who step forward for evaluation; liver anatomical morphology and/or anomalies prohibit donation [53]. Pediatric patients usually receive left lateral segment (segments II and III) while adult recipients may receive right or left lobe depending on the liver volume, size and recipients' weight and height.

Advances in imaging technology allow calculating the liver volume of each lobe and also each segment as desired [54]. Actual knowledge of liver parenchymal, vascular and biliary anatomy is crucial to minimize operative and post-operative complications [55].Computer assisted and image guided surgery have contributed to the safety and precision of the donor operation. Two dimensional CT scans are converted to three dimensional (3D) images that delineate the vascular and biliary anatomy. Pre-operative planning and virtual resection have contributed significantly to liver resection safety. Also 3D pre-operative images guide venous reconstruction and help surgeons avoid venous congestion [56].

In a series of 236 patients who received LDLT for HCC and 172 patients outside Milan criteria; the recurrence rate was 12.7%. One and three year recurrence free survival was 72.7% and 64.7% respectively. Independent risk factors for tumor recurrence were serum alpha feto protein level, tumor size, bilobar distribution, tumor differentiation and vascular invasion. [57]. Vakili et al found that in HCC tumor recurrence is higher in LDLT recipients than in deceased donor recipients; 28.6 % versus 12.1% respectively. Paradoxically one- and five -year patient and graft survival in LDLT were 94% and 81% [58]. This higher HCC recurrence rate in LDLT may be explained by the time lag bias. Longer waiting time for deceased donors liver recipients discloses tumors with aggressive biology and patients drop out from the list. Another explanation may be the milieu of tumor regeneration with outpouring of growth factors that enhances tumor recurrence. Whether LDLT enhances recurrence remains controversial. In a well matched cohort of LDLT and DDLT recipients for HCC; the survival and recurrence rate were similar in the two groups. Microvascular invasion was the only predictor of tumor recurrence using regression analysis [59]. In a series of 221 LDLT for HCC; one of the significant factors for tumor recurrence is tumor size and number. Three-year HCC recurrence rates were 13.6% within Milan criteria, 20% within UCSF criteria and 51.6% beyond UCSF criteria [60].

9. Split livers

Another solution that was improvised to expand the donor pool in face organ shortage is split livers. The deceased donor liver is split to transplant two patients. Usually, the split incurs left lateral segment (segment II and III) for a pediatric recipient and the extended right (segments IV-VIII) for an adult recipient. Survival of split liver transplant is comparable to those of whole graft [61, 62]. *In vivo,* also *in situ,* splitting offers better out comes than *ex vivo* splitting in terms of post-operative complications and graft dysfunction [63]. In a series of six patients with HCC who received split liver grafts with a median follow up of 20 months no recurrence was observed [64]

In both approaches of reduced grafts, LDLT and split liver transplant, size matching is an important consideration in LDLT. A ratio of graft volume to standard liver volume of > 30% is crucial for adequate post-transplant hepatic function [65].

Small for size syndrome has been described in LDLT recipients when the graft liver volume is too small for the recipient [66]. Graft failure was attributed to high portal blood flow. It was described mainly in left lobe recipients. One of the protective strategies is of portal blood modulation. This is achieved by partial diversion of the portal blood flow to the inferior vena cava (IVC) by anastomosing the right portal branch to the right hepatic vein [67].

Also, large for size syndrome is a result of size mismatch when the abdominal cavity of the recipient cannot accommodate comfortably the graft [68]. Graft compression exaggerates the ischemia reperfusion injury. Using synthetic grafts such as gortex mesh or alloderm to close the abdominal wall without tension increase the chances of postoperative infections

10. Immunosuppression

Immunosuppression remains the drawback of transplantation. Immunosuppression entails substantial cost, compliance, vulnerability to a wide scope of infections and side effects and *de novo* malignancies.

Steroids, calcinurin inhibitors (CNIs) including cyclosporine and tacrolimus, mycofenolate mofetil and mammalian target of rapamycin (mTOR) inhibitor (rapamycin) remain the main agents for maintenance therapy. Each of those agents has a myriad of side effects. Usually two to three agents are used in combination in a trial to reduce the dose of each and subsequently minimize size effects. Major side effects of CNIs are renal toxicity, hypertension, diabetes mellitus and neurotoxicity. Serum levels have to be monitored frequently and dose adjusted accordingly. Major side effects of sirolimus are impaired wound healing, hypercholesterolemia, anemia, thrombocytopenia and mouth ulcers.

Steroids have a wide range of side effects including increased susceptibility to infections, diabetes mellitus, hypertension, impaired wound healing and cataracts to name a few. Early withdrawal of steroids is thought to be beneficial especially in HCV patients to control recurrence of viral hepatitis. One study found that early steroid withdrawal had no influence on HCV recurrence but reduced the incidence of post OLT diabetes mellitus [69].

In quest for the holy grail of transplantation, immune tolerance, induction immunosuppressive therapies have evolved to include various biological agents that are either monoclonal (muromonab-CD3, daclizumab, basiliximab, alemtuzumab) or polyclonal antithymocyte globulin [equine] or antithymocyte globulin [rabbit] antibodies. These agents can be further classified to depleting agents and non-depleting agents according to their ability to deplete lymphocyte. Depleting agents include antithymocyte globulin and anti CD52, alemtuzumab (Campath). Antilymphocyte globulin causes T lymphocyte lysis through a complement – dependent manner while alemtuzumab causes lymphocyte lysis by binding to CD 52, a receptor present on virtually all B and T lymphocytes. Non depleting agents include basiliximab (simulect) and Daclizumab (zenapax). Both agents are receptor antagonists that have high affinity to alpha subunits of IL-2 receptor, also known as CD- 25. IL-2 antagonism prevents T lymphocyte activation and proliferation.

The rational of induction immunotherapy is immunomodulation to curb allograft rejection, reduce the steroid and CNIs doses and subsequently minimize the side effects. The initial results are encouraging. In a randomized controlled study using rabbit antithymocyte globulin (RATG) for induction therapy; steroids were avoided, rejection episodes were less and HCV recurrence was decreased [70]. Using interlukin-2 receptor antibody (basiliximab) for induction allowed early withdrawal of the steroids and reduction of the tacrolimus dose. This was associated with fewer incidences of post OLT diabetes and acute cellular rejection [71].

New immunosuppression agents or immunomodulation agents for a better term, are being developed and tested in clinical trials involving mainly kidney transplant. Voclosporin (ISA247) is a novel CNI that proved to have similar effectiveness to Tacrolimus with potential reduction in new onset diabetes mellitus [72]. Belatacept is a chimeric fusion protein that blocks costimulation of T-lymphocytes was comparable to cyclosporine plus an improved renal function and fewer metabolic complications but increased risk of post-transplant lymphoproliferative disease [73]. Everolimus is an mTOR inhibitor, a rapamycin analogue. In a randomized controlled study involving liver transplant recipients, everolimus was found to impart same efficacy and better renal function when used with low dose tacrolimus compared to standard dose tacrolimus [74].

11. Tumor recurrence

Tumor recurrence remains a potential threat to HCC patients who receive liver transplants. HCC recurrence can be as high as 40% following OLT [75]. Researchers at University of Western Ontario, Canada looked at variables that significantly influence HCC recurrence post OLT. In a total of 75 cases 20 cases had recurrence within a follow up mean of 8 years. Tumor criteria were assessed based on the explant pathology. Those patients within UCSF criteria had a recurrence rate of 67% versus 12% of those within Milan criteria ($p < 0.001$). Also, 5-year survival was lower in UCSF group compared to Milan group 15% versus 83% respectively ($p < 0.001$) [76].

Immunosuppression regimen may have an influence on tumor recurrence. Decaens and colleagues found out that induction therapy with lymphocyte antibody (ATG) or anti CD3 antibody is a risk factor for HCC recurrence after OLT [77].

The antiproliferative property of rapamycin (sirolimus) makes it an attractive option for HCC patients in an attempt to reduce tumor recurrence and reduce the long term side effects of CNIs. In an animal model using human HCC tumor (LCI-D20) cell line; rapamycin alone or in combination with sorafineb was found to inhibit primary tumor growth and lung metastasis [78]. In one matched -cohort of HCC patients who underwent OLT; one group received sirolimus and the other group received tacrolimus based immunosuppression. Three-year recurrence free survival in the sirolimus group was 86% compared to 56% in the tacrolimus based group ($p < 0.04$) [79]. This issue remains controversial specially that HCC patients fall under different criteria; Milan, UCSF and beyond UCSF and immunosuppression protocols can vary great deal. Most publications in favor of the hypothesis that using sirolimus for post OLT immunosuppression reduces tumor recurrence are retrospective and level 3-4 evidence according to center for evidence based medicine, Oxford, U.K. [80]. This highlights the need for prospective, well designed, multicenter studies to solve this debate.

In a multivariate analysis involving 109 patients who underwent OLT, Lai et al found that exceeding UCSF criteria ($p = 0.003$) and microvascular invasion ($p = 0.007$) were independent risk factors for recurrence [81].

Up- to -7 criteria was tested in a recent study involving 479 HCC patients who received OLT at two different centers. In 335 patients who met up -to -7 criteria; the calculated recurrence probability at 1-, 3- and 5- year was 4%, 8% and 14%. Multivariate analysis showed that only macrovascular invasion and tumor grade were significant predictors of survival [82].

Many liver transplant centers confirm that tumor biology plays an important role post OLT survival and recurrence. Crude markers such as degree of differentiation (G1-G4) and microvascular invasion are increasingly found to be predictors of recurrence [83]. Also, tumor numbers, diameter of the largest lesion and donor age were significant predictors of recurrence [84]. Another study included 48 patients found that pre transplant AFP slope greater than 50 μg/L per month is associated with higher rate of one year recurrence [85].

The fact that tumor recurs in a subgroup of transplant patients after removal of the only source i.e. HCC bearing liver coupled with the growing evidence of the role or vascular invasion, both micro and macro, as a risk factor for recurrence supports the hypothesis of circulating tumor cells (CTC) role in recurrence [86].

12. Conclusion and future look

In conclusion, the major strides in liver transplantations made it a valuable therapeutic option for a subset of carefully selected HCC patients. Studies continue to identify tumor criteria that yield post-transplant outcomes comparable to those of non-tumor transplant patients. Tumor signature at a molecular level is a promising field to further characterize HCC in the context of liver transplantation. Pre transplant loco-regional therapies, especially for T2 HCC patients who are anticipated to wait more than six months, provide tumor control and possibly improve outcomes. Ongoing research in surgical technology adds new items to the surgical armamentarium such as image guided surgery, Nano knife that makes liver surgery safer and more effective. Advances in immunomodulation are coming up with promising new agents that are more efficient and with fewer side effects.

Author details

Emad H. Asham[1], Howard Mansour[2] and Mark Ghobrial[1*]

*Address all correspondence to: rmghobrial@tmhs.org

1 Transplant & HPB Surgery, Center for Liver Disease and Transplantation, The Methodist Hospital, Texas Medical Center, Houston, Texas, USA

2 Hepatology, Center for Liver Disease and Transplantation, The Methodist Hospital, Texas Medical Center, Houston, Texas, USA

References

[1] Center for Disease Control and Prevention. Morbidity and Mortality Weekly Report 2010; 59 (17):517.

[2] Morgan TR, Mandayam S, Jamal MM. Alcohol and hepatocellular carcinoma. Gastroenterology. 2004 ;127(5 Suppl 1):S87-96.

[3] McCollough. The clinical features, diagnosis and natural history of non-alcoholic fatty liver disease. Clin Liver Dis 2004; 8:521-533.

[4] Shimada M, Hashimoto E, Taniai M, Hasegawa K, Hiroaki Okuda H, Hayashi N, Takasaki K, Ludwig J. Hepatocellular carcinoma in patients with non-alcoholic steatohepatitis. J Hepatol 2002; 37:154-160.

[5] Finch SC, Finch CA, 1995. Idiopathic hemochromatosis and iron storage disease: A. Iron metabolism in hemochromatosis. Medicine 34: 381-430.

[6] Farinati F, Floreani A, De Maria N, Fagiuoli S, Naccarato R, Chiaramonte M.. Hepatocellular carcinoma in primary biliary cirrhosis. J Hepatol. 1994; 21(3):315-6.

[7] Bassendine M, Rushbrook S, Chapman R. In: Sherlock S (ed.) Diseases of the liver and Biliary, Diseases of the Liver and Biliary System. Edinburgh. 12th Edition. Blackwell Science 2011 page 338-342.

[8] Belghiti J, Vilgrain V, Paradis V In: L.H. Blumgart (ed.) Surgery of The Liver and Bilairy Tract and the pancreas. 4th Edition. Edniburgh .Saunders 2007: 1142-1143.

[9] Kuper H, Tzonou A, Kaklamani E, Hsieh C, Lagiou P, Adami H, Trichopoulos D, Stuver S. Tobacco smoking, alcohol consumption and their interaction in the causa-

tion of hepatocellular carcinoma. International Journal of Cancer 2000, 85(4): 498–502.

[10] Liu Y, Chang CC, Marsh GM, Wu F. Population attributable risk of aflatoxin-related liver cancer: Systematic review and meta-analysis. Eur J Cancer. 2012 Mar 8. Epub ahead of print.

[11] Takayasu K, Muramatsu Y, Moriyama N, Wakao F, Makuuchi M, Takayama T, Kosuge T, Okazaki N, Yamada R. Radiological study of idiopathic Budd-Chiari syndrome complicated by hepatocellular carcinoma. A report of four cases. Am J Gastroenterol. 1994 Feb; 89(2):249-53.

[12] Iwatzuki S, Gordon R, M.D., Sahw Jr B, Starzl T. Role of Liver Transplantation in Cancer Therapy. Ann Surg 1985; 202(40: 401-407.

[13] Mazzaferro V, Regalia E, Doci R, Andreola S, Pulvirenti A, Bozzetti F, et al. Liver transplantation for the treatment of small hepatocellular carcinomas in patients with cirrhosis.N Engl J Med 1996;334:693-699.

[14] Yao FY, Ferrell L, Bass. NM, et al. Liver transplantation for hepatocellular carcinoma: expansion of the tumor size limits does not adversely impact survival. Hepatology 2001; 33: 1394– 403.

[15] Adler M, De Pauw F, Vereerstraeten P, et al. Outcome of patients with hepatocellular carcinoma listed for liver transplantation within the Euro transplant allocation system. Liver Transpl 2008; 14: 526–33.

[16] DuBay D, Sandroussi C, Sandhu L, et al. Liver transplantation for advanced hepatocellular carcinoma using poor tumor differentiation on biopsy as an exclusion criterion. Ann Surg. 2011; 253:166-72.

[17] Mazzaferro V, Llovet JM, Miceli R, Bhoori S, Schiavo M, Mariani L, et al. Predicting survival after liver transplantation in patients with hepatocellular carcinoma beyond the Milan criteria: a retrospective, exploratory analysis. Lancet Oncol 2009;10:35-43.

[18] Paradis V, Degos F, Dargere D, Pham N, Belghiti J, Degott C, et al. Identification of a new marker of hepatocellular carcinoma by serum protein profiling of patients with chronic liver diseases. HEPATOLOGY 2005; 41:40-47.

[19] Kim T, Murakami T, Takahashi S, Tsuda K, Tomoda K, Narumi Y, Oi H, Sakon M, Nakamura H. Optimal phases of dynamic CT for detecting hepatocellularcarcinoma: evaluation of unenhanced and triple-phase images. Abdom Imaging 1999; 24: 473–480.

[20] Ito K. Hepatocellular carcinoma: Conventional MRI findings including gadolinium-enhanced dynamic imaging. European Journal of Radiology 2006; 58 (2): 186–199.

[21] Alqahtani SA, Fouad TR, Lee SS. Cirrhotic cardiomyopathy. Semin Liver Dis. 2008 Feb;28(1):59-69.

[22] Møller S, Henriksen J H. Cirrhotic cardiomyopathy: a pathophysiological review of circulatory dysfunction in liver disease. Heart 2002;87:9–15.

[23] Saborido BP, Diaz JC, de Los Galanes SJ, Segurola CL, de Usera MA, Garrido MD, et al. Does preoperative fine needle aspiration-biopsy produce tumor recurrence in patients following liver transplantation for hepatocellular carcinoma? Transplant Proc 2005;37:3874-3877.

[24] Mullhaupt B , Francois Durand, Tanja Roskams,4 Philipp Dutkowski,2 and Markus Heim. Is Tumor Biopsy Necessary? Liver transplantation2011; 17:S14-S25.

[25] Bellis L, Castellacci R, Fabrizio M, Festuccia F, Corvisieri P and Puito C.Hepatic venous pressure gradient determination in patients with hepatitis C virus-related and alcoholic cirrhosis. Euro J of Gastroent & Hepat 2003; 15(10): 1085-1089.

[26] Singhal A, Jayaraman M, Dhanasekaran D, Kohli V. Molecular and serum markers in hepatocellular carcinoma: Predictive tools for prognosis and recurrence. Crit Rev Oncol Hematol. 2012 May; 82(2):116-40.

[27] Llovet JM, Bru C, Bruix J. Prognosis of hepatocellular carcinoma: the BCLC staging classification. Semin Liver Dis 1999; 19: 329–338.

[28] Burix J and Sherman M. Management of Hepatocellular Carcinoma: An Update Hepatology 2011; 53(3):1020-2.

[29] Kashiwagi T. PDG-PET and hepatocellular carcinoma. J Gastroenterol 2004; 39:1017-1018.

[30] Panjalaa C, D. L. Senecalb, M. D. Bridgesc,G. P. Kimd, R. E. Nakhlehe, J. H. H. Nguyenf and D. M. Harnois. The Diagnostic Conundrum and LiverTransplantation Outcome for Combined Hepatocellular-Cholangiocarcinoma. Am J Transpl 2010; 10: 1263–1267.

[31] Tickoo S, Zee S, Obiekwe S, Xiao, Koea, Robiou C ,Blumgart L, Jarnagin, W, Ladanyi M , Klimstra, D. Combined Hepatocellular-Cholangiocarcinoma: A Histopathologic, Immunohistochemical, and In Situ Hybridization Study. Am J Surg Path. 2002; 26 (8): 989-997.

[32] Bolondi L, Gaiani S, Celli N, Golfieri R, Grigioni W, Leoni S, Venturi A, Piscaglia F . Characterization of Small Nodules in Cirrhosis by Assessment of Vascularity: The Problem of Hypovascular Hepatocellular Carcinoma. Hepatology 2005;42(1): 27-34.

[33] Bolondi L, Sofia S, Siringo S, Gaiani S, Casali A, Zironi G, et al. Surveillance programme of cirrhotic patients for early diagnosis and treatment of hepatocellular carcinoma: a cost-effectiveness analysis. Gut 2001;48:251-259.

[34] Rougier P, Mitrya E, Barbareb JC , Taiebc J. Hepatocellular Carcinoma (HCC): An Update. Sem Oncol 2007 ; 34, Supplement 1: S12–S20.

[35] Majno P, Riccardo Lencioni,2 Franc¸oise Mornex,3 Nicolas Girard,3 Ronnie T. Poon,4 and Daniel Cherqui. Is the Treatment of Hepatocellular Carcinoma on the Waiting List Necessary? Liver Transp 2011; 17:S98–S108.

[36] Cilloa U, A. Vitaleb,∗, F. Grigolettoc, E. Gringeria, F. D'Amicoa, M. Valmasonia, A. Brolesea,G. Zanusa, N. Srsena, A. Carraroa, P. Burrad, F. Farinatid, P. Angelie and D. F. D'Amicoa. Intention-to-Treat Analysis of Liver Transplantation in Selected, Aggressively Treated HCC Patients Exceeding the Milan Criteria. American Journal of Transplantation 2007; 7: 972–981.

[37] Graziadei W, Sandmueller H, Waldenberger P, Koenigsrainer A, Nachbaur K, Jaschke W, Margreiter R, Vogel W. Chemoembolization Followed by Liver Transplantation for Hepatocellular Carcinoma Impedes Tumor Progression While on the Waiting List and Leads to Excellent Outcome. Liver Transplantation 2003;l 9,(6): 557-563

[38] Lu D, Yu N, Raman S, Lassman C, Tong M, Britten C, Durazo F, Saab S, Han S, Finn R, Hiatt J, Bussuttil R. Percutaneous radiofrequency ablation of hepatocellular carcinoma as a brigde to liver transplantation. Hepatology 2005; 41(5) 1130- 1137.

[39] Kurokohchi K, S Watanabe, T Masaki, N Hosomi, T Funaki, K Arima, S Yoshida, Y Miyauchi, S Kuriyama. Combined use of percutaneous ethanol injection and radiofrequency ablation for the effective treatment of hepatocelluar carcinoma. Inter J Onc 2002; 21(4):841-6.

[40] Yao F., kerlan R, Hirose R, Davern T, Bass N, Feng S, Peters M, terrault N, Freise C, Ascher N and Roberts J. Excellent Outcome Following Down-Staging of Hepatocellular Carcinoma Prior to Liver Transplantation: An Intention-to-Treat Analysis. Hepatology 2008; 48(3):

[41] Guo Y, Zhang Y, Klein R, Nijm GM, Sahakian AV, Omary RA, et al. Irreversible electroporation therapy in the liver: longitudinal efficacy studies in a rat model of hepatocellular carcinoma. Cancer Res 2010; 70:1555-1563.

[42] Thomas K, Chung W, Ellis S, Frederman D, Kavnoudias H, Loader-Oliver D, Robert S, Evans P, Ball C, Haydon A. Investigation of the Safety of Irreversible Electroporation in Humans. J Vas Interven Rad 2011; 22,(5): 611-621.

[43] Wilhelm SM, Carter C, Tang L, et al. BAY 43-9006 exhibits broad spectrum oral antitumor activity and targets the RAF/MEK/ERK pathway and receptor tyrosine kinases involved in tumor progression and angiogenesis. Cancer Res. 2004; 64: 7099-7109.

[44] Sonnenberg F, Beck R, Markov Models in Medical Decision Making. A Practical Guide. Med Decision Making December 1993; 13(4): 322-338.

[45] Vitale A,1 Michael L. Volk,2 Davide Pastorelli,3 Sara Lonardi,3 Fabio Farinati,4 Patrizia Burra,4 Paolo Angeli, Cillo U. Use of Sorafenib in Patients With Hepatocellular

Carcinoma Before Liver Transplantation: A Cost-Benefit Analysis While Awaiting Data on Sorafenib Safety. Hepatology 2009; 51 (1): 165-173.

[46] Llovet JX, Bruix J, Gores GJ. Surgical resection versus transplantation for early hepatocellular carcinoma. Clues for the best therapy. Hepatology 2000; 31:1019-1021.

[47] Adam,R Azoulay D, Castaing D, Eshkenazy R, Pascal G, Hashizume K, Samuel D and Bismuth H. Liver resection as a bridge to transplantation for Hepatocellular carcinoma on cirrhosis. A reasonable strategy? Ann Surg 2003; 238(4):508-519.

[48] Belghiti J, Cortes A, Abdalla E, Regimbeau J, Parkash K, Durand F, Sommacale D, Dondero F, Lesurtel M, Sauvanet A, Farges O, Kianmanesh R. Resection prior to transplantation for hepatocellular carcinoma. Ann Sur 2003; 238(6):885-893.

[49] Malinchoc M, Kamath P, Gordon F, Peine CJ, Rank J, ter Borg PC. A Model to predict poor survival in patients undergoing transjugular portosystemic shunts. Hepatology 2000;31:864-71.

[50] United Network for Organ Sharing/Organ Procurement and Transplantation Network. UNOS/OPTN policy 3.6.4.4. http://optn.transplant.hrsa.gov/.

[51] Sceintific Registery of Transplant Recepients annual report 2010. www.srtr/annual_reports/2010/flash.

[52] Pomfret EA, Pomposelli JJ, Lewis WD, et al. Live donor adult liver transplantation using right lobe grafts: donor evaluation and surgical outcome. Arch Surg 2001; 136:425–433.

[53] Lee S, Hwang S, Moon D, Ahn C, Kim K, Sung K, Ko G, Park K, Ha T Song G. Expanded Indication Criteria of Living Donor Liver Transplantation for Hepatocellular Carcinoma at One Large-Volume Center. Liver Transpl 2008 14:935-945.

[54] Koichi Urata1, Seiji Kawasaki MD1,*, Hidetoshi Matsunami1, Yasuhiko Hashikura1, Toshihiko Ikegami1, Shinpachi Ishizone3, Yoshitaka Momose3, Atsushi Komiyama2, Masatoshi Makuuchi. Calculation of child and adult standard liver volume for liver transplantation. Hepatology 1995; 21(5): 1317–1321.

[55] Chen YS, Chen CL, Liu PP, Chiang YC.Preoperative evaluation of donors for living related liver transplantation. Transplant Proc 1996; 28:2415–2416.

[56] Lang H, Radtke A, Hindennach M, Schroeder T, Frühauf N, Malagó M, Bourquain H, Peitgen H, Oldhafer K, Broelsch C. Arch Surg. 2005;140:629-638. Impact of Virtual Tumor Resection and Computer-Assisted Risk Analysis on Operation Planning and Intraoperative Strategy in Major Hepatic Resection Br J Surg. 2012; 99(6):855-63.

[57] Todo S and Hiroyuki Furukawa H, on behalf of the Japanese Study Group on Organ Transplantation. Living Donor Liver Transplantation for Adult Patients With Hepatocellular Carcinoma: Experience in Japan. Ann Surg. 2004; 240(3): 251-26.

[58] Vakili K, Pomposelli JJ, Cheah YL, et al. Living donor liver transplantation for hepatocellular carcinoma: increased recurrence but improved survival. Liver Transpl 2009; 15: 1861–6.

[59] Sandhu L, Sandroussi C, Guba M, Selzner M, Ghanekar A, Cattral M, McGLivary I, Levy G, Greig P, Renner E and Grant D. Living Donor Liver Transplantation Versus Deceased Donor Liver Transplantation for Hepatocellular Carcinoma: Comparable Survival and Recurrence. Liver Transpl. 2012 Mar;18(3):315-22.

[60] Lee SG, Hwang S, Moon DB, Ahn CS, Kim KH, Sung KB, Ko GY, park KM, Ha TY, Song GW. Expanded Indication Criteria of Living Donor Liver Transplantation for Hepatocellular Carcinoma at One Large-Volume Center. Liver transpl. 2008; 14: 935-945.

[61] Muller S, Mehrabi A, Schmied B, Welsch T, Engleman F, Schemmer P, Weits J and Schmidt J.Partial liver transplantation-living donor liver transplantation and split liver transplantation. Nephrol Dial Transplant (2007) 22 [Suppl 8]: viii13–viii22.

[62] Rela M, Vougas V, Muiesan P, Valica-Melendez H, Smyrniotis V, Gibbs P, Kaani J, Williams R, Heaton N. Split Liver transplantation: King's College Hospital Experience. Ann Surg 1998; 227(2): 282-288

[63] Busuttil R, Goss J. Split liver transplant. Ann Surg 199; 229(3): 313-321.

[64] Sotiropoulos GC, Lang H, Frühauf NR, Molmenti EP, Omar OS, Radtke A, Paul A, Nadalin S, Frilling A, Broelsch CE, Malagò M.. Split liver transplantation for hepatocellular carcinoma. Hepatogastroenterology. 2006 Sep-Oct;53(71):764-7.

[65] Lo MC, Fan ST, Chan JKF, et al. Minimum graft volume for successful adult to adult living donor liver transplantation for fulminant hepatic failure. Transplantation 1996; 62:696-698.

[66] Dahm F, Georgeiv, Clavien P. Small-for-Size Syndrome After Partial Liver Transplantation: Definition, Mechanisms of Disease and Clinical Implications. Am J Transpl 2005; 5: 2605–2610.

[67] Botha J, Langnas A, Campos D, Grant W, Freise C, Ascher N, Mercer D, Roberts J. Left Lobe Adult-to-Adult Living Donor Liver Transplantation: Small Grafts and Hemiportocaval Shunts in the Prevention of Small-for-Size Syndrome. Liver Transpl. 2010 May;16(5):649-57.

[68] Emond JC, Leib M. The living-related liver transplant evaluation: linking risk factors and outcome. Liver Transpl Surg 1996;2 [5 Suppl 1]: S57–S63.

[69] Klintmalm GB, Davis GL, Teperman L, Netto GJ, Washburn K, Rudich SM, Pomfret EA, Vargas HE, Brown R, Eckhoff D, Pruett TL, Roberts J, Mulligan DC, Charlton MR, Heffron TG, Ham JM, Douglas DD, Sher L, Baliga PK, Kinkhabwala M, Koneru B, Abecassis M, Millis M, Jennings LW, Fasola CG. A randomized, multicenter study comparing steroid-free immunosuppression and standard immunosuppression for

liver transplant recipients with chronic hepatitis C. Liver Transpl. 2011; 17(12): 1394-403.

[70] Eason J, Loss G, Blazek J, Nair S, Mason A. Steroid-Free Liver Transplantation Using Rabbit Antithymocyte Globulin Induction: Results of a Prospective Randomized Trial. Liver Transplantation 2001; 7(8): 693-697

[71] Liu C, Fan S, Lo C, Chan S, Ng I, Lai C, Wong J. Interleukin-2 Receptor Antibody (Basiliximab) for Immunosuppressive Induction Therapy After LiverTransplantation: A Protocol With Early Elimination of Steroids and Reduction of Tacrolimus Dosage. Liver Transplantation 2004; 10, (6): 728–733.

[72] Busque S, Cantarovich M, Mulgaonkar S, Gaston R, Gaber AO, Mayo PR, Ling S, Huizinga RB, Meier-Kriesche HU; PROMISE Investigators. The PROMISE study: a phase 2b multicenter study of voclosporin (ISA247) versus tacrolimus in de novo kidney transplantation. Am J Transplant. 2011 Dec;11(12):2675-84.

[73] Vincenti F, Charpentier B, Vanrenterghem Y, Rostaing L, Bresnahan B, Darji P, et al. A phase III study of belatacept-based immunosuppression regimens versus cyclosporine in renal transplant recipients (BENEFIT study). Am J Transplant 2010;10:535-546.

[74] Saliba F, De Simone P, Nevens F, De Carlis LMetselaar HJ, Beckebaum S, et al. Efficacy and safety of everolimus with early reduction or elimination of tacrolimus in 719 de novo liver transplant recipients: 12 month results of a randomized, controlled study. Hepatology 2011;54 (Suppl);

[75] Marsh JW, Dvorchik I, Subotin M, et al. The prediction of risk of recurrence and ime to recurrence of hepatocellular carcinoma after orthotopic liver transplantation: a pilot study. Hepatology. 1997;26(2):444-450.

[76] Parfitt J, Marotta P, AlGhamdi M, Wall W, Khakhar A, Suskin N, Quan D, McAllister V, Ghent C , Levstik M, McLean C, Chakrabarti S, Garcia B and Driman D. Recurrent Hepatocellular Carcinoma after Transplantation: Use of a Pathological Score on Explanted Livers to Predict Recurrence. Liver Trans 2007; 13:543-551.

[77] Decaens T, Roudot-Thoraval F, Bresson-Handi S, Meyer C, GugenheimJ, Durand F, Bernard P, Boillot O, Compagon P, Calmus Y, Hardwigsen J, Ducef C, Pageaux P, Dharancy S, Chazouilleres O, Cherqui D, Duvoux C. Role of immunosuppression and tumor differentiation in predicting recurrence after liver transplantation for hepatocellular carcinoma: A multicenter study of 412 patients. W J Gastroent 2006; 12(45): 7319-7325.

[78] Wang Z, Zhou J, Fan J, Qiu SJ, Yu Y, Huang XW and Tang ZY. Effect of Rapamycin Alone and in Combination with Sorafenib in an Orthotopic Model of Human Hepatocellular Carcinoma. Clin Cancer Res August 15, 2008 14; 5124.

[79] Vivarelli M, Dazzi A, Zanello M, Cucchetti A, Cescon M, Ravaioli M, Del Gaudio M, Lauro A, Grazi G, Pinna A. Effect of Different Immunosuppressive Schedules on Re-

currence-Free Survival After Liver Transplantation for Hepatocellular Carcinoma. Transplantation 2010; 89 (2): 227-231.

[80] Schnitzbauer A, Schlitt H, and Geissle E. Influence of Immunosuppressive Drugs on the Recurrence of Hepatocellular Carcinoma After Liver Transplantation: A Gap Between Basic Science and Clinical Evidence. Transplantation 2011; 91(11): 1173- 1176.

[81] Lai Q , Merlib M, Ginanni Corradinib S, Menninia G, Gentilib F, Molinarob A, Morabitoa V, Ferrettic G, Pugliesed F, Novellia G, Berlocoa P, Rossia M. Predictive Factors of Recurrence of Hepatocellular Carcinoma After Liver Transplantation: A Multivariate Analysis. Transplantation Proceedings 2009;41(4): 1306–1309.

[82] D'Alco F, Schwartz M, Vltale A, Tabrizian P, Roayale S, Thing A, Guido M, Martin J, Schlano T and Cllio U. Predicting Recurrence After Liver Transplantation in Patients with Hepatocellular Carcinoma Exceeding the Up-To-Seven CriteriaLiver Transpl 15:1278-1287, 2009.

[83] Dudek K, Kornasiewicza O , Remiszewskia P, Kobryńb K, Ziarkiewicz-Wróblewskac B, Górnickac B, Zieniewicza K, Krawczyka M. Impact of Tumor Characteristic on the Outcome of Liver Transplantation in Patients With Hepatocellular Carcinoma. Transplantation Proceedings 2009; 41, (8): 3135–3137.

[84] Sharma P, Welch K, Hussain H, Pelletier S, Fontana R, Marrero J, Merion R. Incidence and risk factors of Hepatocellular carcinoma recurrence after liver transplantation in the MELD era. Dig Dis Sci 2012; 57:806-812.

[85] Han K, Tziman G, Barkun J, Metrakos P, Tchervenkv J, Hilzenrat N, Wong P, Deschenes M. Pre-operative alpha feto protein slope is predeictive of hepatocellular carcinoma recurrence after liver transplantation. Can J Gastroenterol 2007; 21(1): 39-45.

[86] Xu W, Cao L, Chen L, Isolation of circulating tumor cells using a novel cell separation strategy. Clin Cancer Res. 2011; 17: 3783-93.

Chapter 3

Radioembolization for the Treatment of Unresectable Hepatocellular Carcinoma

Hojjat Ahmadzadehfar, Amir Sabet and
Hans Jürgen Biersack

Additional information is available at the end of the chapter

http://dx.doi.org/10.5772/56291

1. Introduction

Nuclear medicine therapy is required to be highly specific and targeted since it always involves administration of unsealed sources of radioactivity. Radionuclides emitting ß-particles are generally used for therapeutic purposes because of their ability to penetrate and depositing cytotoxic energy in tissues. There are several choices of ß emitters with respect to energy of the emission. Lower energy ß particles can travel a few cell diameters, or at most in the sub-millimeter range, whereas higher energy ß particles such as those emitted by yttrium 90 (90Y) have a greater tissue penetration with a range beyond the source of several millimeters. The physical half-life of the therapeutic radionuclide is also an important consideration and underlying principle for therapy planning. For therapeutic purposes, radionuclides are usually, except in thyroid treatment, attached to a drug or particle that controls the biodistribution. The ideal therapeutic radiopharmaceutical is one that remains attached to the parent drug or its metabolites, and is excreted rapidly through a known simple route[1].

1.1. Concepts and principles

Along with the significant progress in hepatobiliary surgery in the last 30 years, various innovative liver-directed treatments have been developed [2] including conformal radiation, hepatic arterial infusion chemotherapy (HAI), transarterial chemoembolization (TACE), radiofrequency ablation (RFA) and radioembolization (RE) with radionuclide microspheres [3].

Conformal and stereotactic radiation therapy techniques can be used to deliver high radiation doses in cases with focal involvement [4]; however, since hepatic primary neoplasms are often multifocal and irregular in shape, and potentially replacing large parts of the liver volume, only a small minority of patients are optimal candidates for such therapies[5].

Radioembolization (RE), also named selective internal radiation therapy (SIRT), is a promising catheter based liver-directed modality for patients with primary and metastatic liver cancer. RE provides several advantages over traditional treatment methods including its low toxicity profile[6, 7].

Its rationale arises from the anatomic and physiological aspects of hepatic tumors being exploited for the delivery of therapeutic agents. The prominent feature is the dual blood supply of liver tissue, from the hepatic artery and the portal vein. Observations on vascular supply to hepatic malignancies have demonstrated that metastatic hepatic tumors >3 mm derive 80–100% of their blood supply from the arterial rather than the portal hepatic circulation[8]. Normal liver tissue, in contrary, is predominantly fed by the portal vein (60-70%). Apart from RE with 90Y microspheres, being an approved therapy by the Food and Drug Administration (FDA), various other radionuclides has also been used or investigated for treatment of liver tumors including Phosphorus-32, Rhenium-188 and holmium-166[9-12]. In this chapter, however, we focus only on the therapeutic indications, usefulness and methods of treatment with ^{90}Y-microspheres.

1.2. Physical characteristics of ^{90}Y and microspheres

^{90}Y is a pure β emitter, produced by neutron bombardment of yttrium-89 in a reactor, with a limited tissue penetration (mean 2.5 mm, max 11 mm), and short half-life (64 h), making it an ideal transarterial liver-directed agent. The size of the microspheres ranges between 20-40 μm. The upper size limit of the microspheres allows delivery to the tumours via the hepatic artery, while the lower size limit prevents the microspheres from passing from the arterial circulation into the venous circulation. The microspheres remain trapped within the vasculature of the tumours and deliver a selective radiation dose to the tumour tissue [13].

The mean tissue penetration of 2.5 mm of ß particles emitted from the selectively delivered yttrium allows an extremely high local tumour doses ranging from 50 to 150 Gy [14-17] to > 1000 Gy to the tumour tissue while sparing normal liver parenchyma. This is in contrast to traditional whole liver external beam radiation where radiation doses have to be limited to 30 Gy to prevent serious hepatic dysfunction [18].

Two 90Y microsphere products are commercially available: TheraSphere® (glass microspheres) and Sirsphere® (resin microsphere). There are some distinct differences in properties between the two products as shown in Table 1.

1.3. Patient selection criteria

The selection process of patients referred for RE involves several aspects to be taken into account. Patients considered for RE should have especially (*1*) unresectable hepatic tumour, (*2*) liver-dominant tumour burden, (*3*) a life expectancy of at least 3 months and (4) an ECOG performance score of ≤2[19]. The general clinical condition, as described by the ECOG or Karnofsky performance score is an important aspect for patient selection prior to RE. Patients with a significantly reduced performance status are at higher risk of developing severe side effects, including radiation induced liver failure[20, 21] and generally have worse treatment outcome.

Y90 microspheres	SIR-Spheres	TheraSphere
Company	Sirtex Medical, Sydney, Australia	MDS Nordion, Ottawa, Ontario, Canada
material	resin-based	glass-based
Diameter	20–60 μm	20–30 μm
Activity per particle	50 Bq	2500 Bq
Number of microspheres per 3-GBq vial	40–80 X 106	1.2 X 106
Specific gravity	1.6 g/mL	3.2 g/mL
Maximal prescribed dose (GBq)	3	20
Relative embolic potential	Higher	Lower
Relative pressure for infusion	Lower	Higher
Contrast injection during infusion	possible	Not possible

Table 1. Properties of resin and glass yttrium-90 microspheres

These lead to questioning the rationale of posing the patient at such costly and potentially harmful treatment measure. Contraindications for RE include pretreatment angiogram indications of flow to the gastrointestinal tract which can not be corrected by coilc embolization techniques, an excessive shunting to the lungs that would result in > 30 Gy lung dose on a single administration as quantified by the tc-99m macroaggregated albumin (Tc-MAA) scan, excessive tumour burden with limited hepatic reserve, and biochemical evidence of reduced liver function as potentially indicated by elevated levels of bilirubin (widely suggested cut-off: 2 mg/dl), highly elevated liver enzymes (AST or ALT > 5x upper normal limit), significantly altered INR or PTT, or reduced serum albumin. Patients with prior radiotherapy involving the liver should be carefully reviewed on a case-by-case basis (Table 2) [7, 19].

1. Absent surgical (resection, liver transplantation) or ablative options (RFA)
2. Preserved liver function (intact liver synthesis)
a Bilirubin (< 2 mg/dl) b. Albumin (≥ 3 mg/dl) c. PT/PTT (no endogenous severe impairment) d. AST/ALT ≤ 5 x normal
3. Adequate general condition (ECOG performance score ≤ 2)
4. Liver-dominant tumor burden 5. Life-expectancy ≥ 3 months 6. Acceptable LSF (≤20% for resin and ≤30Gy for glass microspheres)

Table 2. Basic requirements for radioembolization

The renal status should be adequate to accommodate for any concurrent chemotherapy that is part of the treatment plan[22], as well as for the use of contrast agents during the diagnostic and the therapeutic angiogram. Hemodialysis patients may be treated with RE, however, dialysis has to be planned and timed before and after the intervention.

The decision to perform RE should be based on an interdisciplinary consent, ideally after discussion in an adequate tumor board with participation of specialists in surgery, gastroenterology, oncology, radiology, nuclear medicine and radiation therapy. Especially patients not fulfilling the common inclusion criteria should only be accepted as RE candidates after appropriate consent from such interdisciplinary tumor board.

1.4. Imaging modalities before radioembolization

The imaging includes a three-phase contrast computed tomography (CT) and/or gadolinium-enhanced magnetic resonance imaging (MRI) of the liver for assessment of tumour and non-tumour volume, main portal vein patency, and extent of extrahepatic disease.

18F-Fluorodeoxyglucose positron emission tomography/computed tomography (18F-FDG-PET/CT) is a very sensitive functional imaging modality for tumours with high glucose metabolism such as colorectal carcinoma, melanoma, head and neck tumors, and breast cancer. However, it is not a satisfactory imaging choice for pre- and post treatment evaluation of patients with HCC as these tumours except for their aggressive types, show no or a very low grade FDG uptake. This results in the suboptimal sensitivity of 18F-FDG-PET for HCC, ranging between 50% and 70% [23, 24]. Nevertheless, 18F-FDG-PET may provide prognostic information (metabolic grading) as patients with a negative FDG-PET have a better prognosis than those with high FDG uptake. Furthermore, addition of a metabolic imaging to the anatomical imaging modalities before performing RE leads to a more accurate follow up and therapy response assessment[25].

1.5. Angiogram with selective visceral catheterization and therapy simulation

Once a patient has been selected as a candidate for RE, an initial angiographic evaluation, known as test-angiogram, has to be performed as the first step, It is well known that the anatomy of the mesenteric system and the hepatic arterial bed has a high degree of variation, with "normal vascular anatomy" being present in only 60% of cases. Therefore, in order to perform any kind of therapeutic transarterial procedure in the liver in a safe and efficient manner it is essential to be acquainted with the hepatic arterial anatomy[26].

A feature of the neoplastic vasculature within tumours is the formation of arteriovenous anastomoses or shunts. Shunts allow microspheres to directly enter the venous return by bypassing the terminal arterioles in the tumour. This will deposit the shunted microspheres into the lung, resulting in radiation pneumonitis [22, 27].

Dystopic spread of microspheres to other extrahepatic visceral sites such as stomach, duodenum or pancreas, may also be associated with the risk of severe radiation damage leading to pain, ulceration and possibly perforation, pancreatitis, cholecystitis, skin necrosis and other non-target radiation complications[28].

Avoiding extrahepatic deposition of microspheres requires prophylactic embolization of all extrahepatic vessels including the gastroduodenal, right gastric and pancreaticoduodenal branches. If embolization is not possible, the catheter for treatment can alternatively be placed beyond the respective origins of these vessels. The angiogram must be accomplished with Tc-MAA injected into the hepatic artery similar to the application during microsphere treatment [19]. Scintigraphy should be performed within 1 hour of Tc-MAA injection to prevent false-positive extrahepatic activity due to free ^{99m}technetium (^{99m}Tc). The unwanted uptake of ^{99m}Tc-pertechnetate in the thyroid and stomach can be avoided using perchlorate. For this purpose patients should receive 600 mg perchlorate orally 30 minutes before angiography [29, 30].

It is of note that these vessels/organs can revascularize quickly, and therefore the embolization should be performed close to the intended time of RE, with a check arteriogram required before RE to ensure that such revascularization has not occurred[19].

Determining the possibility of lung damage due to liver-to-lung shunting is relatively simple as described by Lau et al.[31] Following infusion of 100-400 MBq Tc-MAA in the hepatic arterial branches, a whole body scan in anterior and posterior projections is sufficient to calculate the percentage of lung shunting and, consequently, the possibility of pulmonary side effects. The percentage of lung shunting can be determined from the total counts within regions of interest (ROIs) over both lobes of the lung and the liver, using the geometric mean of ventral and dorsal images. Depending on the shunt rate, a reduction of the total administered dose to the liver may be necessary. The highest tolerable dose to the lungs after treatment with RE is considered to be up to 30 Gy with a single injection, and up to 50 Gy for multiple injections[27]. The estimated dose (Gy) to the lungs is equal to A (GBq) x LSF x 50, assuming the total mass of both lungs to be 1 kg. Where A is the activity infused and LSF is the lung shunt fraction. The cumulative absorbed lung radiation dose can be calculated with the following equation [32] [33]:

$$\text{Cumulative absorbed lung radiation dose} = 50 \times \text{ lung mass} \sum_{i=1}^{n} Ai \times \text{LSF}_i$$

Where Ai = activity infused, LSFi = lung shunt fraction during infusion, n = number of infusions, and approximate vascular lung mass = 1 kg.

Another way is recommended by SIRTex Company as shown in table 3. According to SIRTex recommendations, the amount of microspheres delivered to the patient should be reduced if the lung shunting is more than 10% and RE should not be performed if there is a shunt more than 20% of the administered dose[22].

Percent Lung Shunting	Activity of SIR-Spheres microspheres
<10%	Deliver full amount of SIR-Spheres
10% to 15%	Reduce amount of SIR-Spheres by 20%
15% to 20%	Reduce amount of SIR-Spheres by 40%
>20%	Do not give SIR-Spheres microspheres

Table 3. The percent lung shunting may alter the activity that can be safely implanted commensurate with acceptable risk of radiation pneumonitis.

Extrahepatic hot spots in Tc-MAA images indirectly mark the possible locations of microspheres misplaced during therapy. However, detection and accurate localisation of extrahepatic hot spots using only two-dimensional planar scintigraphic images is not always possible, mainly due to the low spatial resolution. Furthermore, the localization of several different organs within a relatively small region of upper abdomen demands the analysis of tomographic images in order to accurately distinguish whether the Tc-MAA has accumulated in the liver or in some adjacent organ [30] as planar images cannot always make this distinction due to organ superposition.

If an extrahepatic tracer accumulation is detected by the Tc-MAA scan, angiogram and coil-embolization of aberrant arteries should be repeated prior to the RE until no extrahepatic accumulation is detectable[30]. In this setting, Tc-MAA SPECT/CT imaging has been shown to provide valuable additional information compared to planar and SPECT images and is the imaging modality of choice [30, 34, 35]. It significantly increases the sensitivity and negative predictive value of Tc-MAA scan compared to planar and SPECT alone[30, 34]. The sensitivity, specificity, positive predictive value and negative predictive value of SPECT/CT in the diagnosis of abdominal extrahepatic shunting has been found to be as high as100%, 93 %, 89 % and 100 % respectively [30].

2. Dose calculation and therapy planning

In addition to the selective distribution of the microspheres to the liver, the distribution within the liver plays a critical role in the planning of RE. The treatment should result in low radiation doses to normal liver tissue and a lethal dose to the tumor tissue. Abnormal high radiation doses to normal tissue may result in radiation induced hepatitis with potential risk of liver failure[36].

The required activity for treatment of each patient is to be calculated differently according to

whether glass or resin microspheres are to be used and their significant physical differences should be considered (Table 1). Selection of the optimal activity of microspheres for an individual patient is a complex and challenging task. There are some methods for dose calculation which are briefly introduced here.

2.1. Glass ^{90}Y microsphere activity calculation

TheraSphere® consists of insoluble glass microspheres, where ^{90}Y is an integral constituent of the glass. The mean sphere diameter ranges from 20 to 30 μm. Each milligram contains between 22,000 and 73,000 microspheres[37].

The dose determination for glass microspheres is based on a nominal average target dose (80-150 Gy/kg) and the patient's liver mass which determined from the CT or MRI data and assumes the uniform distribution of the microsphere throughout liver volume as [38]:

$$A(GBq)_{glass} = \frac{D(Gy) \times M(Kg)}{50}$$

In this equation, A is the activity, D the nominal target dose, and M is the mass of the targeted liver tissue.

It is recommended that the cumulative lung dose be kept to < 50 Gy to prevent radiation pneumonitis. The target dose for any given solid tumor is not known; however, it is believed that doses of 100–120 Gy balance response rates and hepatic fibrosis risk when glass microspheres are used[19].

When lung shunt fraction and residual activity in the vial after treatment are taken into account, the actual dose delivered to the target mass (Gy) becomes:

D (in Gy) = [A (in GBq)×50×(1 – [LSF – R])]/M (in kg)

where A is net activity delivered to the liver, D is the radiation absorbed dose to the target liver mass, M is target liver mass, LSF is lung shunt fraction, and R is percentage residual activity in the vial[21].

2.2. Resin ^{90}Y microsphere activity calculation

There are two methods for prescribed activity determination provided by the resin microsphere user's manual[22] (*1*) the empiric method and (2) the partition method.

2.2.1. The empiric method

The empiric method recommends a standard amount of activity which is varied only according to the size of the tumour within the liver. The recommended activity to be implanted for different degrees of tumour involvement of the liver is as follow:

Tumor <= 25% of the total mass of the liver by CT scan = 2 GBq whole-liver delivery

Tumor > 25% but < 50% of liver mass by CT scan = 2.5 GBq whole-liver delivery

Tumor > 50% of liver mass by CT scan = 3 GBq for whole-liver Delivery

2.2.2. The Body Surface Area (BSA) method

BSA method is a variant of the empiric method that is to adjust the activity implanted according to the size of the tumor within the liver and the size of the patient. The BSA method is calculated as follows:

First BSA is calculated from a weight/height chart

$$BSA(m^2) = 0.20247 \times height(m)^{0.725} \times weight(kg)^{0.425}$$

The activity of resin microspheres can be calculated with following formula:

Activity of resin microspheres in

GBq= $(BSA - 0.2) + [\frac{volume\ of\ tumour}{volume\ of\ tumour + volume\ of\ normal\ liver}]$

The BSA method is recommended for patients having concurrent systemic chemotherapy or for particularly small patients[22].

2.2.3. The partition model

This method involves implanting the highest possible activity to the tumour while maintaining radiation dose to sensitive tissues such as the lung and the normal liver. The partition model was developed from basic MIRD methodology to provide an estimate of the radiation dose separately to tumour and to normal liver. The partition model considers the liver and tumour to be effectively separate organs from the MIRD point of view. This model relies on accurate information relating to the degree of lung shunting, liver mass, tumour mass and tissue/normal (T/N) ratio.

Use of the partition model requires two measurements to be made:

1. measurement of the volume of tumour and normal liver determined from a CT or MRI scan and

2. measurement of the proportion of Tc-MAA activity that lodges in the tumour, normal liver and lung.

To determine the T/N the following equation should be used:

$$T \Big/ N = \frac{(A_{tumour} / M_{tumour})}{A_{liver} / M_{liver}}$$

Where

A Tumor is the activity in tumor

M Tumor is the mass of tumor

A Liver is the activity in the normal liver

M Liver is the mass of the normal liver

The activity could be calculated as shown by the equation below:

$$A(GBq)_{resin} = \frac{D_{liver}(\{T : N \times M_{tumour}\} + M_{liver})}{49670(1 - LSF / 100)}$$

Where

D_{liver} = nominal dose (Gy) to the liver

LSF = shunt fraction (%) of microspheres from liver to lung based on MAA scan

M_{liver} = total mass of liver (kg) from CT volume

The partition model has been described in detail in the SIRTex user manual[22].

The activity prescribed can be reduced if the hepatic function is compromised. There is no consensus guideline regarding the needed rate of reduction in the activity if a patient's liver function or estimated reserve is only just good enough to be a candidate. Generally, more experienced users reduce dose by 30% for patients with poorer liver function who are still candidates for this approach according to established eligibility criteria[19]. The amount of 90Y should be also reduced according to the dose adjustment of lung shunt (table 3) if the percentage lung shunting is greater than 10%[39].

3. Radioembolization

3.2. Complications and side effects

3.2.2. Intrahepatic complications

Before performing the RE some pre medications should be administered.

1. Gastrointestinal (GI) prophylaxis to prevent GI inflammation and ulceration:

Due to the possibility of small unrecognized arterial vessels coursing to the GI system the routine use of prophylactic antiulcer medications in all patients is recommended. A proton pump inhibitor (e.g. omeprazole or pantoprazole) or H2-blocker (e.g. ranitidine) commencing 1 week prior to RE and continuing for at least 4 weeks post treatment is to be administered.

2. Anti-nausea prophylaxis

Anti-emetics (e.g. ondansetron or granisetron) are recommended prior to and after RE to reduce post-treatment nausea.

2. Post embolization syndrome prophylaxis

Fever, malaise and lethargy can occur due to the radiation injury and embolic effect of the RE on the tumour neo-vasculature. Provided the patient is not diabetic – and oral steroids are not otherwise contra-indicated – a tapering 5-day steroid dose pack of oral corticosteroids is recommended. However, this is not a routine practice at all centres.

2. Pain control

Oral analgesia may be required for 1 week following treatment to relieve pain from radiation injury and the embolic effect of microspheres, as well as liver capsular pain from tumour edema[22]. Using slow infusion of an i.v. analgesia (e.g. pethidin) and a corticosteroid during therapy with resin microspheres could be helpful against embolization symptoms.

3.1. Application of the calculated dose

On the treatment day, the calculated activity is injected after confirming the absence of collateral vessels connecting to the gastrointestinal tract. Administration is performed in an angiography suite, primarily by an interventional radiologist. The catheter is usually positioned in essentially the same location as that used at arteriography for therapy planning. There are two different administration sets for application of resin and glass microspheres. The preparation of these sets and the method of injection have been described in detail in the respective instructions manuals [22, 32].

During the application direct tracking of microspheres distribution is not feasible and not required when using glass microspheres. But, it should be performed if resin microspheres are administered because the resin microspheres have an embolic tendency. In this case the radiologist must repeatedly check with fluoroscopy to make sure that resin microspheres are being delivered to the liver and no reflux is occurring back down the artery as this will result in spillage into other organs such as the stomach and duodenum.

It is highly recommended to perform Bremsstrahlung (BS) scintigraphy up to 24 hours after application of the microspheres to document the distribution of microspheres within the liver. Accidental extrahepatic spread of microspheres can also be visualized on post-therapeutic BS images. In case of adverse events this may allow for a faster diagnosis and early initiation of treatment. Although whole body and planar BS scans can detect diffuse extrahepatic ^{90}Y microspheres accumulations in the lungs, intestinal tract or along HFA, their analysis may be difficult and even misleading due to the low spatial resolution and organ superposition. Distinguishing between the accumulation of 90Y in the liver and in some adjacent organ demands the analysis of tomographic images. In a study obtained by our group the sensitivity, specificity, positive predictive value, negative predicative value and accuracy of SPECT and SPECT/CT in prediction of GI ulcer were 13 %,88%,8%,92%, 82 % and 87%,100%,100%,99 %, 99% respectively[40].

Overall, the incidence of complications after RE, if patients are selected appropriately and target delivery is performed meticulously, is low[5]. The complications can be divided into extrahepatic and intrahepatic.

There is also frequent observation of post embolization symptoms that are not addressed as complications. It is quite common for patients undergoing RE with resin microspheres to experience mild post embolization syndrome during the therapy, on the day of treatment and for up to 1-2 weeks after treatment. These symptoms include fatigue, nausea, and abdominal pain[19]. The most prominent aspect of post embolization syndrome is fatigue, occurring in over 50% of the patients[13].

3.2.1. Extrahepatic complications

Serious complications have been reported when microspheres were inadvertently deposited in excessive amounts in organs other than liver. Reported conditions include gastrointestinal ulceration/bleeding, gastritis/duodenitis, cholecystitis, pancreatitis, and radiation pneumonitis [5, 7, 27, 41-43].

Delayed cases of gastroduodenal ulceration were observed despite a standard pre-treatment evaluation and the contribution of experienced interventional radiologists [31]. These cases that would be associated with small amounts of Tc-MAA misplaced into the stomach and undetected by conventional scintigraphic planar images could have been avoided by the use of SPECT/CT [34, 44].

One important complication is affection of the non tumorous hepatic parenchyma by radiation. Cases of veno-occlusive disease, radiation hepatitis and hepatic fibrosis have been described. To avoid liver complication the therapeutic doses should be adjusted as accurately as possible and careful dosimetric studies should be carried out. Transient elevation in liver function tests may occur in patients following RE, specifically a mild increase in alanine transaminase, alkaline phosphatise and bilirubin[22]. As expected, the likelihood of toxicity is often related to the patient's pretreatment liver condition and bilirubin level [5, 21, 45, 46].

3.2.2.1. Radioembolization Induced Liver Disease (REILD)

This mechanism involves the irradiation of normal parenchyma beyond its tolerance (30 Gy) [47]. REILD is a rare complication of RE,occurring in about 0%-4% of the patients, since this technique allows the safe delivery of radioactive particles to liver tumours sparing healthy liver tissue and induce 4-6 times higher tumour absorbed doses from 90Y-microsphere comparing those to the normal liver tissue[48, 51]. REILD may result in various degrees of hepatic decompensation and is hard to distinguish from hepatic veno-occlusive disease. In contrast to radiation induced liver disease from external radiation characterized by symptomatic ascites and elevated liver enzymes but usually not bilirubin, radioembolization-induced liver disease presents with ascites, usually with non-elevated transaminases (except for ALP and GGPT), and significant bilirubin increase.

Kennedy et al studied the incidence of REILD after 680 RE with resin microspheres. REILD was observed after 28 treatments (4%). Their data suggest an association between the amount of activity delivered to the patient and REILD [52]. There may also be an association between the use of the empiric method for the calculation of the dose (for resin microspheres) and toxicity [39].

In another study, age, bilirubin at baseline, treatment approach (whole-liver vs. unilobar), and the amount of activity administered relative to the total volume treated were found to be independent risk factors for the development of REILD[53, 54].

To reduce the possibility of REILD, prophylactic administration of corticosteroid, ursodeoxycholic acid, low-molecular weight heparin, glutamine infusion, prostaglandin-E1, pentoxyfilline and defibrotide may be of benefit [55-57].

High doses of corticosteroids traditionally are administered in an attempt to decrease intrahepatic inflammation. Treatment results are variable and mostly not gratifying, as the condition progresses in some patients to hepatic insufficiency of various degrees[5]. In most patients the only treatment needed is the use of diuretics and sodium restriction to maintain water and sodium balance. Hepatotoxic drugs should be avoided and infections should be identified and treated promptly.

4. Follow up

The most appropriate length of follow-up and the time points to technical success are not yet well defined and follow up schedules vary depending on the treatment plan of each patient.

Continual monitoring of liver function tests is recommended to determine the outcome of treatment. This includes monitoring for stabilization in liver function tests implying the control of disease[22]. A biweekly assessment in order to rule out REILD is recommendable in the first two months after RE.

Abdominal and whole body imaging should be performed for response evaluation as well as for evaluation of extra hepatic metastases. The frequency and the interval of post-RE imaging tests should be planned according to the tumour type and individual treatment plan. In our department patients receive the first post-RE imaging consisted of abdomen MRI and a metabolic imaging, normally FDG-PET/CT if the HCC was FDG avid, 4 weeks after the therapy. The next series of imaging are performed 3, 6, 9 and 12 months after therapy unless there are some other reasons for further imaging studies such as disease progression or performing other therapies such as chemotherapy.

5. Clinical results of the radioembolization in HCC

All the evidence that supports the use of RE in HCC is based on retrospective series or non-controlled prospective studies (levels of evidence II-2 and II-3) and no randomized controlled trials have been published comparing RE with other loco-regional, systemic therapies or best supportive care[58]. Most series of RE for HCC have reported on the outcome of patients at different stages that had progressed or relapsed after TACE or were considered poor candidates for TACE due to the presence of portal vein invasion or bulky tumors.

Geschwind et. al. [59, 60] published a comprehensive analysis on using glass microspheres for HCC which showed improved survival in Okuda I when compared to Okuda II. In this study patients classified as Okuda stage I (n= 54) and II (n= 26) had median survival durations and 1-year survival rates of 628 days and 63%, and 384 days and 51%, respectively (P=.02)[60].

In a prospective study on 291 patients, 526 treatments with glass microspheres were performed and response rates were 42% and 57% based on WHO and EASL criteria, respectively. The overall time to progression was 7.9 months and survival times differed between Child-Pugh A and B patients (A:17.2 months, B:7.7 months, P=0.002). Child-Pugh A patients, with or without PVT, benefited most from treatment and Child-Pugh B patients with PVT had the worst outcomes[61]. They survived for only 5.6 months (95% CI:4.5–6.7).

In a multicenter analysis 325 patients were treated with a median activity of 1.6 GBq resin microspheres[62]. Typically, patients were Child-Pugh class A (82.5%) had underlying cirrhosis (78.5%) and good (ECOG) performance status (ECOG 0-1; 87.7%). Over half of the patients had advanced BCLC staging (BCLC C,56.3%) and one-quarter had intermediate staging (BCLC B, 26.8%). The median overall survival was 12.8 months but varied significantly between the patients with different disease stages (BCLC A, 24.4 months; BCLC B, 16.9 months; BCLC C, 10.0 months). Consistent with this finding, survival varied significantly by ECOG status, hepatic function (Child-Pugh class, ascites, and baseline total bilirubin), tumor burden (number of nodules, alpha-fetoprotein), and presence of extrahepatic disease. In this study the most significant independent prognostic factors for survival upon multivariate analysis were ECOG status, tumor burden (nodules >5), INR >1.2 and extrahepatic disease. Common adverse events were: fatigue, nausea/vomiting, and abdominal pain. Grade 3 or higher increases in bilirubin were reported in 5.8% of patients. All-cause mortality was 0.6% and 6.8% at 30 and 90 days, respectively[62].

In a retrospective analysis, Salem et al. [63]compared RE with TACE regarding time to progression and toxicity. RE resulted in longer time-to-progression and less toxicity in this study. The survival times of the patients were similar for both treatment modalities, however; post-hoc analyses of sample size indicated that a randomized study with more than1000 patients would be required to establish equivalence of survival times between patients given the different therapies.

In a recently published meta analysis of 14 papers, Venti et. al[64] showed almost 80 % any response (AR =(CR+PR+SD)) for a total of 325 patients with HCC. In this meta analysis treatment with resin microspheres was associated with a significantly higher proportion of AR compared to that of glass microsphere treatment (0.89 vs. 0.78 (p=0.02)). Median survival from RE varied between 7.1 and 21.0 months, and median survival from diagnosis or recurrence was 9.4– 24.0 months.

In a study of 108 patients with advanced HCC and liver cirrhosis[65] complete responses were determined in 3% of patients, partial responses in 37%, stable disease 53%, and primary progression in 6% of patients. Time to progression was 10.0 months and the median overall survival was 16.4 months.

5.1. Radioembolization of patients with portal vein thrombosis

A compromised portal vein blood flow is usually considered a contraindication for TACE[66].

Due to the lack of significant macroembolic effect causing liver decompensation, portal vein thrombosis is not an absolute contraindication to RE. However, patients with main portal vein thrombosis have a poor prognosis after RE with a median overall survival ranging from 3 to 6 months[67, 68]. On the Contrary, patients with branch (segmentary or lobar) portal vein thrombosis may achieve an unforeseeable median survival post-RE of 10 to 14 months[67, 69].

5.2. Treating and Downsizing of HCC as a bridging to transplantation or resection

Patients with HCC are only conferred the United Network for Organ Sharing (UNOS) priority status upgrade if they meet the Milan (T2) criteria [70]. Therefore, if a patient can be down-staged from T3 to T2, the immediate advantage is a significant gain in status and therefore much quicker access to a potentially life-saving organ. Lewandowski et al.[71] treated 86 patients with either TACE (n = 43) or RE (n = 43). The patients treated with RE achieved a median dose of 110 Gy. Median tumor size was similar in both groups. Partial response rates favored RE versus TACE (61% vs. 37%). Downstaging to UNOS T2 was achieved in 31% of TACE and 58% of RE patients. Time to progression according to UNOS criteria was similar for both groups. Event-free survival was significantly greater for RE than TACE (17.7 vs. 7.1 months, p =0.0017). Overall survival favored RE compared to TACE (censored 35.7/18.7 months; p = 0.18; uncensored 41.6/19.2 months; p = 0.008). The authors concluded that RE may outperform TACE for downstaging HCC from UNOS T3 to T2. There was also a significant difference between these two groups considering the median number of hospitalization days, being two days for TACE and 0 for RE (p < 0.001)[71].

Author, year	n	Response rate	Median survival
Lau[31], 1998	71	PR:27%, SD:65%	9.4 months
Goin[77], 2005	121		Low risk: 15.5 months High risk: 3.6 months
Salem[21], 2005	43	PR: 47 %	Okuda I: 24 months Okuda II: 13 months
Young[51], 2007	41		Okuda I: 21.7 months Okuda II: 14.2 months
Kulik[67], 2008	108	PR: 42% SD: 35 %	No PVT: 15.4 months Branch PVT: 10.0 months Mail PVT: 4.4 months
Inarrairaegui[78], 2010	62		13 months < 5 nodules: 19 months > 5 nodules: 8 months
Hilgard[65], 2010	108	CR: 3% PR: 37 % SD: 53%	16.4 months
Salem, 2010	291	CR: 23 % PR: 34 %	BCLC A: 26.9 months BCLC B: 17.2 months BCLC C: 7.3 months BCLC D: 2.5 months
Sangro[62], 2011	325		12.8 months BCLC A:24.4 months BCLC B: 16.9 months BCLC C: 10.0 months

PR: partial response; CR: complete response; SD: stable disease; PVT: portal vein thrombosis;

Table 4. Response rate and median survival of patients with HCC underwent RE

HCC arising from the caudate lobe is rare and has a poorer prognosis than HCC arising from the other hepatic lobes[72, 73]. In a retrospective study by Ibrahim et al[74] the effect of RE of unresectable HCC in caudate lobe was investigated in 8 patients who received a median radiation dose of 117 Gy. All patients presented with both cirrhosis and portal hypertension. Four patients were UNOS stage T3. One patient (13%) showed complete tumor response by WHO criteria, and three patients (38%) showed complete response using EASL guidelines. Serum AFP decreased by more than 50% in most patients (n = 6, 75%). Four patients (50%) were UNOS downstaged from T3 to T2, three of who underwent transplantation. One specimen showed histopathologic evidence of 100% complete necrosis, and two specimens demonstrated greater than 50% necrosis. Thus, RE seems to be a feasible, safe, and effective treatment option for patients with unresectable caudate lobe HCC.

Kulik et al.[75] reported a study of 35 patients with T3 unresectable HCC with RE with the intention of downstaging to resection or RFA. The study showed that RE can be used as a bridge to transplantation, surgical resection, or RFA. This allows the patients more time to wait for donor organs and thus increase their chance to undergoing liver transplantation[59]. Post RE downstaging followed by tumor resection or transplantation provides the possibility of long-term survival in a select subgroup (UNOS T3 stage) with otherwise limited options[76].

In Table 4 a summary of literatures on RE of HCC with more than 40 patients is demonstrated.

6. Conclusion

RE is a promising treatment modality to achieve regional tumour response and disease control in HCC. It offers survival benefit with a low toxicity profile. Recent investigations showed favorable survival outcomes even in patients with limited hepatic reserve and portal vein thrombosis that were excluded from most therapeutic options. However, Caution regarding patient selection, treatment preparation and performance is particularly important to prevent serious toxicity. Improvements in predicting dosimetry will lead to optimization of treatment outcome even in borderline treatment candidates.

RE has also been successfully used to bridge and downstage patients to resection, ablation or transplantation. With the sustained accumulation of promising clinical results, RE is moving forward from the salvage setting indication to the use in earlier stages of metastatic disease. Clinical trials should further define the precise role of RE in the treatment paradigm.

Author details

Hojjat Ahmadzadehfar*, Amir Sabet and Hans Jürgen Biersack

*Address all correspondence to: hojjat.ahmadzadehfar@ukb.uni-bonn.de or nuclearmedicine@gmail.com

Department of Nuclear Medicine, University Hospital Bonn, Germany

References

[1] Eary, J. Principles of Therapy with Unsealed Sources. In: Eary J, Brenner W, eds. NUCLEAR MEDICINE THERAPY (2007).

[2] Jarnagin, W. R, Gonen, M, Fong, Y, Dematteo, R. P, Ben-porat, L, et al. Improvement in perioperative outcome after hepatic resection: analysis of 1,803 consecutive cases over the past decade. Ann Surg (2002). discussion-7., 236, 397-406.

[3] Mulcahy, M. F, Lewandowski, R. J, Ibrahim, S. M, Sato, K. T, Ryu, R. K, et al. Radioembolization of colorectal hepatic metastases using yttrium-90 microspheres. Cancer (2009). , 115, 1849-58.

[4] Greco, C, & Catalano, G. Di Grazia A, Orecchia R. Radiotherapy of liver malignancies. From whole liver irradiation to stereotactic hypofractionated radiotherapy. Tumori (2004). , 90, 73-9.

[5] Murthy, R, Nunez, R, Szklaruk, J, Erwin, W, Madoff, D. C, et al. Yttrium-90 microsphere therapy for hepatic malignancy: devices, indications, technical considerations, and potential complications. Radiographics (2005). Suppl 1: S, 41-55.

[6] Campbell, A. M, Bailey, I. H, & Burton, M. A. Analysis of the distribution of intraarterial microspheres in human liver following hepatic yttrium-90 microsphere therapy. Phys Med Biol (2000). , 45, 1023-33.

[7] Salem, R, & Thurston, K. G. Radioembolization with 90Yttrium microspheres: a state-of-the-art brachytherapy treatment for primary and secondary liver malignancies. Part 1: Technical and methodologic considerations. J Vasc Interv Radiol (2006). , 17, 1251-78.

[8] Lien, W. M, & Ackerman, N. B. The blood supply of experimental liver metastases. II. A microcirculatory study of the normal and tumor vessels of the liver with the use of perfused silicone rubber. Surgery (1970). , 68, 334-40.

[9] Vente, M. A, Nijsen, J. F, De Wit, T. C, Seppenwoolde, J. H, Krijger, G. C, et al. Clinical effects of transcatheter hepatic arterial embolization with holmium-166 poly(L-lactic acid) microspheres in healthy pigs. Eur J Nucl Med Mol Imaging (2008). , 35, 1259-71.

[10] Lin, Y. C, Tsai, S. C, Hung, G. U, Lee, J. C, Huang, Y. S, et al. Direct injection of (188)Re-microspheres in the treatment of hepatocellular carcinoma: compared with traditional percutaneous ethanol injection: an animal study. Nuklearmedizin (2005). , 44, 76-80.

[11] Liu, L, Jiang, Z, Teng, G. J, Song, J. Z, Zhang, D. S, et al. Clinical and experimental study on regional administration of phosphorus 32 glass microspheres in treating hepatic carcinoma. World J Gastroenterol (1999). , 5, 492-505.

[12] Amoui, M, Pirayesh, E, Akhlaghpoor, S, Tolooee, B, Poorbeigi, H, et al. Correlation Between CT/MRI and Bremsstrahlung SPECT of 32P After Radioembolization of Hepatic Tumors. Iran J Radiol (2010). , 7, 1-5.

[13] Ahmadzadehfar, H, Biersack, H. J, & Ezziddin, S. Radioembolization of liver tumors with yttrium-90 microspheres. Semin Nucl Med (2010). , 40, 105-21.

[14] Sarfaraz, M, Kennedy, A. S, Lodge, M. A, Li, X. A, Wu, X, et al. Radiation absorbed dose distribution in a patient treated with yttrium-90 microspheres for hepatocellular carcinoma. Med Phys (2004). , 31, 2449-53.

[15] Sarfaraz, M, Kennedy, A. S, Cao, Z. J, Sackett, G. D, Yu, C. X, et al. Physical aspects of yttrium-90 microsphere therapy for nonresectable hepatic tumors. Med Phys (2003). , 30, 199-203.

[16] Dancey, J. E, Shepherd, F. A, Paul, K, Sniderman, K. W, Houle, S, et al. Treatment of nonresectable hepatocellular carcinoma with intrahepatic 90Y-microspheres. J Nucl Med (2000). , 41, 1673-81.

[17] Stubbs, R. S, Cannan, R. J, & Mitchell, A. W. Selective internal radiation therapy (SIRT) with 90Yttrium microspheres for extensive colorectal liver metastases. Hepatogastroenterology (2001). , 48, 333-7.

[18] Lawrence, T. S, Robertson, J. M, Anscher, M. S, Jirtle, R. L, Ensminger, W. D, et al. Hepatic toxicity resulting from cancer treatment. Int J Radiat Oncol Biol Phys (1995). , 31, 1237-48.

[19] Kennedy, A, Nag, S, Salem, R, Murthy, R, Mcewan, A. J, et al. Recommendations for radioembolization of hepatic malignancies using yttrium-90 microsphere brachytherapy: a consensus panel report from the radioembolization brachytherapy oncology consortium. Int J Radiat Oncol Biol Phys (2007). , 68, 13-23.

[20] Lewandowski, R. J, Thurston, K. G, Goin, J. E, Wong, C. Y, Gates, V. L, et al. Y microsphere (TheraSphere) treatment for unresectable colorectal cancer metastases of the liver: response to treatment at targeted doses of 135-150 Gy as measured by [18F]fluorodeoxyglucose positron emission tomography and computed tomographic imaging. J Vasc Interv Radiol (2005). , 16, 1641-51.

[21] Salem, R, Lewandowski, R. J, Atassi, B, Gordon, S. C, Gates, V. L, et al. Treatment of unresectable hepatocellular carcinoma with use of 90Y microspheres (TheraSphere): safety, tumor response, and survival. J Vasc Interv Radiol (2005). , 16, 1627-39.

[22] Eiber, H. B, Goldbloom, A. A, Boyd, L. J, Chapman, I, & Deutschberger, O. Newer clinical and laboratory studies in the aged. II. Correlated serum lipid partitions and

lipoprotein molecules (Sf 0-400) in patients 80-100 years of age: preliminary report. Bull N Y Acad Med (1954). , 30, 719-20.

[23] Ramirez de Molina ARodriguez-Gonzalez A, Gutierrez R, Martinez-Pineiro L, Sanchez J et al. Overexpression of choline kinase is a frequent feature in human tumor-derived cell lines and in lung, prostate, and colorectal human cancers. Biochem Biophys Res Commun (2002). , 296, 580-3.

[24] Hara, T, Kosaka, N, & Kishi, H. PET imaging of prostate cancer using carbon-11-choline. J Nucl Med (1998). , 39, 990-5.

[25] Roedl, J. B, Halpern, E. F, Colen, R. R, Sahani, D. V, Fischman, A. J, et al. Metabolic tumor width parameters as determined on PET/CT predict disease-free survival and treatment response in squamous cell carcinoma of the esophagus. Mol Imaging Biol (2009). , 11, 54-60.

[26] Covey, A. M, Brody, L. A, Maluccio, M. A, Getrajdman, G. I, & Brown, K. T. Variant hepatic arterial anatomy revisited: digital subtraction angiography performed in 600 patients. Radiology (2002). , 224, 542-7.

[27] Leung, T. W, Lau, W. Y, Ho, S. K, Ward, S. C, Chow, J. H, et al. Radiation pneumonitis after selective internal radiation treatment with intraarterial 90yttrium-microspheres for inoperable hepatic tumors. Int J Radiat Oncol Biol Phys (1995). , 33, 919-24.

[28] Liu, D. M, Salem, R, Bui, J. T, Courtney, A, Barakat, O, et al. Angiographic considerations in patients undergoing liver-directed therapy. J Vasc Interv Radiol (2005). , 16, 911-35.

[29] Sabet, A, Ahmadzadehfar, H, Muckle, M, Haslerud, T, Biermann, K, et al. Significance of Oral Administration of Natrium Perchlorate in Planning of Liver Directed Radioembolisation. 23rd Annual EANM Congress. Vienna, Austria (2010).

[30] Ahmadzadehfar, H, Sabet, A, Biermann, K, Muckle, M, Brockmann, H, et al. The significance of 99mTc-MAA SPECT/CT liver perfusion imaging in treatment planning for 90Y-microsphere selective internal radiation treatment. J Nucl Med (2010). , 51, 1206-12.

[31] Lau, W. Y, Ho, S, Leung, T. W, Chan, M, Ho, R, et al. Selective internal radiation therapy for nonresectable hepatocellular carcinoma with intraarterial infusion of 90yttrium microspheres. Int J Radiat Oncol Biol Phys (1998). , 40, 583-92.

[32] Eiber, I. S. Biologic reaction for pregnancy with male frogs Rana ridibunda.]. Akush Ginekol (Mosk) (1951). , 4, 40-2.

[33] Salem, R, & Hunter, R. D. Yttrium-90 microspheres for the treatment of hepatocellular carcinoma: a review. Int J Radiat Oncol Biol Phys (2006). S, 83-8.

[34] Hamami, M. E, Poeppel, T. D, Muller, S, Heusner, T, Bockisch, A, et al. SPECT/CT with 99mTc-MAA in Radioembolization with 90Y Microspheres in Patients with Hepatocellular Cancer. J Nucl Med (2009). , 50, 688-92.

[35] Denecke, T, Ruhl, R, Hildebrandt, B, Stelter, L, Grieser, C, et al. Planning transarterial radioembolization of colorectal liver metastases with Yttrium 90 microspheres: evaluation of a sequential diagnostic approach using radiologic and nuclear medicine imaging techniques. Eur Radiol (2008). , 18, 892-902.

[36] Moroz, P, Anderson, J. E, Van Hazel, G, & Gray, B. N. Effect of selective internal radiation therapy and hepatic arterial chemotherapy on normal liver volume and spleen volume. J Surg Oncol (2001). , 78, 248-52.

[37] Lewandowski, A, & Salem, R. Yttrium-90 Radioembolization of Hepatocellular Carcinoma and Metastatic Disease to the Liver. SEMINARS IN INTERVENTIONAL RADIOLOGY (2006). , 23, 64-72.

[38] Murthy, R, Habbu, A, & Salem, R. Trans-arterial hepatic radioembolisation of yttrium-90 microspheres. Biomedical Imaging and Intervention Journal (2006).

[39] Riaz, A, Lewandowski, R. J, Kulik, L. M, Mulcahy, M. F, Sato, K. T, et al. Complications Following Radioembolization with Yttrium-90 Microspheres: A Comprehensive Literature Review. J Vasc Interv Radiol (2009).

[40] Ahmadzadehfar, H, Muckle, M, Sabet, A, Wilhelm, K, Kuhl, C, et al. The significance of bremsstrahlung SPECT/CT after yttrium-90 radioembolization treatment in the prediction of extrahepatic side effects. Eur J Nucl Med Mol Imaging (2011).

[41] Murthy, R, Brown, D. B, Salem, R, Meranze, S. G, Coldwell, D. M, et al. Gastrointestinal complications associated with hepatic arterial yttrium-90 microsphere therapy. Journal of Vascular and Interventional Radiology (2007). , 18, 553-62.

[42] Carretero, C, Munoz-navas, M, Betes, M, Angos, R, Subtil, J. C, et al. Gastroduodenal injury after radioembolization of hepatic tumors. Am J Gastroenterol (2007). , 102, 1216-20.

[43] Salem, R, Parikh, P, Atassi, B, Lewandowski, R. J, Ryu, R. K, et al. Incidence of radiation pneumonitis after hepatic intra-arterial radiotherapy with yttrium-90 microspheres assuming uniform lung distribution. Am J Clin Oncol (2008). , 31, 431-8.

[44] Ahmadzadehfar, H, Sabet, A, Biermann, K, Brockmann, H, Kuhl, C, et al. The significance of Tc-99m-MAA SPECT-CT liver perfusion imaging in treatment planning for yttrium 90 microsphere selective internal radiation treatment. J NUCL MED MEETING ABSTRACTS (2009). , 50, 1662.

[45] Kennedy, A. S, Coldwell, D, Nutting, C, Murthy, R, Wertman, D. E, et al. Resin 90Y-microsphere brachytherapy for unresectable colorectal liver metastases: modern USA experience. Int J Radiat Oncol Biol Phys (2006). , 65, 412-25.

[46] Goin, J. E, Salem, R, Carr, B. I, Dancey, J. E, Soulen, M. C, et al. Treatment of unresectable hepatocellular carcinoma with intrahepatic yttrium 90 microspheres: factors associated with liver toxicities. J Vasc Interv Radiol (2005). , 16, 205-13.

[47] Ingold, J. A, Reed, G. B, Kaplan, H. S, & Bagshaw, M. A. Radiation Hepatitis. Am J Roentgenol Radium Ther Nucl Med (1965). , 93, 200-8.

[48] Fox, R. A, Klemp, P. F, Egan, G, Mina, L. L, Burton, M. A, et al. Dose distribution following selective internal radiation therapy. Int J Radiat Oncol Biol Phys (1991). , 21, 463-7.

[49] Sangro, B, Bilbao, J. I, Boan, J, Martinez-cuesta, A, Benito, A, et al. Radioembolization using 90Y-resin microspheres for patients with advanced hepatocellular carcinoma. Int J Radiat Oncol Biol Phys (2006). , 66, 792-800.

[50] Kennedy, A. S, Nutting, C, Jakobs, T, Cianni, R, Notarianni, E, et al. A First Report of Radioembolization for Hepatic Metastases From Ocular Melanoma. Cancer Invest (2009).

[51] Young, J. Y, Rhee, T. K, Atassi, B, Gates, V. L, Kulik, L, et al. Radiation dose limits and liver toxicities resulting from multiple yttrium-90 radioembolization treatments for hepatocellular carcinoma. J Vasc Interv Radiol (2007). , 18, 1375-82.

[52] Kennedy, A. S, Mcneillie, P, Dezarn, W. A, Nutting, C, Sangro, B, et al. Treatment parameters and outcome in 680 treatments of internal radiation with resin 90Y-microspheres for unresectable hepatic tumors. Int J Radiat Oncol Biol Phys (2009). , 74, 1494-500.

[53] Seidensticker, R, Seidensticker, M, Damm, R, Mohnike, K, Schutte, K, et al. Hepatic toxicity after radioembolization of the liver using (90)y-microspheres: sequential lobar versus whole liver approach. Cardiovasc Intervent Radiol (2012). , 35, 1109-18.

[54] Sangro, B, Gil-alzugaray, B, Rodriguez, J, Sola, I, Martinez-cuesta, A, et al. Liver disease induced by radioembolization of liver tumors: description and possible risk factors. Cancer (2008). , 112, 1538-46.

[55] Senzolo, M, Germani, G, Cholongitas, E, Burra, P, & Burroughs, A. K. Veno occlusive disease: update on clinical management. World J Gastroenterol (2007). , 13, 3918-24.

[56] Bayraktar, U. D, Seren, S, & Bayraktar, Y. Hepatic venous outflow obstruction: three similar syndromes. World J Gastroenterol (2007). , 13, 1912-27.

[57] Chopra, R, Eaton, J. D, Grassi, A, Potter, M, Shaw, B, et al. Defibrotide for the treatment of hepatic veno-occlusive disease: results of the European compassionate-use study. Br J Haematol (2000). , 111, 1122-9.

[58] Sangro, B, Inarrairaegui, M, & Bilbao, J. I. Radioembolization for hepatocellular carcinoma. J Hepatol (2012). , 56, 464-73.

[59] Riaz, A, Lewandowski, R. J, Kulik, L, & Salem, R. Yttrium-90 radioembolization using Thera- Sphere(R) in the management of primary and secondary liver tumors. Q J Nucl Med Mol Imaging (2009). , 53, 311-6.

[60] Geschwind, J. F, Salem, R, Carr, B. I, Soulen, M. C, Thurston, K. G, et al. Yttrium-90 microspheres for the treatment of hepatocellular carcinoma. Gastroenterology (2004). S, 194-205.

[61] Salem, R, Lewandowski, R. J, Mulcahy, M. F, Riaz, A, Ryu, R. K, et al. Radioembolization for hepatocellular carcinoma using Yttrium-90 microspheres: a comprehensive report of long-term outcomes. Gastroenterology (2009).

[62] Sangro, B, Carpanese, L, Cianni, R, Golfieri, R, Gasparini, D, et al. Survival after yttrium-90 resin microsphere radioembolization of hepatocellular carcinoma across Barcelona clinic liver cancer stages: a European evaluation. Hepatology (2011). , 54, 868-78.

[63] Salem, R, Lewandowski, R. J, Kulik, L, Wang, E, Riaz, A, et al. Radioembolization results in longer time-to-progression and reduced toxicity compared with chemoembolization in patients with hepatocellular carcinoma. Gastroenterology (2011). e2., 140, 497-507.

[64] Vente, M. A, Wondergem, M, & Van Der Tweel, I. van den Bosch MA, Zonnenberg BA et al. Yttrium-90 microsphere radioembolization for the treatment of liver malignancies: a structured meta-analysis. Eur Radiol (2009). , 19, 951-9.

[65] Hilgard, P, Hamami, M, Fouly, A. E, Scherag, A, Muller, S, et al. Radioembolization with yttrium-90 glass microspheres in hepatocellular carcinoma: European experience on safety and long-term survival. Hepatology (2010). , 52, 1741-9.

[66] Bruix, J, & Sherman, M. Management of hepatocellular carcinoma: an update. Hepatology (2011). , 53, 1020-2.

[67] Kulik, L. M, Carr, B. I, Mulcahy, M. F, Lewandowski, R. J, Atassi, B, et al. Safety and efficacy of 90Y radiotherapy for hepatocellular carcinoma with and without portal vein thrombosis. Hepatology (2008). , 47, 71-81.

[68] Woodall, C. E, Scoggins, C. R, Ellis, S. F, Tatum, C. M, Hahl, M. J, et al. Is selective internal radioembolization safe and effective for patients with inoperable hepatocellular carcinoma and venous thrombosis? J Am Coll Surg (2009). , 208, 375-82.

[69] Inarrairaegui, M, Thurston, K. G, Bilbao, J. I, Avola, D, & Rodriguez, D. M et al. Radioembolization with use of yttrium-90 resin microspheres in patients with hepatocellular carcinoma and portal vein thrombosis. J Vasc Interv Radiol (2010). , 21, 1205-12.

[70] Mazzaferro, V, Regalia, E, Doci, R, Andreola, S, Pulvirenti, A, et al. Liver transplantation for the treatment of small hepatocellular carcinomas in patients with cirrhosis. N Engl J Med (1996). , 334, 693-9.

[71] Lewandowski, R. J, Kulik, L. M, Riaz, A, Senthilnathan, S, Mulcahy, M. F, et al. A Comparative Analysis of Transarterial Downstaging for Hepatocellular Carcinoma: Chemoembolization Versus Radioembolization. Am J Transplant (2009).

[72] Takayama, T, & Makuuchi, M. Segmental liver resections, present and future-caudate lobe resection for liver tumors. Hepatogastroenterology (1998)., 45, 20-3.

[73] Takayasu, K, Muramatsu, Y, Shima, Y, Goto, H, Moriyama, N, et al. Clinical and radiologic features of hepatocellular carcinoma originating in the caudate lobe. Cancer (1986)., 58, 1557-62.

[74] Ibrahim, S. M, Kulik, L, Baker, T, Ryu, R. K, Mulcahy, M. F, et al. Treating and downstaging hepatocellular carcinoma in the caudate lobe with yttrium-90 radioembolization. Cardiovasc Intervent Radiol (2012)., 35, 1094-101.

[75] Kulik, L. M, Atassi, B, Van Holsbeeck, L, Souman, T, Lewandowski, R. J, et al. Yttrium-90 microspheres (TheraSphere) treatment of unresectable hepatocellular carcinoma: downstaging to resection, RFA and bridge to transplantation. J Surg Oncol (2006)., 94, 572-86.

[76] Inarrairaegui, M, Pardo, F, Bilbao, J. I, Rotellar, F, Benito, A, et al. Response to radioembolization with yttrium-90 resin microspheres may allow surgical treatment with curative intent and prolonged survival in previously unresectable hepatocellular carcinoma. Eur J Surg Oncol (2012)., 38, 594-601.

[77] Goin, J. E, Salem, R, Carr, B. I, Dancey, J. E, Soulen, M. C, et al. Treatment of unresectable hepatocellular carcinoma with intrahepatic yttrium 90 microspheres: a risk-stratification analysis. J Vasc Interv Radiol (2005)., 16, 195-203.

[78] Inarrairaegui, M, Martinez-cuesta, A, Rodriguez, M, Bilbao, J. I, Arbizu, J, et al. Analysis of prognostic factors after yttrium-90 radioembolization of advanced hepatocellular carcinoma. Int J Radiat Oncol Biol Phys (2010)., 77, 1441-8.

Chapter 4

Image-Guided Therapies for Hepatocellular Carcinoma in Hepatocelluar Carcinoma — Future Outlook

Bruno C. Odisio, Ravi Murthy and Michael J. Wallace

Additional information is available at the end of the chapter

http://dx.doi.org/10.5772/56794

1. Introduction

The use of image-guided locoregional therapies (LRTs) plays a key role in the management of patients with hepatocellular carcinoma (HCC). These therapies, classically used for palliation, are now more frequently being used with curative intent either as a bridge before the definitive therapy (surgical resection or orthotopic liver transplantation) or as a sole or combined therapy in selected patients for whom surgical options are precluded [1-3]. The refinement and development of new imaging technologies combined with recent advances in catheter technology, embolic agents, chemotherapeutic drugs, and delivery systems have been linked to further improved patients' outcomes, thus increasing the interest in this approach. In the first part of this chapter, an overview of the current available image-guided LRTs will be given. In the second part, indications for different LRTs according to tumor stage will be discussed. The third section will discuss the pivotal role of follow-up diagnostic imaging in the pre- and post-procedural care of patients with HCC. Finally, future directions with regard to the use of LRTs will also be presented and discussed.

2. Overview of currently available image-guided LRT options

2.1. Transarterial therapies

2.1.1. Chemoembolization

Hepatic transarterial embolization for the treatment of liver tumors was first performed in the 1970s to improve local disease control. The rationale behind this approach emerged from the peculiarities of blood flow to HCC, which is supplied preferentially via the hepatic artery owing to the intense angiogenesis during disease progression. For transarterial chemoembolization (TACE), first described in 1977 by Yamada [4], one or more chemotherapeutic drugs are added to the embolic agent, on the basis of the theory that tumor ischemia caused by embolization of the dominant arterial supply has a synergistic effect with the chemotherapeutic drugs. Several chemotherapeutic agents are used for TACE, the two most commonly used doxorubicin and cisplatin, which can be mixed with one or several different embolic agents. Recently, the development of calibrated microparticles loaded with doxorubicin (DEBDOX-TACE) have gained acceptance. These drug-eluting microspheres allow more reliable distal occlusion of small vessels and delivery of high-dose chemotherapy to the tumor with a very low systemic circulation of the chemotherapeutic agent. A randomized phase II study [6] comparing conventional TACE with DEBDOX-TACE demonstrated a significant reduction in liver toxicity and serious adverse drug events in the latter arm and an insignificant trend of better antitumoral effect [5, 6].

2.1.2. Yttrium-90 microsphere radioembolization

Transarterial radioembolization (TARE) is the transcatheter arterial delivery of microspheres loaded with yttrium-90 (^{90}Y), a pure beta emitter with a physical half-life of 64.2 hours, after which it decays into stable zirconium. Like other transarterial therapies, TARE relies on the preferential arterial supply and enhanced microvascular density of hepatic neoplasms [7, 8]. Acting as carriers, these biocompatible microspheres can conceptually deliver radiation preferentially to tumors following hepatic artery delivery via embolization in the tumor-related arterioles. Additionally, employing high-energy beta radiation instead of traditional gamma radiation can potentially create an intense local radiotherapeutic effect that is proportional to the density of microsphere distribution. Hence, compared to nonselective extracorporeal x-ray radiotherapy, TARE allows the particles to be deposited predominantly within the tumor vasculature, thereby leading to tumor damage while preserving the surrounding liver parenchyma. This critical feature allows the delivery of substantially higher radiation doses than those that can be safely delivered via external beam radiotherapy.

In the United States, two Food and Drug Administration (FDA)-approved ^{90}Y microsphere products are in current clinical use: TheraSphere® (MDS Nordion Inc., Kanata, Ontario, Canada), which consists of glass microspheres, and the resin-based SIR-Spheres™ (SIRTeX Medical Ltd., Sydney, New South Wales, Australia). The glass ^{90}Y microspheres are approved in the United States for use in radiation treatment or as a neoadjuvant treatment before surgery or liver transplantation in patients with HCC under the auspices of a humanitarian device FDA exemption for orphan devices. TheraSphere has been used for neoplasia other than HCC under compassionate circumstances after adherence to FDA-related guidelines. The resin ^{90}Y microspheres have premarket approval for the treatment of hepatic metastasis from colorectal primary cancers with adjuvant hepatic arterial infusion of floxuridine. However, globally, the regulatory approval of both products is more generic, and they also commonly used for HCC therapy. The use of resin microspheres for an indication not included in the US FDA-specific labeling is considered off-label use. Clinicians should consult and adhere to their institutional and regulatory agencies before prescribing the treatment for off-label use with either device.

2.1.3. Embolization with ^{131}iodine

The use of radioactive iodine (^{131}I) has been proposed for internal radiotherapy for HCC. In this technique, ethiodized oil is tagged to the ^{131}I via an atom-atom exchange. ^{131}I-lipiodol then emits gamma radiation with energy of 374 KeV and penetration of up to 0.4 mm. The retention of lipiodol inside the HCC tumor cells allows a targeted dose-intensified radiation therapy to be delivered. Despite the reported efficacy of ^{131}I-lipiodol [9, 10], its use in routine daily practice is limited owing to the lack of additional data and the complexity of this procedure when compared with other available therapies such as TACE and TARE. Patients are also required to be isolated for several days after the procedure for radiation safety. An initial randomized study comparing internal ^{131}I-lipiodol radiation therapy versus supportive care in patients with HCC and portal vein thrombosis suggested the former conferred a survival benefit [9]. Considering the lack of clinical evidence and the possible severe side effects such as liver failure and pneumonia related to its use, this treatment method deserves further analysis.

2.2. Percutaneous ablative therapies

2.2.1. Ethanol injection

Percutaneous ethanol injection (PEI) is the prototypical technique used for percutaneous ablation. On this technique, absolute ethanol is injected inside the tumor and around it using a guiding needle inducing coagulative necrosis as a result of cell dehydration, protein denaturation and chemical occlusion of small vessels. PEI is a well-established technique for treating nodular types HCCs with the extent of necrosis obtained via this technique intrinsically correlated with the size of the lesions with complete necrosis achieved in 90%, 70%, and 50% of tumors measuring <2 cm, 2-3 cm, and 3-5 cm, respectively [11-13]. A possible explanation for the suboptimal response of larger tumors to PEI is the presence of intratumoral septa and/or a capsule that blocks the diffusion of ethanol. Recently, the introduction of a specific multipronged injection needle (Quadrafuse, RexMedical, Philadelphia, PE) for single-session PEI has resulted in a sustained complete response rate of 80%-90% in tumors measuring < 4cm [14].

2.2.2. Radiofrequency ablation

Radiofrequency ablation (RFA) has become the first-line choice for percutaneous ablation and has superseded PEI as the method of choice for ablative LRT mainly because it yields complete necrosis with fewer sessions than required for PEI, especially in larger tumors, thus leading to better local disease control [15-19]. This technology relies on its physical characteristics to deliver an alternating electrical current within the lesion via an electrode needle placed directly into the tumor. The resulting frictional heat and movement of electrons within the lesion and surrounding tissues generate heat in the immediate vicinity of the electrode which is then conducted to the surrounding environment, thereby resulting in the coagulative necrosis of a predetermined volume of tissue. RFA is performed by connecting a generator that provides an electric current to a metallic applicator probe (needle), which is inserted into the tumor percutaneously via computed tomography, fluoroscopy, magnetic resonance imaging, or ultrasound guidance. Thermal energy is applied to tissues through the tip of the probe. The tissues surrounding the tip are destroyed within seconds as temperatures reach 55°- 60°C. Care is taken to avoid charring tissues, which limits heat propagation. Ideally, the ablation zone should encompass the tumor and a 5-10-mm margin of normal tissue, which might eliminate small, undetected satellite lesions. The size and shape of the ablation zone vary depending on the amount of energy, the type and number of electrodes, the duration of ablation, and inherent tissue characteristics [20].

Initial RFA indications included the treatment of small lesions (<3cm) in patients who were not surgical candidates and the palliation of large lesions. However, owing to the efficacy and safety profile of the technique, its use has greatly expanded and it is now offered to patients who are surgical candidates with comparable 5 year survival outcomes to resection [21]. The limitations of the technique include a "heat-sink" effect, whereby adjacent blood vessels produce perfusion-mediated attenuation of thermal energy deposition, potentially leading to incomplete ablation; large (>5 cm) lesions; and proximity to thermal sensitive structures, such as the gastrointestinal wall, gallbladder, diaphragm, and nerves.

2.2.3. Microwave ablation

Microwave ablation (MW) is an emerging hyperthermic ablative therapy that is a valuable alternative to RFA for the ablation of HCC. Several MW systems have been approved for clinical use in the United States [22], comprised by an energy generator that is connected via a coaxial cable to a percutaneous needle(s) that functions as an active antenna that delivers energy within the tumor. The application of electromagnetic microwaves in the matter creates heat by agitating water molecules in the surrounding tissue, thereby producing friction and heat and inducing cellular destruction via coagulative necrosis [23]. Compared with other available ablative technologies, MW creates larger tumor ablation volumes with consistently higher intratumoral temperatures, has faster ablation times, and an improved and a more favorable convection profile [22], thus resulting in a reduction in the "heat sink" effect created by vessels in proximity to the ablated zone [24]. Recent advances in MW engineering have resulted in better MW systems with the potential for creating more effective ablation zones.

2.2.4. Cryoablation

The application of freezing temperatures to tumors can be also utilized to cause tissue destruction. Similarly to RFA and MW, a cryoablation probe is directly inserted into the target lesion. Argon circulates through the probe, causing a rapid drop in the local temperature around the probe, promoting local ischemia and a disruption of the cellular membrane. Ice crystals form within the cells and adjacent interstitium, causing cell dehydration and surrounding vascular thrombosis. Subsequently, when the tissues thaw, vascular occlusion leads to further ischemic injury [25]. Consistent tumor cell death is accomplished when the tissues are exposed to temperatures of at least -20ºC within an area of approximately 3 mm inside the margins of the ice ball. As with RFA, the main limitations of cryoablation include proximity of the lesion to blood vessels, gastrointestinal organs, nerves, and skin. Treatment of large tumor volumes with cryoablation can lead to the development of rare but serious systemic complications, such as 'cryoshock', a cytokine-mediated inflammatory response associated with coagulopathy and multiorgan failure, myoglobinuria, and severe thrombocytopenia [26-28]. Otherwise, most complications of cryotherapy are generally similar to those of RFA, such as hemorrhage and injury to adjacent organs.

2.3. Combination therapies

The use of combined therapies, either a combination of different LRTs or LRT combined with systemic therapies, has gained particular attention in the last decade. Combining different modalities of LRT such as RFA and chemoembolization could increase the treatment success rate, particularly in large HCCs [29]. The rationale for this approach lies in the devascularization of large HCCs via embolization or chemoembolization, which reduces the possibility of having a deleterious "heat sink" effect in hypervascular tumors treated with RFA and thereby increases its therapeutic effect. This approach has been validated in several studies that demonstrated larger ablation zones when bland embolization or chemoembolization was performed before the ablative treatment [30-32]. Moreover, performing RFA before chemoembolization has been shown to increase the deposition of the chemoembolic agent in the periphery of the ablated tumor, the most common area for disease recurrence [33].

It is also suggested that the hypoxic environment after TACE may trigger the expression of neoangiogenic factors such as the vascular endothelial growth factor (VEGF), possibly leading to tumor growth and progression. Therefore, to avoid the development of a neoangiogenesis cascade and, by consequence, tumor progression systemic therapies in the form of chemotherapy or antiangiogenic drugs with the intent of acting in different fronts of neoangiogenesis have been proposed.

3. LRT for HCC according to disease stage

To review the available LRTs according to different stages of disease, we used the Barcelona Clinic Liver Cancer (BCLC) staging system, which has emerged in recent years as the standard means of classifying HCC. In this system, cases are classified into 5 different stages – very early (0), early (A), intermediate (B), advanced (C), and terminal (D) – according to pre-estabilished prognostic variables, thereby allowing therapies to be allocated according to treatment-related status (Figure 1). Terminal-stage treatment options are beyond the scope of this chapter, as LRTs are not administered in that setting.

3.1. Very early stage (0)

Patients diagnosed with very early-stage disease (performance status: 0, Child-Pugh score: A, single HCC <2 cm) on the BCLC staging system have the highest potential for cure. Surgical resection is the modality of choice for this stage and yields a 5-year survival rate of around 75% in these patients, with the anatomic resection–defined as the en bloc removal of a portion of liver supplied by a major branch of the portal vein and the hepatic artery

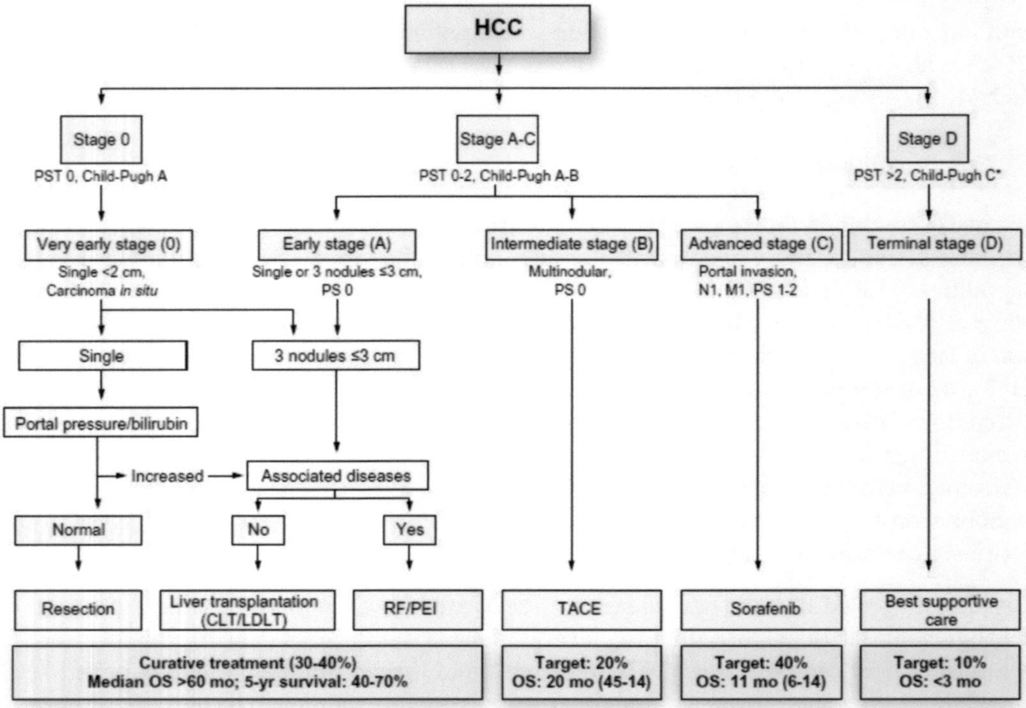

Figure 1. BCLC staging system and treatment strategy, 2011 [2]

utilized as the preferred surgical technique [34, 35]. Despite the improvements achieved with recent refinements in surgical technique and postoperative care, which resulted in a low mortality rate of 1%-3%, anatomic resection in patients with very early HCC is still limited depending on the volume of segments that need to be resected. Nodules smaller than 2 cm that are not subcapsular, perivascular, or adjacent to the gallbladder are the ideal indication for ablative therapies, and RFA is the standard technique in many institutions [2, 36, 37]. In a recent study, Cho and colleagues [38] concluded that RFA and hepatic resection are equally effective for the treatment of stage 0 HCC. Livraghi and colleagues [19] reported a complete response rate of 97.2% and a 5-year survival rate of 68% in 218 patients with very early-stage HCC treated using RFA. In another recent study [39] of 83 patients with very early HCC who were treated using different modalities of percutaneous ablation (33 PEI, 19 MW, and 31 RFA), the complete response rate was 95%, and the 5-year survival rate was 78%. Therefore, RFA is suggested by some authors as first-line therapy for very early-stage HCC, and surgical resection is reserved for when individual patient variables render RFA unfeasible or unsafe [40]. In selected cases of very early-stage HCC, when surgery or RFA cannot be offered because of increased bilirubin level, signs of portal hypertension, and risky tumor location, such as pericholecystic lesions and lesions near the hilum, PEI can still be offered as an alternative.

3.2. Early stage (A)

Patients with a solitary HCC or up to three lesions measuring less than 3 cm without associated diseases are the ideal candidates to be effectively treated with liver transplantation. On those where associated disease exists or where bridge therapy is required before liver transplantation, percutaneous ablation (PEI/RFA) is the modality of choice. Compared with PEI, RFA is consistently more effective and renders better local disease control. It also offers a survival benefit compared with PEI, as demonstrated by three independent meta-analyses that revealed 5-year survival rates of 51%-64% in patients who met the BCLC criteria for surgical resection [41-43].

MW ablation is emerging as a viable alternative to RFA in patients with early-stage HCC owing to its larger tumor ablation volumes, because the inherent characteristics of this technique are less affected by the "heat-sink" effect created by vessels in proximity to the tumor. To date, the only randomized control trial comparing RFA and MW ablation did not reveal any differences in the effectiveness of the two techniques, with a trend toward RFA in respect achieving tumor ablation in fewer sessions [44]. Nevertheless, the recent advances in MW engineering along with improvements in the learning curve of this technology will potentially create a more effective ablation zone and better local disease control when compared to RFA.

Although not specified in the BCLC guidelines, a combination of ablative and transarterial treatments could be considered for cases in which the target lesion measures between 3 and 5 cm in its longest axis in view of the suboptimal response of larger lesions to ablative therapies alone [30, 31, 45, 46]. The recent results of a randomized control trial [46] accessing the efficacy of combining RFA with subsequent conventional TACE (lipiodol plus epirubicin at 30-50 mg followed by introduction of gelatin sponge) in patients with HCCs measuring 3.1-5.0 cm showed that the rate of tumor progression was significantly lower in the combination group than in the ablation-only group (39% versus 6%, P=0.012) [46]. DEB-TACE administered after RFA has also been studied and yielded a potential increase of 60.9%+-39.0 in treatment-induced necrosis on imaging [33]. Further studies to determine the ideal sequence of techniques and the real impact of this approach are needed.

When percutaneous ablative therapies such as RFA and MW are not feasible or safe, TACE can be performed as an alternative. This can be a valuable tool in patients with solitary large (>5 cm) lesions, for whom the benefits of combining different LRTs seems negligible. In a recent study, DEB-TACE administered before liver transplantation yielded complete necrosis in 77% of treated tumors on pathology (mean size: 3.2 cm+/-1.54 cm) with no serious adverse events observed.

3.2.1. Intermediate stage (B)

TACE is the standard of care for patients with stage B disease, according to BCLC guidelines. This indication is based on the improved survival rates demonstrated in a meta-analysis of six randomized clinical trials that compared TACE with the best supportive care or suboptimal therapies [47]. Of note, however, the studies included in this meta-analysis were considerably heterogeneous (particularly with regard to the patient populations and the TACE techniques used), and the cases of intermediate-stage HCC comprised a heterogeneous population of patients whose liver function and tumor burden varied widely. Therefore, not all patients included in BCLC stage B will have the same benefits from TACE, as demonstrated by a recent meta-analysis of randomized control trials [48]. On a recent study by Burrel et al [49], a median survival of 42.8 months was achieved with the use of DEB-TACE in patients classified as BCLC-B after censoring follow-up at the time of liver transplantation, sorafenib treatment and TARE. A sub-stratification of this patient population, along with the comparison of TACE with other LRTs and systemic therapies, should be encouraged in future research.

The combination of DEB-TACE with sorafenib in patients with intermediate-stage HCC was assessed in a phase II randomized, double-blind, placebo-controlled trial. Patients who received sorafenib combined with DEB-TACE had a longer time to progression than did the control group, to whom DEB-TACE was administered in combination with placebo (hazard ratio: 0.797). Nonetheless, the difference in median survival was only 3 days in favor of the sorafenib group (169 versus 166 days), and the difference in overall survival between two groups was 6 days in favor of the placebo group (562 versus 554 days). Evidence from ongoing phase III trials is expected to clarify the clinical efficacy of this combination.

The use of radioembolization with ^{90}Y in patients with intermediate to advanced stage HCC has been investigated in a phase II study [50]. In this study, 17 patients with intermediate-stage HCC without portal vein thrombosis were treated with a lobar delivery of 120 Gy. Nine (52.9%) patients had complete response (CR) or partial response (PR) accordingly to the European Association for the Study of Liver (EASL) criteria. Disease control (CR, PR or stable disease [SD]) was achieved in 15 patients (88.2%). Time to progression was 13 months, and overall survival was 18 months (range, 12–38 months) [50]. In a recent multicenter trial [51] assessing the use of radioembolization with ^{90}Y in patients with HCC, 87 patients with BCLC stage B HCC treated with ^{90}Y had a median survival of 16.9 months (95% CI 12.8-22.8). Of note, this study demonstrated that radioembolization with ^{90}Y appears to be particularly promising for the subset of patients with intermediate-stage HCC who are considered poor candidates for TACE (median survival: 15.4-16.6 months) as well for those for whom prior TACE or bland embolization was ineffective (median, 15.4 months). The results of this study emphasize the possibility of using radioembolizaiton as a complementary therapy to TACE in the HCC armamentarium.

3.3. Advanced stage (Stage C)

According to the BCLC guidelines, the use of the systemic multi tyrosine-kinase inhibitor, sorafenib, is the cornerstone for patients with advanced HCC [2]. The benefit of this therapy was demonstrated in two randomized control trials [52, 53] in which this new therapy was compared with placebo. Both studies revealed an improvement in the median overall survival and the median time to disease progression on imaging. Although LRTs are not recommended for patients with BCLC stage C disease, many patients who undergo LRT in the form of TACE or radioembolization are in fact classified as having advanced-stage disease according to the aforementioned criteria. This subclass of patients is characterized by the presence of tumoral invasion of a branch vein with or without limited extra-hepatic disease and a performance status 1-2. Combination therapy using TACE and sorafenib is technically feasible and generally well tolerated in patients with unresectable HCC [54-56]. In a recent phase II study of concurrent conventional TACE and sorafenib, Park et al. [55] demonstrated a median time to progression of 7.3 and 5 months for patients with BCLC stage B and C disease, respectively. Compared with unpublished data from the same group, the combination of sorafenib with conventional TACE yielded increased time to progression in both patients with BCLC stages B and C when compared with conventional TACE (cTACE) alone (4.5 and 2.8 months, respectively).

Concurrent therapy with DEB-TACE and sorafenib has also been investigated [56]. DEB-TACE promotes a lesser degree of serum aminotransferase elevation than does conventional TACE, which is the most common cause for delaying therapy with sorafenib. Of note, sorafenib should ideally be administered as soon as possible after TACE is administered to to prevent an early surge of vascular endothelial growth factor and other angiogenic factors. Pawlik et al. [56] assessed the safety and response rate of combination therapy using DEB-TACE and sorafenib in patients with advanced-stage HCC. The results of this study demonstrated that the combination of sorafenib and DEB-TACE was well tolerated and safe, and most toxic effects related to sorafenib were manageable with dose adjustment. Disease control was achieved in 95% of patients (SD+PR), according to Response Evaluation Criteria in Solid Tumors (RECIST) with an objective response of 58% (according to the EASL).

4. Imaging response assessment for LRT

The RECIST and the world health organization (WHO) criteria are the standard criteria for assessing imaging response in patients who undergo systemic therapies using cytotoxic drugs. These criteria assess the response of target lesions solely on the basis of their measurement in diameters and their changes after systemic therapy. In the setting of LRT, tumor response as determined via by simple measurement in diameters is not accurate enough since tumor necrosis, a common endpoint for all LRTs, is not taken into consideration.

The inconsistency of using these response evaluation criteria for systemic therapy in patients undergoing LRTs was first addressed by a panel of experts on HCC from the European Association Study of Liver in 2000, which suggested that response assessment should be based on the estimation of the reduction in viable tumor, as recognized by arterial-phase enhancement on radiologic imaging. The concept of achieving complete necrosis (complete response) after LRT is a good surrogate for excellent outcome and has been confirmed by a number of different studies [57-60].

More recently, the addition of molecular targeted therapies such as sorafenib, bevacizumab, and erlotinib to the anticancer armamentarium rendered an improvement in overall survival without showing any significant imaging response rate according to the RECIST criteria [54, 61]. This finding can also be explained by the ability of these new agents to cause necrosis in the target lesions without any significant significantly affecting the reduction of the size of the lesions. In fact, it is now known that some lesions tend to increase in volume after the use of molecularly targeted therapies owing to the presence of massive necrosis and edema on their interior.

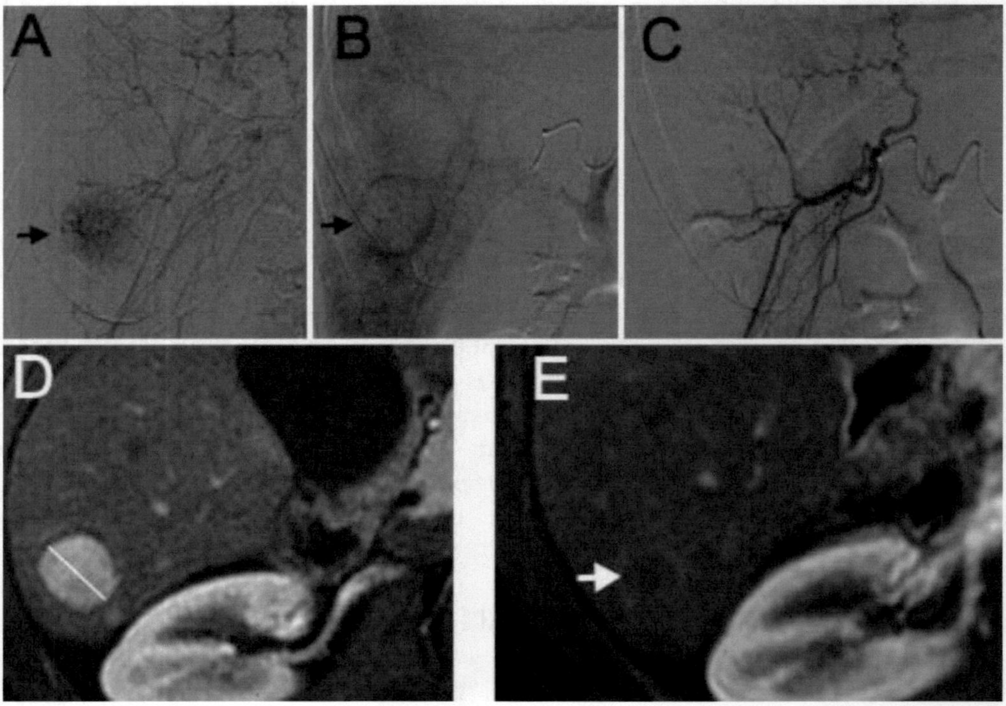

Figure 2. TACE and magnetic resonance imaging follow-up utilizing the mRECIST: (A) Digital subtraction angiography (DSA) demonstrating the hypervascular lesion (black arrow) located in the segment VI. (B) Parenchymal phase showing the encapsulated pattern of the lesion (black arrow). (C) post DEB-TACE DSA no longer characterizing the hypervascular tumor. (D)Baseline magnetic resonance imaging (MRI) showing the hypevascular tumor in the arterial phase (white line) measuring 3.2 cm. (D) post DEB-TACE MRI arterial phase, showing the absence of arterial enhancement at the lesion (white arrow) after the DEB-TACE, configuring acomplete response according to the mRECIST. Liver explant analysis confirmed complete necrosis of the treated

To address all the limitations associated with the RECIST criteria in assessing therapy response, especially that of HCC, novel imaging correlative endpointswere proposed by different investigators [61-63]. One of the initial proposals created was the amendment of enhancement criteria to the WHO criteria (EASL criteria), which use the enhancement observed in the arterial phase by the intravenous contrast as a surrogate for viable tumor, whereas the absence of arterial enhancement within the tumor indicates tumor necrosis. Despite the initial enthusiasm, recent studies have demonstrated that these criteria cannot provide prognostic data to enable differentiation between the survival outcomes of patients who achieved partial response and those who had stable disease. This is possibly explained by the different thresholds for therapy response extrapolated from the WHO criteria. Therefore, a new proposal suggested for assessing therapy response for HCC was made by the modification of the conventional RECIST criteria with the incorporation of the concept of viable tumor (Figure

2). These criteria, also known as the modified RECIST (mRECIST) [63], have been demonstrated to be an accurate tool for assessing response for both locoregional and systemic therapies [59, 60, 64] and should be used as the method of choice for assessing treatment response in patients with HCC [2]. Although mRECIST helps to predict survival outcomes in patients undergoing LRTs, further data are needed to establish these criteria for assessing survival in the setting of systemic therapies with molecularly targeted drugs. A summary of the different response criteria are summarized in Figure 3.

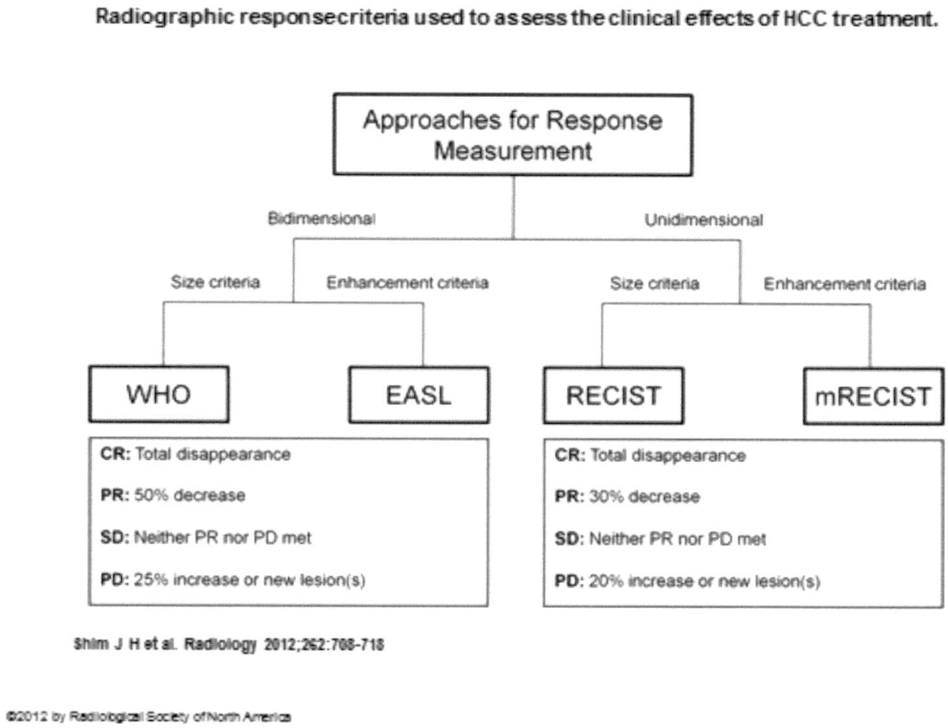

Figure 3. Radiographic response criteria used to assess the clinical effects of HCC treatment [59]. Adapted from: Shim, J.H., et al., Which response criteria best help predict survival of patients with hepatocellular carcinoma following chemoembolization? A validation study of old and new models. Adapted from Radiology, 2012. 262(2): p. 708-13.

5. Future directions

The last few decades were characterized by establishing the limits of outcomes of liver directed therapies for HCC. Recent therapeutic advances exploiting molecular biological pathways have created new vistas in our collective approaches towards this disease. Certain distinct clinical scenario will remain the focus of future endeavors such as recurrence and cancer prevention. Tumor recurrences are a major drawback in patients with very early and early stages HCC submitted to ablative therapies or resection. Effective preventive agents in the form of better ablative technologies or combined loco-regional and systemic therapies are needed given the projected increase in patients at risk for developing HCC. Irreversible electroporation (IRE) is a new ablative therapy that increases cell membrane permeability by changing the transmembrane potential and subsequently disrupts the lipid bilayer integrity resulting in cell death [65, 66]. Currently there is one IRE system available on the market. Similarly to an RFA system, this system consists of two major components: a generator that delivers energy of up to 3000 V and a needle-like electrical probe. Compared with other available ablative technologies, this technology can create a sharper boundary between the treated and untreated area in vivo within microsecond or milliseconds; moreover, because it is a non-thermal technique, issues associated with perfusion-mediated tissue cooling or heating are not relevant. Preclinical investigations [67] focused on HCC have demonstrated the great potential of this technology for targeted ablation of HCC and have prompted its clinical evaluation.

Light-activated drug therapy uses light-emitting diodes to activate talaporfin sodium, a small molecule synthesized from a chlorophyll derivate that has the ability to concentrate within the tumors when administered intravenously and activated by placing a percutaneous light emitter intratumorally under imaging guidance. Talaporfin is capable of absorbing long-wavelength light, resulting in singlet oxygen that causes apoptotic cell death through oxidation and permanent tumor vessel occlusion. Preclinical animal studies suggested that the production of large apoptotic masses in tumor with light-activated drug therapy yields tumor-specific clones of CD8+ T cells which infiltrate distant, untreated tumors. A phase III clinical trial is currently assessing the use of talaporfin for HCC.

In patients with advanced-stage HCC, future research will hopefully better delineate the indications for TACE and TARE, either in the form of isolated therapy or combined with sorafenib with possible improvements in slowing disease progression. Finally, advances in molecular cell biology will identify new therapeutic strategies for patients with advanced-stage HCC. For these advances to take place, a multidisciplinary continuous clinical and experimental research is vital.

Author details

Bruno C. Odisio*, Ravi Murthy and Michael J. Wallace

*Address all correspondence to: bcodisio@mdanderson.org

Section of Interventional Radiology, Division of Diagnostic Imaging, University of Texas MD Anderson Cancer Center Houston, Houston, USA

References

[1] Bruix, J. and M. Sherman, *Management of hepatocellular carcinoma: an update.* Hepatology, 2011. 53(3): p. 1020-2.

[2] *EASL-EORTC clinical practice guidelines: management of hepatocellular carcinoma.* J Hepatol, 2012. 56(4): p. 908-43.

[3] Yao, F.Y., et al., *A prospective study on downstaging of hepatocellular carcinoma prior to liver transplantation.* Liver Transpl, 2005. 11(12): p. 1505-14.

[4] Yamada, R., et al., *Hepatic artery embolization in 32 patients with unresectable hepatoma.* Osaka City Med J, 1980. 26(2): p. 81-96.

[5] Lammer, J., et al., *Prospective randomized study of doxorubicin-eluting-bead embolization in the treatment of hepatocellular carcinoma: results of the PRECISION V study.* Cardiovasc Intervent Radiol, 2010. 33(1): p. 41-52.

[6] Vogl, T.J., et al., *Liver, gastrointestinal, and cardiac toxicity in intermediate hepatocellular carcinoma treated with PRECISION TACE with drug-eluting beads: results from the PRECISION V randomized trial.* AJR Am J Roentgenol, 2011. 197(4): p. W562-70.

[7] Breedis, C. and G. Young, *The blood supply of neoplasms in the liver.* Am J Pathol, 1954. 30(5): p. 969-77.

[8] Ridge, J.A., et al., *Perfusion of colorectal hepatic metastases. Relative distribution of flow from the hepatic artery and portal vein.* Cancer, 1987. 59(9): p. 1547-53.

[9] Raoul, J.L., et al., *Randomized controlled trial for hepatocellular carcinoma with portal vein thrombosis: intra-arterial iodine-131-iodized oil versus medical support.* J Nucl Med, 1994. 35(11): p. 1782-7.

[10] Chua, T.C., et al., *Intra-arterial iodine-131-lipiodol for unresectable hepatocellular carcinoma.* Cancer, 2010. 116(17): p. 4069-77.

[11] Lencioni, R., *Loco-regional treatment of hepatocellular carcinoma.* Hepatology, 2010. 52(2): p. 762-73.

[12] Livraghi, T., et al., *Percutaneous ethanol injection in the treatment of hepatocellular carcinoma in cirrhosis. A study on 207 patients.* Cancer, 1992. 69(4): p. 925-9.

[13] Sala, M., et al., *Initial response to percutaneous ablation predicts survival in patients with hepatocellular carcinoma.* Hepatology, 2004. 40(6): p. 1352-60.

[14] Kuang, M., et al., *Ethanol ablation of hepatocellular carcinoma Up to 5.0 cm by using a multipronged injection needle with high-dose strategy.* Radiology, 2009. 253(2): p. 552-61.

[15] Shiina, S., et al., *A randomized controlled trial of radiofrequency ablation with ethanol injection for small hepatocellular carcinoma.* Gastroenterology, 2005. 129(1): p. 122-30.

[16] Lin, S.M., et al., *Randomised controlled trial comparing percutaneous radiofrequency thermal ablation, percutaneous ethanol injection, and percutaneous acetic acid injection to treat hepatocellular carcinoma of 3 cm or less.* Gut, 2005. 54(8): p. 1151-6.

[17] Brunello, F., et al., *Radiofrequency ablation versus ethanol injection for early hepatocellular carcinoma: A randomized controlled trial.* Scand J Gastroenterol, 2008. 43(6): p. 727-35.

[18] Lencioni, R.A., et al., *Small hepatocellular carcinoma in cirrhosis: randomized comparison of radio-frequency thermal ablation versus percutaneous ethanol injection.* Radiology, 2003. 228(1): p. 235-40.

[19] Livraghi, T., et al., *Sustained complete response and complications rates after radiofrequency ablation of very early hepatocellular carcinoma in cirrhosis: Is resection still the treatment of choice?* Hepatology, 2008. 47(1): p. 82-9.

[20] Ahrar, K., et al., *Percutaneous radiofrequency ablation of renal tumors: technique, complications, and outcomes.* J Vasc Interv Radiol, 2005. 16(5): p. 679-88.

[21] Cho, Y.K., et al., *Hepatic resection versus radiofrequency ablation for very early stage hepatocellular carcinoma: a Markov model analysis.* Hepatology. 51(4): p. 1284-90.

[22] Lubner, M.G., et al., *Microwave tumor ablation: mechanism of action, clinical results, and devices.* J Vasc Interv Radiol, 2010. 21(8 Suppl): p. S192-203.

[23] Simon, C.J., D.E. Dupuy, and W.W. Mayo-Smith, *Microwave ablation: principles and applications.* Radiographics, 2005. 25 Suppl 1: p. S69-83.

[24] Yu, N.C., et al., *Microwave liver ablation: influence of hepatic vein size on heat-sink effect in a porcine model.* J Vasc Interv Radiol, 2008. 19(7): p. 1087-92.

[25] Gage, A.A. and J. Baust, *Mechanisms of tissue injury in cryosurgery.* Cryobiology, 1998. 37(3): p. 171-86.

[26] Bageacu, S., et al., *Cryosurgery for resectable and unresectable hepatic metastases from colorectal cancer.* Eur J Surg Oncol, 2007. 33(5): p. 590-6.

[27] Seifert, J.K., et al., *Large volume hepatic freezing: association with significant release of the cytokines interleukin-6 and tumor necrosis factor a in a rat model.* World J Surg, 2002. 26(11): p. 1333-41.

[28] Sheen, A.J., G.J. Poston, and D.J. Sherlock, *Cryotherapeutic ablation of liver tumours.* Br J Surg, 2002. 89(11): p. 1396-401.

[29] Wang, W., J. Shi, and W.F. Xie, *Transarterial chemoembolization in combination with percutaneous ablation therapy in unresectable hepatocellular carcinoma: a meta-analysis.* Liver Int, 2010. 30(5): p. 741-9.

[30] Veltri, A., et al., *Radiofrequency thermal ablation (RFA) after transarterial chemoembolization (TACE) as a combined therapy for unresectable non-early hepatocellular carcinoma (HCC).* Eur Radiol, 2006. 16(3): p. 661-9.

[31] Rossi, S., et al., *Percutaneous radio-frequency thermal ablation of nonresectable hepatocellular carcinoma after occlusion of tumor blood supply.* Radiology, 2000. 217(1): p. 119-26.

[32] Yamasaki, T., et al., *Percutaneous radiofrequency ablation therapy for patients with hepatocellular carcinoma during occlusion of hepatic blood flow. Comparison with standard percutaneous radiofrequency ablation therapy.* Cancer, 2002. 95(11): p. 2353-60.

[33] Lencioni, R., et al., *Doxorubicin-eluting bead-enhanced radiofrequency ablation of hepatocellular carcinoma: a pilot clinical study.* J Hepatol, 2008. 49(2): p. 217-22.

[34] Llovet, J.M., J. Fuster, and J. Bruix, *Intention-to-treat analysis of surgical treatment for early hepatocellular carcinoma: resection versus transplantation.* Hepatology, 1999. 30(6): p. 1434-40.

[35] Huo, T.I., et al., *The model for end-stage liver disease based cancer staging systems are better prognostic models for hepatocellular carcinoma: a prospective sequential survey.* Am J Gastroenterol, 2007. 102(9): p. 1920-30.

[36] Gervais, D.A., et al., *Society of Interventional Radiology position statement on percutaneous radiofrequency ablation for the treatment of liver tumors.* J Vasc Interv Radiol, 2009. 20(1): p. 3-8.

[37] Lencioni, R., et al., *Loco-regional interventional treatment of hepatocellular carcinoma: techniques, outcomes, and future prospects.* Transpl Int, 2010. 23(7): p. 698-703.

[38] Cho, Y.K., et al., *Hepatic resection versus radiofrequency ablation for very early stage hepatocellular carcinoma: a Markov model analysis.* Hepatology, 2010. 51(4): p. 1284-90.

[39] Kuang, M., et al., *Long-term outcome of percutaneous ablation in very early-stage hepatocellular carcinoma.* J Gastrointest Surg, 2011. 15(12): p. 2165-71.

[40] Lencioni, R. and L. Crocetti, *Local-regional treatment of hepatocellular carcinoma.* Radiology, 2012. 262(1): p. 43-58.

[41] Cho, Y.K., et al., *Systematic review of randomized trials for hepatocellular carcinoma treated with percutaneous ablation therapies.* Hepatology, 2009. 49(2): p. 453-9.

[42] Germani, G., et al., *Clinical outcomes of radiofrequency ablation, percutaneous alcohol and acetic acid injection for hepatocelullar carcinoma: a meta-analysis.* J Hepatol, 2010. 52(3): p. 380-8.

[43] Bouza, C., et al., *Meta-analysis of percutaneous radiofrequency ablation versus ethanol injection in hepatocellular carcinoma.* BMC Gastroenterol, 2009. 9: p. 31.

[44] Shibata, T., et al., *Small hepatocellular carcinoma: comparison of radio-frequency ablation and percutaneous microwave coagulation therapy.* Radiology, 2002. 223(2): p. 331-7.

[45] Morimoto, M., et al., *Radiofrequency ablation combined with transarterial chemoembolization for subcapsular hepatocellular carcinoma: A prospective cohort study.* Eur J Radiol, 2012.

[46] Morimoto, M., et al., *Midterm outcomes in patients with intermediate-sized hepatocellular carcinoma: a randomized controlled trial for determining the efficacy of radiofrequency ablation combined with transcatheter arterial chemoembolization.* Cancer, 2010. 116(23): p. 5452-60.

[47] Llovet, J.M. and J. Bruix, *Systematic review of randomized trials for unresectable hepatocellular carcinoma: Chemoembolization improves survival.* Hepatology, 2003. 37(2): p. 429-42.

[48] Cabibbo, G., et al., *A meta-analysis of survival rates of untreated patients in randomized clinical trials of hepatocellular carcinoma.* Hepatology, 2010. 51(4): p. 1274-83.

[49] Burrel, M., et al., *Survival of patients with hepatocellular carcinoma treated by transarterial chemoembolisation (TACE) using Drug Eluting Beads. Implications for clinical practice and trial design.* J Hepatol, 2012. 56(6): p. 1330-5.

[50] Mazzaferro, V., et al., *Yttrium(90) radioembolization for intermediate-advanced hepatocarcinoma: A phase II study.* Hepatology, 2012.

[51] Sangro, B., et al., *Survival after yttrium-90 resin microsphere radioembolization of hepatocellular carcinoma across Barcelona clinic liver cancer stages: a European evaluation.* Hepatology, 2011. 54(3): p. 868-78.

[52] Llovet, J.M., et al., *Sorafenib in advanced hepatocellular carcinoma.* N Engl J Med, 2008. 359(4): p. 378-90.

[53] Cheng, A.L., et al., *Efficacy and safety of sorafenib in patients in the Asia-Pacific region with advanced hepatocellular carcinoma: a phase III randomised, double-blind, placebo-controlled trial.* Lancet Oncol, 2009. 10(1): p. 25-34.

[54] Abou-Alfa, G.K., et al., *Phase II study of sorafenib in patients with advanced hepatocellular carcinoma.* J Clin Oncol, 2006. 24(26): p. 4293-300.

[55] Park, J.W., et al., *Phase II study of concurrent transarterial chemoembolization and sorafenib in patients with unresectable hepatocellular carcinoma.* J Hepatol, 2012. 56(6): p. 1336-42.

[56] Pawlik, T.M., et al., *Phase II trial of sorafenib combined with concurrent transarterial chemoembolization with drug-eluting beads for hepatocellular carcinoma.* J Clin Oncol, 2011. 29(30): p. 3960-7.

[57] Lam, V.W., et al., *Incomplete ablation after radiofrequency ablation of hepatocellular carcinoma: analysis of risk factors and prognostic factors.* Ann Surg Oncol, 2008. 15(3): p. 782-90.

[58] Shim, J.H., et al., *Complete necrosis after transarterial chemoembolization could predict prolonged survival in patients with recurrent intrahepatic hepatocellular carcinoma after curative resection.* Ann Surg Oncol, 2010. 17(3): p. 869-77.

[59] Shim, J.H., et al., *Which response criteria best help predict survival of patients with hepatocellular carcinoma following chemoembolization? A validation study of old and new models.* Radiology, 2012. 262(2): p. 708-18.

[60] Gillmore, R., et al., *EASL and mRECIST responses are independent prognostic factors for survival in hepatocellular cancer patients treated with transarterial embolization.* J Hepatol, 2011. 55(6): p. 1309-16.

[61] Llovet, J.M., et al., *Design and endpoints of clinical trials in hepatocellular carcinoma.* J Natl Cancer Inst, 2008. 100(10): p. 698-711.

[62] Thomas, M.B., et al., *Hepatocellular carcinoma: consensus recommendations of the National Cancer Institute Clinical Trials Planning Meeting.* J Clin Oncol, 2010. 28(25): p. 3994-4005.

[63] Lencioni, R. and J.M. Llovet, *Modified RECIST (mRECIST) assessment for hepatocellular carcinoma.* Semin Liver Dis, 2010. 30(1): p. 52-60.

[64] Edeline, J., et al., *Comparison of tumor response by Response Evaluation Criteria in Solid Tumors (RECIST) and modified RECIST in patients treated with sorafenib for hepatocellular carcinoma.* Cancer, 2012. 118(1): p. 147-56.

[65] Davalos, R.V., I.L. Mir, and B. Rubinsky, *Tissue ablation with irreversible electroporation.* Ann Biomed Eng, 2005. 33(2): p. 223-31.

[66] Edd, J.F., et al., *In vivo results of a new focal tissue ablation technique: irreversible electroporation.* IEEE Trans Biomed Eng, 2006. 53(7): p. 1409-15.

[67] Guo, Y., et al., *Irreversible electroporation therapy in the liver: longitudinal efficacy studies in a rat model of hepatocellular carcinoma.* Cancer Res, 2010. 70(4): p. 1555-63.

Chapter 5

Neoadjuvant Chemotherapy for Hepatocellular Carcinoma

Xin-yu Huang, Qi Zheng and Zhou Yuan

Additional information is available at the end of the chapter

http://dx.doi.org/10.5772/56289

1. Introduction

Hepatocellular carcinoma (HCC), a primary fatal malignancy of the liver, is the sixth most common cancer and the third most common cause of cancer death worldwide [1]. The estimated incidence of HCC is about 500,000–1000, 000 per year worldwide, causing 600,000 deaths globally per year [2]. It varies widely according to geographic location, with the highest incidence in sub-Saharan Africa and China, where chronic hepatitis B virus (HBV) infection remains the leading cause [3]. In the United States and Europe, the incidence of HCC is on the rise and is expected to increase over the next two decades because the number of patients with chronic hepatitis C virus (HCV) infection gradually increased in the past two decades [4]. Liver cirrhosis, especially after chronic infection with hepatitis B or C virus, remains the main risk factor that predisposes to the development of HCC, although rarely can HCC develop in a patient without cirrhotic liver. Despite of major progress in diagnosis and therapeutic options of HCC in the past two decades, the prognosis of HCC is still dismal and 5-year survival rate is less than 5%.

Of the therapies aiming at cure, surgical resection or liver transplantation are the optimal treatments with better outcomes in well-selected patients HCC. Unfortunately, more than 50% of all HCCs are diagnosed at locally advanced tumor stage or extrahepatic metastasis and therefore not eligible for potentially curative therapy such as surgical resection and liver transplantation [5]. In addition, some patients with early HCC are not eligible for curative hepatic resection because of poor liver function. Thus, only 10%-30% of patients with early HCC at diagnosis are amenable to curative surgical treatment and the rest of patients with have to receive non-curative treatment. Furthermore, after curative resection, tumor recurrence rates can be as high as 25% per year and 50-90% of postoperative death is due to recurrent disease. Therefore, despite curative treatment options for patients with early stage HCC, survival rate after curative treatment has been as low as 50% at 3 years and 20-30% at 5 years

[6-8]. Tumor recurrence is the main drawback of resection and intra-hepatic recurrence is frequently the only site of recurrence. HCC commonly arises from chronic hepatitis viral or alcoholic liver diseases, which are likely to harbor multiple and independent clones of premalignant cells. When these clones are further exposed to continuous carcinogenic insults, multicentric carcinogenesis follow. Thus, intra-hepatic recurrence may represent either "de novo" tumor formation in a cirrhotic liver, or intra-hepatic metastasis from a clonally identical neoplasm. In other word, recurrent HCC can result from intrahepatic dissemination of the primary tumor (true recurrence) or by new "de novo" carcinogenesis. No matter how the recurrence happens, it is generally believed that recurrences arise not because of inadequate resection but because of pre-existing microscopic tumor foci that are undetected by imaging modalities, or because malignant cells have been disseminated during surgical manipulation[9-10]. Therefore, neoadjuvant or adjuvant therapy could potentially delay or decrease the incidence of intrahepatic recurrence, which could improve patients' prognosis after hepatic resection.

Liver transplantation is an optimal treatment to manage end-stage liver disease with HCC, because this procedure cures not only the tumor but also the underlying cirrhosis. Liver transplantation achieves excellent results in selected patients with HCC. Patients with solitary HCC of less than 5 cm or with up to three nodules of less than 3 cm with no macroscopic vascular invasion (the Milan criteria) have a 5-year survival of 70% after liver transplantation, with recurrence in less than 10% [11]. Compared with surgical resection, liver transplantation is associated with better overall and disease-free survival in well-selected patients [12].Unfortunately, the majority of HCC patients are diagnosed at a late stage and therefore not eligible for liver transplantation. Furthermore, patients drop off the transplant list owing to tumor progression during the long waiting time, resulting from shortage of liver donor worldwide. Thus, it is pivotal to decrease the rate of dropout by using neoadjuvant therapy for those patients during the waiting time. In addition, neoadjuvant therapy for HCC beyond the Milan criteria may downstage HCC tumors within the Milan criteria to expand liver transplantation candidates.

Neoadjuvant therapy is used preoperatively with the aim to reduce tumor recurrence in the past two decades. The aims of neoadjuvant therapy are to reduce the tumor mass thus making curative surgery more feasible and to reduce postoperative recurrence. Thus, the administration of neoadjuvant chemotherapy may offer several theoretical advantages. First, neoadjuvant therapy can reduce the tumor burden and shrink the tumor so patients are amenable to curative and negative-margin resection. Second, it can potentially eliminate "circulating cancer cells" or "disseminated cancer cells", which is regarded as the source of tumor recurrence. Third, neoadjuvant chemotherapy potentially reduces intraoperative tumor cells spread. Fourth, the delivery of treatment agents before surgical manipulation may provide better tissue oxygenation, facilitating the distribution of chemotherapy agents into the tumor, and increasing normal tissue tolerance. Fifth, the administration of chemotherapy before surgery allows an in-vivo assessment of tumor chemo-sensitivity through analyzing resected tissue samples. Finally, neoadjuvant chemotherapy may also lead to more definitive surgical resections by reducing the risk of tumoral infiltration of lymph nodes and of resection margins in the surgical specimen.

However, neoadjuvant therapy has the disadvantage of delaying the surgery. This can be detrimental if the tumor fails to respond to the therapy and continues to grow and becomes inoperable. Moreover, neoadjuvant therapy also has the potential to adversely affecting the liver function, with an increased risk of liver failure after partial hepatectomy [13-14]. In recent decades, more light has been shed on the role of neoadjuvant or adjuvant therapy for HCC.

2. Neoadjuvant therapy for resectable hepatocellular carcinoma

Surgical resection offers the only hope for cure and is the preferred option for patients with HCC. For those noncirrhotic HCC patients, surgical resection is the optimal curative treatment. They are likely to tolerate extended hepatic resection without liver failure. Moreover, the noncirrhotic residual liver is less likely to develop de-novo HCC. Unfortunately, the majority of patient develops HCC in the context of cirrhosis, so the selection criteria of liver resection depend not only on tumor-related parameters (tumor size, numbers, location and vascular invasion) but also on preserved liver function. Meanwhile, the long-term survival remains poor owing to high incidence of recurrence and metastasis after hepatectomy. Recurrences, in particular, intrahepatic recurrences are the most common and are found in up to 68-96% of patients undergoing resection [15-16]. Therefore, neoadjuvant HCC therapy, which can decrease or delay the incidence of intra-hepatic recurrence, may improve the results of liver resection.

Large HCC, tumor with a diameter of 5 cm or more, are relatively common, especially when HCC screening is not a routine practice in patients at risk. Generally speaking, patients with large HCC are not eligible for liver transplantation or ablation. Hepatic resection thus remains the only surgical treatment option for these patients. Despite improvements in preoperative assessment and intraoperative techniques in liver resection over the past 10 years, major liver resection in diseased liver is still considered a risky procedure [17-18], because of the potential risk of developing liver dysfunction after hemihepatectomy or hepatic trisegmentectomy. Thus, portal vein embolization (PVE) is used prior to extended hepatectomy to increase future remnant liver volume and to prevent postoperative liver dysfunction.

The primary goal of neoadjuvant HCC therapy is to eradicate residual microscopic HCC foci and to reduce the incidence of a second HCC from developing within the live remnant after partial hepatectomy and thus to reduce death from recurrent HCC. Recently published reviews concluded that there are little or no evidence to show that neoadjuvant therapy added benefit after curative hepatectomy for HCC so far. However, neoadjuvant therapy is continuously evolving and gaining importance in the treatment of HCCs. At present, the most popular techniques include transarterial chemo-embolization(TACE), portal vein embolization (PVE), and target therapy. Herein, we review the rationale behind each strategy and the studies on neo-adjuvant treatments for HCC before partial hepatectomy.

2.1. TACE

Since transarterial chemoembolization (TACE) was introduced during the late 1970s as a palliative treatment for patients with unresectable hepatocellular carcinoma (HCC), it has been applied more frequently in patients with unresectable HCC. In contrast to the normal liver which has dual blood supply, mainly from the portal venous system, hepatocellular carcinoma tumor is supplied almost exclusively by arterial supply. By direct infusion of the lipiodol and chemotherapy through the hepatic artery, it allows a high dose of chemotherapy to be delivered directly to the tumor. This provides the rationale for therapeutic local chemotherapy and hepatic artery selective obstruction of HCC via TACE. The embolization of the hepatic artery reduces the blood flow of tumor, creates ischemia and increases the contact time between the chemotherapeutic agent and the tumor cells, resulting in synergetic effect and complete tumor necrosis.

A meta-analysis including seven randomized clinical trials was undertaken in the late 1990s to investigate the usefulness of TACE for treating unresectable HCC, which demonstrated an improvement in 2-year survival ($P = 0.017$) compared with control patients who were treated conservatively or received suboptimal management [19]. According to the guidelines published by the American Association for Study of Liver Diseases (AASLD) [20] and the European Association for the Study of the Liver (EASL) [21], TACE is recommended as first-line non-curative therapy for non-surgical patients with large/multifocal HCC who do not have vascular invasion or extrahepatic spread (level I). Given the promising results in its palliative role, TACE has been evaluated as a neoadjuvant therapy with the hope of reducing tumor size, inducing tumor necrosis, and preventing tumor dissemination. Preoperative TACE is not only intended to prevent recurrence by controlling intrahepatic spread via the portal system, but also to facilitate surgery by reducing tumor bulk. The use of TACE as a neoadjuvant treatment for HCC was first described in the early 1990s, where its use was proposed in a variety of settings; palliatively for unresectable recurrent HCC, to increase the rate of resectability of unresectable HCC, and to downstage the primary tumor for liver transplantation [22].

Whether preoperative TACE is beneficial for survival of patients with resectable HCC remains a controversy owing to the numerous conflicting reports. A few studies suggested that preoperative TACE may be beneficial for overall survival and/or disease-free survival in patients with resectable HCC [23-24]. In contrast, several studies have shown that neoadjuvant TACE had no significant influence on postoperative survival [25-26]. A randomized controlled trial from China indicated that preoperative TACE did not improve surgical outcome and five patients lost the chance of undergoing a curative liver resection owing to disease progression and hepatic failure [27]. Furthermore, several studies have found that preoperative TACE negatively affected survival of patients postoperatively [28-29]. A meta-analysis including three randomized clinical trials is undertaken to evaluate the definitive effect of preoperative TACE on both disease-free survival rate and overall survival rate following curative resection in resectable HCC patients, which demonstrated no significant benefits for 5-year overall survival and disease-free survival[30]. However, the number of patients was small in these trials, which limited the ability to draw frim conclusions. Another systemic analysis indicates that there appears to be no DFS advantage by using TACE as a neoadjuvant therapy for resectable HCC, although it is a safe procedure [31].

Can we predict which kind of HCC will develop necrosis after neoadjuvant TACE owing to its heterogeneity or does it benefit the subgroup of patients according to tumor size, tumor stage, frequency of TACE, the interval between TACE and operation, etc.? The answer to these questions is very important to evaluate the role of neoadjuvant TACE. In conclusion, current evidence indicates that there appears to be no DFS advantage despite its safety and feasibility. In future, a well-designed prospective multi-institutional randomized controlled trials (RCTs), with a clearly defined protocol for concealed allocation, eligibility criteria, TACE intervention regimen and endpoints will be potentially meaningful.

2.2. PVE+TACE

Hepatic resection is considered to be the only curative treatment for patients with large HCC and preserved liver functions, because these patients are not amenable to liver transplantation or ablative therapy. For these patients, major hepatic resection is feasible in theory and technique to achieve complete resection and provide the possibility of cure, but, most of them will develop postoperative liver failure, a fatal complication, owing to no enough remnant liver volume. In addition, most patients with hepatitis B or C virus–associated liver cirrhosis increase the risk of postoperative live failure.

Preoperative portal vein embolization (PVE), first reported by Makuuchi, is a technique to induce atrophy of the embolized lobe to be removed with compensatory hypertrophy of the nonembolized future liver remnant (FLR). This technique was first applied to patients with hilar bile duct tumors (Klatskin tumors) [32], then has been introduced in major hepatic resection. The aim of PVE is to preserve enough remnant liver volume and to prevent post-hepatectomy liver failure, which is the predominant cause of death in cirrhotic patients. However, the major limitation of PVE is a compensatory increase in the hepatic arterial flow to the embolized segments, thus resulting in insufficient nonembolized liver hypertrophy or rapid tumor growth because most HCCs are hypervascular tumors fed mainly by arterial blood flow [33]. To overcome the shortcoming of PVE, sequential preoperative TACE combined with PVE has been evolved. The new technique has recently shown promising results for increasing the rate of hypertrophy in HCC patients with chronic liver disease, as it decreases arterial flow and thus increases parenchymal damage in the embolized liver and suppresses arterioportal shunts [34]. In addition, it may have a strong anticancer effect by obstructing tumor feeding vessels and suppressing intrahepatic spread by portal vein invasion from HCC and arterio-portal shunts in HCC patients. Thus, preoperative TACE+PVE may increase the probability of resectability for major hepatectomy and may decrease the risk of postoperative hepatic failure. However, sequential TACE and PVE may have the theoretical drawback of increased risk of liver damage caused by double occlusion of the blood supply. The data from Yoo shows that incidence of hepatic failure is higher in the PVE-only group than in the TACE + PVE group ($P = 0.185$) after operation and overall ($P = 0.028$) and recurrence free ($P = 0.001$) survival rates are significantly higher in the TACE + PVE group than in the PVE-only group[35]. Other studies also show that preoperative sequential TACE and PVE is a safe and feasible technique and the short and long-term survival outcomes are satisfactory [36-37].

2.3. Sorafenib

Sorafenib is an oral multi-kinase inhibitor, which simultaneously inhibits molecular components of the Raf–MEK–ERK signaling pathway, abrogating tumor growth and VEGFR-1,

VEGFR-2, VEGFR-3, and PDGFR-β, thus inhibiting neoangiogenesis [38]. By targeting two key pathways that are reported to play an important role in the pathogenesis of hepatocellular carcinoma, sorafenib is likely to delay disease progression [39]. Furthermore, sorafenib exhibited growth-inhibitory effects, induction of apoptosis, and down-regulation of the anti-apoptotic proteins in a wide range of tumor models.

Recently, Sorafenib was approved and regarded as the first and so far the only drug which shows an increase in overall survival in patients with advanced, unresectable HCC. In the large randomized phase III study (SHARP), median overall survival (OS) increased from 7.9 months in the placebo group to 10.7 months in the sorafenib group. Sorafenib showed a significant benefit also in terms of time to progression (TTP), with a median of 5.5 months in the sorafenib group and 2.8 months in the placebo group. On the basis of these findings, FDA has approved sorafenib for advanced HCC treatment [40]. Thus, for patients with unresectable HCC, sorafenib is the first systemic therapy to significantly prolong survival and is now considered standard of care for patients with Child A cirrhosis and good performance status. Could sorafenib downstage HCC and thus represent a bridge to surgery, as a neoadjuvant therapy for advance HCC? The phase III SHARP study reported a partial response of only 2% with complete remission given the cytostatic nature of sorafenib effect. However, Irtan et al reported two cases of locally advanced HCC with portal vein tumor thrombosis (PVTT) who complete regression by sorafenib treatment allowed curative resection with good long-term outcome [41]. Another study also reports two cases with large HCC in the right liver with venous neoplastic thrombi undergo curative resection after sorafenib treatment [42]. However, no large clinical experiences have been reported in neoadjuvant therapy with the use of sorafenib. Thus, large scale RCT clinical trials should be undertake to investigate the role of sorafenib as a neoadjuvant treatment in advanced HCC, preferably in combination with local therapy modalities to increase the chances of down-sizing.

In summary, further randomized controlled studies need to be carried out. Currently, there is no consensus on a standard neoadjuvant therapy in partial hepatectomy for HCC.

3. Neoadjuvant therapy for hepatocellular carcinoma before liver transplantation

Liver transplantation is a potentially curative treatment for HCC for those patients with early HCC in the setting of cirrhosis. It has two principle advantages to remove the tumor as well as the underlying liver cirrhosis, restoring both liver function and decreasing the risk of de novo HCC. Compared with surgical resection, liver transplantation is associated with better overall and disease-free survival in well-selected patients (5 year-DFS >75% vs. 50%) [43]. Patients with solitary HCC of less than 5 cm or with up to three nodules of less than 3 cm, with no macroscopic vascular invasion (the Milan criteria) have a 5-year survival of 70% after liver transplantation, with recurrence in less than 10% [11]. In addition, the survival matches post-transplant survival of most other indications for liver transplantation, such as end-stage liver cirrhosis disease. As evidence accumulated of good outcomes in some patients outside the

http://dx.doi.org/10.5772/56289

Milan criteria, there was a drive to identify expanded criteria and to increase the number of eligible candidates for liver transplantation. Among the many proposals, only the University of California San Francisco (UCSF) criteria (one tumor ≤6 5 cm, three nodules at most with the largest ≤4 5 cm, and total tumor diameter ≤8 cm) have been prospectively validated with long-term survival comparable to patients with Milan criteria [44]. At present, the Milan criteria have been adopted as the guideline of liver transplantation for HCC worldwide. Unfortunately, the majority of HCC patients are diagnosed in a late stage and therefore not eligible for liver transplantation. Meanwhile, shortage of available graft is still a very stringent problem worldwide so that many patients will drop off the transplant list owing to tumor progression during the long waiting time. Historical data suggest that the median doubling time in HCC is about 3 to 6 months, but the waiting time for live transplantation continues to increase and is up to 24 months in the United States [45]. So, many eligible patients with HCC will drop out if they are not given some effective therapy to stop tumor progression during the waiting time. Thus, neoadjuvant therapy has been proposed as a strategy to treat HCC before liver transplantation.

Neoadjuvant therapy for HCC beyond the Milan criteria has been performed with the purpose of downstaging HCC to parameters within the Milan criteria. This enables substantially the expansion of liver transplantation candidates with potential good outcomes after transplantation. It is defined as 'downstaging therapy'. Another aim of neoadjuvant therapy is to delay tumor progression and decrease dropout for those patients within Milan criteria HCC. It is defined as 'bridging therapy'. The last aim of neoadjuvant therapy can decrease or even eliminate circulating cancer cells, which are the mainstay source of recurrence and metastasis. Although associated with good results, around 10% of within Milan criteria HCC patients will exhibit post-transplant recurrence. Recurrence is either due to the growth of occult metastases or to the engraftment of circulating tumor cells. Thus, pre-transplant neoadjuvant therapy may serve a pivotal role in improving survival following liver transplantation. At present, neoadjuvant therapy is gradually evolving and gaining importance in the treatment of HCC patients undergoing liver transplant.

Locoreginal therapy, such as TACE, transarterial radio-embolization (TARE) and radiofrequency ablation (RFA), and systemic chemotherapy are most common used as neoadjuvant therapy for patients with HCC before liver transplantation. Herein, we evaluate the rationale of each strategy for HCC before liver transplantation.

3.1. TACE

The rationale for using TACE as a neoadjuvant therapy prior to liver transplantation is to control tumor growth while the patient awaits an organ and to cause significant tumor necrosis, which may reduce tumor dissemination during surgery. In addition, TACE can be used to downstage tumor and make them eligible for transplantation[46]. In a case-control study, researchers showed that the high rate of tumor necrosis observed in the pretransplant TACE group was not associated with difference in overall survival [47]. In the French multicenter case-control study, the patients in the TACE group in which more than 80% of the tumor was necrotic at the time of transplantation and their matched controls had 5-year survival rate of 63% and 54%, respectively (p = 0.9) [48]. Thus, although preoperative TACE can lead to tumor necrosis in about one third of cases and reduces tumor size in half of the patients, there was no sufficient evidence to support the concept that it can improve long-term survival for patients with within Milan criteria HCC after transplantation.

Success in downstaging has been reported in many studies, although most of these are uncontrolled observational studies. As a downstaging tool in his study, Graziadei et al. included 15 advanced HCC patients not eligible for transplantation received TACE (range, 2–12). 11 patients had a partial response with >50% necrosis and 1 < 50%. 10 patients underwent OLT and and found to have 30% HCC recurrence rate. Thus, despite successful downstaging before OLT, patients with primarily advanced HCC had a significantly less favorable outcome in the intent-to-treat analysis as well as in the post-transplantation survival compared with patients with early-stage HCC (31% vs. 94% at 5 years, $p < 0.001$ and 41% vs. 94% at 5 years, $p < 0.001$) [49]. Downstaging of HCC by TACE is possible in most of candidates; however, these patients tend to have higher dropout rates, higher recurrence rates, and unfavorable outcomes compared with early stage patients. Therefore, there is currently no sufficient evidence that pretransplant TACE may delineate the possibility of expanding current selection criteria for liver transplantation in patients with HCC.

3.2. RFA

Radiofrequency ablation appears to be equivalent to surgical resection inducing total tumor necrosis in tumor < 3 cm [50]. Subsequently, RFA is used as the second most popular neoadjuvant therapy before liver transplantation after TACE. In transplant candidates, RFA has been used mainly as a bridge therapy rather than for downstaging before transplantation owing to its limited efficacy for large tumors. However, RFA can have sever side effect, including tumor dissemination in subcapsular HCC. Pretransplant RFA for HCC as a strategy to reduce dropout has been addressed in some studies [51]. More than 80% of patients were in the Milano criteria treated by FRA with approximately 1 year on the waiting list. The dropout rate ranged from 0 to 14%. However, the effect of preoperative RFA should be carefully evaluated by more randomized clinical trials

In summary, the lack of controlled clinical trials, some uncontrolled studies support the use of RFA as a safe and effective bridge therapy in patients who meet the Milan criteria.

3.3. Transarterial Radio-Embolization (TARE)

Radioembolization involves the transarterial administration of embolic microspheres labeled with Yttrium-90 (Y90). TARE has been used as a primary therapy for unresectable HCC. For patients with unresectable HCC, retrospective studies found similar efficacy and toxicity between radio embolization and TACE. For patients with main portal vein thrombosis, radioembolization may be considered advantageous over TACE, owing to its relatively decreased embolic effect. Radioembolization has also demonstrated favorable outcomes for downstaging tumors to meet the Milan criteria. Lewandowski et al retrospectively compared transarterial radioembolization with Y90 (TARE-90) with TACE in patients with T3 disease. The

TARE-90 group demonstrated a trend toward higher partial response and higher percentage of downstaging from T3 to T2 (58 vs. 31%, P <.028), thus falling within the Milan criteria [52].

3.4. Sorafenib

HCC is highly refractory to traditional cytotoxic chemotherapy, with no evidence to date of a survival benefit from its use. Sorafenib, a small molecule multi-kinase inhibitor acting via inhibition of tumor-cell proliferation and tumor angiogenesis, has been widely used in most solid tumor. Recently, Sorafenib is regarded as the first and so far the only drug which shows an increase in overall survival in patients with advanced, unresectable HCC. Can sorafenib be used as a tool to bridge or downstage HCC for patients before transplantation? At present, there are no reported randomized clinical trials in this setting. However, a few case reports show a promise of HCC tumor response to neoadjuvant sorafenib therapy, with effective downstaging to allow for liver transplant listing [53].

3.5. How to select neoadjuvant therapy?

Patient-individualized treatment strategy should be based on the performance status, hepatic reserve, tumor burden and tumor vascularity pattern. Generally speaking, for single HCC <3 cm, RFA may be appropriate. For larger or multifocal HCC, TACE would be indicated. In cases of thrombosis of the main or large branches of the portal vein, TARE appears to be better tolerated because of its less embolic nature. Moreover, these therapies might be implemented alone or via a combined approach. In addition, the benefit of the thoughtful concept of combining locoregional therapy with systemic therapies such as sorafenib has to be proven. In addition, the combination of locoreginal therapy strategy, such as TACE+RFA and TACE +sorafenib, has been used in some transplantation communities and the outcome is promising. However, due to the lack of prospective data, the most appropriate treatment protocol has not yet been defined.

In summary, more light has been shed on the role of neoadjuvant therapy for HCC in recent decades, although the benefits of the therapy remain marginal so far. One of the possible reasons is tumor heterogeneity. Who will benefit from neoadjuvant therapy? The outcome after neoadjuvant therapy will be better if we can predict who will respond to the neoadjuvant therapy before the treatment.

4. Role of circulating tumor cells in recurrence

The term circulating tumor cells (CTC) defines specifically the tumor cells spontaneously disseminating from primary or metastatic sites and invading into peripheral blood or lymphatic vessels. They are also called disseminated tumor cells (DTCs). CTC may remain silent, in a dormant state, for variable periods of time, or grow into clinically detectable metastases. The presence of CTC reflects the aggressiveness characteristic feature of a solid tumor. The major difficulty in the CTC studies is that an extremely small number of CTCs exists in the bloodstream [54] and common serological, imaging and pathological approaches are not sensitive enough to effectively capture CTC. Approximately less than 10 CTCs may be found among one billion blood cells in early stage cancers; therefore highly sensitive methods are required to detect and isolate these cells from the bloodstream. Although CTC detection has been applied and well documented in different types of cancer, especially in breast cancer [55], CTC detection is not routinely performed in HCC and remains in the experimental field. The clinical results suggest CTC detection and identification can be used to evaluate prognosis and may serve as an early marker to assess antitumor activity of treatment [56]. In addition, CTC detection might bring new interesting information of metastatic process and might be used as diagnostic tool of early recurrence after HCC resection or transplant, and may allow a better patient selection.

A major factor in tumor recurrence after a potentially curative treatment for HCC is CTC. Although tumor recurrence in the liver after tumor resection or transplantation may be explained by either intrahepatic tumor cell spreading or de novo tumor development, intrahepatic tumor recurrence after liver transplantation can be explained only by the homing of systemically disseminated and circulating tumor cells. CTC have the potential to migrate and engraft in multiple organs, including the newly implanted liver, where significant recurrences are observed. The tumor response to preoperative treatment might be predictable prior to surgery by a drop in CTC count and this allows improved choice of the best timing of surgery. After surgery, CTCs can be examined in terms of pharmacodynamic biomarkers to choose the most sensitive chemotherapy agents and assist in deciding the duration of adjuvant therapy.

There are so many questions to answer in future. Is CTC a transient or recurrent phenomenon? Does locoreginal therapy in HCC affect the number of CTC? Can the number of CTC be used as criteria of liver transplantion? Which pharmacological and/or surgical protocols might be successful in eliminating or restricting tumor-cell circulation and spread? Thus, the detailed analysis and characterization of CTC in HCC patients may give us new insights into their biology and may lead to new therapeutic strategies for their elimination.

Author details

Xin-yu Huang, Qi Zheng and Zhou Yuan*

*Address all correspondence to: zhouyuan851@163.com

Department of General Surgery, The Sixth People's Hospital Affiliated to Shanghai Jiao Tong University, Shanghai, China

References

[1] Parkin, D. M, Bray, F, Ferlay, J, & Pisani, P. Global cancer statistics, 2002. CA Cancer J Clin (2005). , 55, 74-108.

[2] El-Serag, H. B, & Rudolph, K. L. Hepatocellular carcinoma: epidemiology and molecular carcinogenesis. Gastroenterology (2007). , 132, 2557-2576.

[3] Munoz, N, & Bosch, X. Epidemiology of hepatocellular carcinoma, in Okuda K, Ishak KG (eds). Neoplasm of the Liver: Tokyo, Springer, (1989).

[4] Davila, J. A, Morgan, R. O, Shaib, Y, et al. Hepatitis C infection and the increasing incidence of hepatocellular carcinoma: A population-based study. Gastroenterology (2004). , 127, 1372-1380.

[5] Bosch, F. Global epidemiology of hepatocellular carcinoma. In: Okuda K, Tabor E, (Eds). Liver cancer. New York: Churchill Livingstone, (1997). , 1997, 13-28.

[6] Lai, E. C, Fan, S. T, Lo, C. M, et al. Hepatic resection for hepatocellular carcinoma: an audit of 343 patients. Ann Surg (1995). , 221, 291-98.

[7] Bismuth, H, Chiche, L, Adam, R, et al. Liver resection versus transplantation for hepatocellular carcinoma in cirrhotic patients.Ann Surg (1993). , 218, 145-51.

[8] Bathe, O, Scudamore, C, Caron, N. R, & Buczkowski, A. Resection of hepatocellular carcinoma. In: Okuda K, Tabor E, (Eds). Liver cancer. New York: Churchill Livingstone, (1997). , 1997, 511-29.

[9] Shi, M, Zhang, C. Q, Zhang, Y. Q, Liang, X. M, & Li, J. Q. Micrometastases of solitary hepatocellular carcinoma and appropriate resection margin. World J Surg (2004). , 28, 376-381.

[10] Wong, I. H, Lau, W. Y, Leung, T, Yeo, W, & Johnson, P. J. Hematogenous dissemination of hepatocytes and tumor cells after surgical resection of hepatocellular carcinoma: a quantitative analysis. Clin Cancer Res (1999). , 5, 4021-4027.

[11] Mazzaferro, V, Regalia, E, Doci, R, et al. Liver transplantation for the treatment of small hepatocellular carcinomas in patients with cirrhosis. N Engl J Med (1996). , 334, 693-9.

[12] Bismuth, H, Chiche, L, Adam, R, et al. Liver resection versus transplantation for hepatocellular carcinoma in cirrhotic patients. Ann Surg (1993). , 218, 145-51.

[13] Lau, W. Y, Lai, E. C, & Lau, S. H. The current role of neoadjuvant/adjuvant/chemoprevention therapy in partial hepatectomy for hepatocellular carcinoma: a systematic review. Hepatobiliary Pancreat Dis Int. (2009). Apr; , 8(2), 124-33.

[14] Rein, M. Neoadjuvant treatment for resectable pancreatic cancer: time for phase III testing? WJG (2010). Oct 21; , 16(39), 4883-7.

[15] Lau, W. Y. Primary hepatocellular carcinoma. In Blumgart LH & Fong Y. (2nd eds.) Surgery of The Liver and Biliary Tract Volume II, W.B. Saunders, London; (2000). , 2000, 1423-1450.

[16] Llovet, J. M, Burroughs, A, & Bruix, J. Hepatocellular carcinoma. Lancet (2003). , 362, 1907-1917.

[17] Fan, ST, Lo, CM, Liu, CL, Lam, CM, & Yuen, . . Hepatectomy for hepatocellular carcinoma: toward zero hospital deaths. Ann Surg 1999; 229: 322-330.

[18] Imamura, H, Seyama, Y, Kokudo, N, Maema, A, Sugawara, Y, & Sano, K. One thousand fifty-six hepatectomies without mortality in 8 years. Arch Surg (2003). , 138, 1198-1206.

[19] Llovet, J. M, & Bruix, J. Systematic review of randomized trials for unresectable hepatocellular carcinoma: chemoembolization improves survival. Hepatology (2003). , 37, 429-42.

[20] Bruix, J, & Sherman, M. Practice Guidelines Committee, American Association for the Study of Liver Diseases. Management of hepatocellular carcinoma. Hepatology (2005). , 42(5), 1208-36.

[21] Bruix, J, Sherman, M, Llovet, J. M, et al. EASL Panel of Experts on HCC. Clinical management of hepatocellular carcinoma. Conclusions of the Barcelona-2000 EASL conference. European Association for the Study of the Liver. J Hepatol (2001). , 35(3), 421-30.

[22] Morino, M, Miglietta, C, Grosso, M, De Giuli, M, & Bismuth, H. Preoperativ chemoembolization for hepatocellular carcinoma. J Surg Oncol (1993). Suppl.):, 91-3.

[23] Gerunda, G. E, Neri, D, Merenda, R, Barbazza, F, Zangrandi, F, Meduri, F, Bisello, M, Valmasoni, M, & Gangemi, A. Faccioli AM: Role of transarterial chemoembolization before liver resection for hepatocarcinoma. Liver Transpl (2000). , 6, 619-626.

[24] Lise, M, & Bacchetti, S. Da Pian P, Nitti D, Pilati PL, Pigato P: Prognostic factors affecting long term outcome after liver resection for hepatocellular carcinoma: results in a series of 100 Italian patients. Cancer (1998). , 82, 1028-1036.

[25] Choi, G. H, Kim, D. H, Kang, C. M, Kim, K. S, Choi, J. S, & Lee, W. J. Kim BR: Is preoperative transarterial chemoembolization needed for a resectable hepatocellular carcinoma? World J Surg (2007). , 31, 2370-2377.

[26] Lu, C. D, Peng, S. Y, Jiang, X. C, & Chiba, Y. Tanigawa N: Preoperative transcatheter arterial chemoembolization and prognosis of patients with hepatocellular carcinomas: retrospective analysis of 120 cases. World J Surg (1999). , 23, 293-300.

[27] Zhou, W. P, Lai, E. C, Li, A. J, et al. A prospective, randomized, controlled trial of preoperative transarterial chemoembolization for resectable large hepatocellular carcinoma. Ann Surg (2009). , 249, 195-202.

[28] Sasaki, A, Iwashita, Y, Shibata, K, Ohta, M, & Kitano, S. Mori M: Preoperative transcatheter arterial chemoembolization reduces long-term survival rate after hepatic resection for resectable hepatocellular carcinoma. Eur J Surg Oncol (2006). , 32, 773-779.

[29] Kim, I. S, Lim, Y. S, Lee, H. C, Suh, D. J, & Lee, Y. J. Lee SG: Pre-operative transarterial chemoembolization for resectable hepatocellular carcinoma adversely affects postoperative patient outcome. Aliment Pharmacol Ther (2008). , 27, 338-345.

[30] Wang, X, Li, J, Peng, Y, Dai, Y, & Xu, W. Influence of preoperative transarterial chemoembolization on the prognosis for patients with resectable hepatocellular carcinoma: a meta-analysis of randomized trials. Hepatogastroenterology. (2011). May-Jun; 58(107-108):869-74.

[31] Chua, T. C, Liauw, W, Saxena, A, Chu, F, Glenn, D, Chai, A, & Morris, D. L. Systematic review of neoadjuvant transarterial chemoembolization for resectable hepatocellular carcinoma. Liver Int (2009). , 30, 166-74.

[32] Makuuchi, M, Takayasu, K, Takuma, T, et al. Preoperative transcatheter embolization of the portal venous branch for patients receiving extended lobectomy due to the bile duct carcinoma. J Jpn Soc Clin Surg. (1984). , 45, 14-20.

[33] Gruttadauria, S, Luca, A, Mandala, L, Miraglia, R, & Gridelli, B. Sequential preoperative ipsilateral portal and arterial embolization in patients with colorectal liver metastases. World J Surg. (2006). , 30, 576-8.

[34] Gruttadauria, S, Luca, A, Mandala, L, Miraglia, R, & Gridelli, B. Sequential preoperative ipsilateral portal and arterial embolization in patients with colorectal liver metastases. World J Surg. (2006). , 30, 576-8.

[35] Yoo, H, Kim, J. H, Ko, G. Y, Kim, K. W, Gwon, D. I, Lee, S. G, & Hwang, S. Sequential transcatheter arterial chemoembolization and portal vein embolization versus portal vein embolization only before major hepatectomy for patients with hepatocellular carcinoma. Ann Surg Oncol. (2011). May; , 18(5), 1251-7.

[36] Ogata, S, Belghiti, J, Farges, O, Varma, D, Sibert, A, & Vilgrain, V. Sequential arterial and portal vein embolizations before right hepatectomy in patients with cirrhosis and hepatocellular carcinoma. Br J Surg. (2006). , 93, 1091-8.

[37] Aoki, T, Imamura, H, Hasegawa, K, et al. Sequential preoperative arterial and portal venous embolizations in patients with hepatocellular carcinoma. Arch Surg (2004). , 139, 766-774.

[38] Wilhelm, S. M, Carter, C, & Tang, L. BAY 43-9006 exhibits broad spectrum oral antitumor activity and targets the RAF/MEK/ERK pathway and receptor tyrosine kinases involved in tumor progression and angiogenesis. Cancer Res (2004). , 64, 7099-109.

[39] Ito, Y, Sasaki, Y, Horimoto, M, et al. Activation of mitogen-activated protein kinases/extracellular signal-regulated kinases in human hepatocellular carcinoma. Hepatology (1998). , 27, 951-8.

[40] Llovet, J. M, Ricci, S, Mazzaferro, V, Hilgard, P, Gane, E, Blanc, J. F, De Oliveira, A. C, Santoro, A, Raoul, J. L, Forner, A, Schwartz, M, Porta, C, Zeuzem, S, Bolondi, L, Greten, T. F, & Galle, P. R. SHARP Investigators Study Group. Sorafenib in advanced hepatocellular carcinoma. N Engl J Med. (2008). , 359, 378-390.

[41] Irtan, S, Chopin-laly, X, Ronot, M, Faivre, S, Paradis, V, & Belghiti, J. Complete regression of locally advanced hepatocellular carcinoma induced by sorafenib allowing curative resection. Liver Int. (2011). May; , 31(5), 740-3.

[42] Barbier, L, & Muscari, F. Le Guellec S, Pariente A, Otal P, Suc B. Liver resection after downstaging hepatocellular carcinoma with sorafenib. Int J Hepatol. (2011).

[43] Onaca, N, Davis, G. L, Goldstein, R. M, et al. Expanded criteria for liver transplantation in patients with hepatocellular carcinoma: a report from the international registry of hepatic tumors in liver transplantation. Liver Transpl (2007). , 13, 391-9.

[44] Yao, F. Y, Ferrell, L, Bass, N. M, Watson, J. J, Bacchetti, P, Venook, A, et al. Liver transplantation for hepatocellular carcinoma: expansion of the tumor size limits does not adversely impact survival. Hepatology (2001). , 33, 1394-1403.

[45] Sheu, J. C, Sung, J. L, Chen, D. S, Yang, P. M, Lai, M. Y, Lee, C. S, et al. Growth rate of asymptomatic hepatocellular carcinoma and its clinical implications. Gastroenterology (1985). , 89, 259-266.

[46] Lesurtel, M, Müllhaupt, B, Pestalozzi, B. C, Pfammatter, T, & Clavien, P. A. Transarterial chemoembolization as a bridge to liver transplantation for hepatocellular carcinoma: an evidence-based analysis. Am J Transplant (2006). , 6(11), 2644-50.

[47] Oldhafer, K. J, Chavan, A, Fruhauf, N. R, et al. Arterial chemoembolization before liver transplantation in patients with hepatocellular carcinoma: marked tumor necrosis, but no survival benefit? J Hepatol (1998). , 29, 953-9.

[48] Decaens, T, & Roudo-thoraval, F. Bresson Hadni S, et al. Impact of pretransplantation transarterial chemoembolization on survival and recurrence after liver transplantation for hepatocellular carcinoma. Liver Transpl (2005). , 11, 767-75.

[49] Graziadei, I. W, Sandmueller, H, Waldenberger, P, et al. Chemoembolization followed by liver transplantation for hepatocellular carcinoma impedes tumor progression while on the waiting list and leads to excellent outcome. Liver Transpl (2003). , 9, 557-63.

[50] Lencioni, R. A, Allgaier, H. P, Cioni, D, et al. Small hepatocellular carcinoma in cirrhosis: randomized comparison of radio-frequency thermal ablation versus percutaneous ethanol injection. Radiology (2003). , 228, 235-40.

[51] Mazzaferro, V, Battiston, C, Perrone, S, et al. Radiofrequency ablation of small hepatocellular carcinoma in cirrhotic patients awaiting liver transplantation: a prospective study. Ann Surg (2004). , 240, 900-9.

[52] Lewandowski, R. J, Kulik, L. M, Riaz, A, et al. A comparative analysis of transarterial downstaging for hepatocellular carcinoma: chemoembolization versus radioembolization. Am J Transplant (2009). , 9, 1920-8.

[53] Vagefi, P. A, & Hirose, R. Downstaging of hepatocellular carcinoma prior to liver transplant: is there a role for adjuvant sorafenib in locoregional therapy? J Gastrointest Cancer. (2010). , 2010(41), 4-217.

[54] Guo, J, Yao, F, Lou, Y, Xu, C, Xiao, B, Zhou, W, Chen, J, Hu, Y, & Liu, Z. Detecting carcinoma cells in peripheral blood of patients with hepatocellular carcinoma by immunomagnetic beads and RT-PCR, J. Clin. Gastroenterol. (2007). , 41(2007), 783-788.

[55] Stathopoulou, A, Vlachonikolis, I, & Mavroudis, D. Molecular detection of cytokeratin-19-positive cells in the peripheral blood of patients with operable breast cancer: evaluation of their prognostic significance. J.Oncol. (2002). , 2002, 20-3404.

[56] Pantel, K, Brakenhoff, R. H, & Brandt, B. Detection clinical relevance and specific biological properties of disseminating tumour cells. Nat Rev Cancer. (2008). May; , 8(5), 329-40.

Chapter 6

Targets and Approaches to Control Hepatocellular Carcinoma in Future

Mukherjee Biswajit,
Hossain Chowdhury Mobaswar ,
Bhattacharya Sanchari and Shampa Ghosh

Additional information is available at the end of the chapter

http://dx.doi.org/10.5772/56867

1. Introduction

Cancer is uncontrolled proliferation of cells, which results from the loss of proper balance between cell death and cell growth. The transformed phenotypes of cancer cells are caused by the accumulation of mutations in a variety of genes, products of which normally play a role in the biochemical pathways that regulate cell death and cell proliferation. Cancer is a broad term used to define a group of more than 250 different diseases (Roncalli et al. 2010). It is a slow multi-stage, multi-step process (Cammà et al. 2008; Calvisi et al. 2009; Sherman 2011). In the first instance, these cells, derived initially from a normal cell, form a primary tumor which comprises a growth-transformed population of cells. The cells acquire a set of mutations to a set of genes which allow them to divide repeatedly in a way that normal cells cannot (Besaratinia et al. 2009; Calvisi et al. 2009). Histologically, cancer is characterized by several morphological alterations, including changes in tissue architecture, cytological abnormalities of both the nucleus and cytoplasm and the presence of abnormal mitoses. A stepwise several biochemical, genetic and biological alterations eventually result in a cancer.

Primary liver cancer or hepatocellular carcinoma (HCC) is a very common malignant hepatobiliary disease and it represents the fifth most frequent neoplastic disease which causes approximately 1 million deaths per year (Yang and Roberts, 2010, Cha et al. 2010). HCC is the third leading cause of cancer related death worldwide (Raphael 2012). Viruses and chemicals have been identified as the most important etiological factor associated with the development of human liver cancer (Carr et al. 2010). The most common cause of HCC is hepatitis B and C (Woo et al. 2008; Masuzaki et al. 2008, Gouas et al. 2010; Iavarone and Colombo 2011) and a number of risk factors that have been identified (Shariff et al. 2009; Sherman 2010; Gomaa et al. 2008 and 2009). Most of HCC cases develop from a cirrhotic liver (Bartolomeo et al. 2011; Chagas et al. 2009; Orlando et al.2009; Cammà et al. 2008) with an annual incidence of 2-6% for hepatitis B virus carriers (Kew 2010; Lim et al. 2009; Hadziyannis 2011) and 3-5% for hepatitis C virus-infected patients (Masuzaki et al. 2008; Rosen 2011). Males are more susceptible to HCC.

Despite the advances in cancer treatments there is no effective chemotherapeutic protocol to treat HCC (Andreana et al. 2009; Arii et al. 2010). Advanced HCC has a poor prognosis (Simile et al. 2011; Sonja et al. 2010). Historically, no effective systemic chemotherapy treatment options have been available for patients with advanced HCC (Bruix and Sherman 2011). Thus, proper understanding of the molecular basis of pathogenesis of HCC can lead us to plan for proper therapeutic strategies to combat the notorious disease.

Accumulating epidemiological evidence suggests that a pronounced predisposition to develop cancer as a consequence of a mutation in a single gene is rare (approximately 1-5%) (Frau et al. 2010). One possible explanation for this finding is that carcinogenesis is a multistage process involving a number of different genes and environmental factors (Chung et al. 2008; Forner et al. 2010; Frau et al. 2010). In connection with many distinct subtypes of cancer, some functional alterations are required for malignant transformation. They are, namely, sufficiency with respect to growth signals, insensitivity to growth-inhibitory signals, evasion of programmed cell death (apoptosis), the potential for unlimited replication, sustained angiogenesis, tissue invasion and metastasis (Bergers and Hanahan 2008; Bartolomeo et al. 2011; Cao et al. 2010; Frau et al. 2010; Gouas et al. 2010). The exact number of distinct stages involved may vary from tumor to tumor, since some of these acquired characteristics probably interact with other processes (Roncalli 2010). Indeed, the heterogeneity of tumors, both with regards to morphology and pattern of gene expression, may even indicate the participation of many more sequential steps.

A highly regulatory network controls cellular proliferation in multicellular organisms. Normally cells in many tissues and organs remain in a non-proliferative state. In response to external stimuli such as growth factors, hormones or antigens, cells are stimulated to begin DNA synthesis and cellular proliferation according to the need of the living system. As soon as the need is fulfilled, the cell division stops. However, cancerous cells are characterized by the unrestrained cellular proliferation due to the alteration of normal cellular signalling process and they acquire complete or partial independence of mitogenic signals through production of growth factors (Garrett et al. 2008; Hironaka et al. 2009) and /or alteration in number or structure of cellular receptors (Lachenmayer et al. 2010) and/ or modulation in the activity of post receptor signalling pathway (Cavard et al. 2008; Chen et al. 2009). The communication of extracellular signals to the cells, then to the nucleus to modulate gene expression is governed by phosphorylation regulated signal transduction cascades which act to amplify the events generated at the cellular membrane by ligand-receptor interaction or cell stress. Therefore, identification of the extracellular factors that modulate cell proliferation and elucidation of the cellular molecular mechanism during the development of cancer can answer many fundamental questions in cancer cell biology. It is important to understand in details the receptors and the signal transduction pathways involved in the pathogenesis of cancer to provide potential target for therapeutic intervention. Many studies have focused to identify molecular pathways to elicit cancer cell proliferation, including HCC. Here many of them have been highlighted to identify fundamental targets of hepatocellular oncogenesis. Thus, the present chapter has been projected to the molecular targets and approaches to intervene the targets for the management of HCC in humans in coming years.

2. Therapeutic targets for HCC

Three generally considered fundamental but interrelated targets of controlling oncogenesis are regulation of deregulated energy metabolism and ion homeostasis; signal transduction, oncogenes and growth factors; and immunomodulation. One of the most characteristic phenotypes of rapidly growing cancer cells is their propensity to catabolise glucose at high rates. Rapidly growing activity to cancer cells has a reduced number of mitochondria and increased glycolytic activity with a shift from respiratory to fermentative ATP supply to cover most of their energy requirement. The stimulation of the K^+, H^+ and Na^+ fluxes is a general early response in most of the quiescent cells stimulated to proliferate by multiple combinations of growth promoting factors. Growth factors, cytokines exert their action on cell proliferation by modulation of cell signalling process. There is a strong relationship between the immune system and cell proliferation. Immune suppressive agents have a powerful effect on hepatocyte growth regulation in HCC.

Reviewing current literature, a selection of therapeutic targets of HCC has been described below.

Like most other cancers, growth factors, their receptors, and downstream signalling proteins play a pivotal role in the development and maintenance of HCC and are of significant interest for future therapeutic approaches. In foetal liver, a large number of growth factors such as epidermal growth factor (EGF), fibroblast growth factor (FGF), hepatocyte growth factor (HGF), insulin-like growth factors (IGFs), platelet-derived growth factor (PDGF), transforming growth factors-α and $-\beta$ (TGF-α, TGF-β), and vascular endothelial growth factor (VEGF) (Höpfner et al. 2008; Hoshida et al. 2008 and 2009) are produced. Their secretion either declines or shuts down in adult liver. However, during hepatic regeneration due to the cause of hepatic injury or damage many such growth factors (Böhm et al. 2010), namely, EGF, TGF-α, IGFs, and VEGF are upregulated in normal hepatocytes. The transient upregulation of those factors is dysregulated in the chronic injured liver leading to sustained mitogenic/ oncogenic signalling, during the development of HCC. FGF and PDGF released from non-hepatocyte sources such as activated hepatic stellate cells, myofibroblasts, endothelial cells, Kupffer cells, and bile duct epithelia have been shown to play important roles in promoting hepatic fibrosis and HCC growth (Friedman 2008). The ubiquitin-proteasome pathway has emerged as a key player in the regulation of several diverse cellular processes. Inhibition of poly-ubiquitination using proteasome inhibitors has shown some light in HCC treatment. Besides, immunomodulation has been found to be effective in stabilizing HCC growth in patients. Number of immunomodulators has been investigated and few of them have been found to be effective. They have been discussed below under immunomodulation agents. Signal transduction, and growth factors; inhibitors of proteasome pathway, immunomodulation and antisense oligomer-mediated inhibition of targeted oncogenes have been projected as future targets and approaches of HCC (Table 1).

Molecular targets in HCC	Inhibitors / Modulators / Antisense oligonucleotides
Growth factors, e.g., EGFR, EGF, TGF-α, TGF-β, VEGF	Cetuximab, Gefitinib, Erlotinib, Vandetanib.
mTOR	Rapamycin, Temsirolimus, Salirasib, RAD001
Multikinase	Sorafenib, Everolimus, AP23573, RAD001.
Proteasome	Bortezomeb
Immunomodulators used in HCC	Thymostimulin, Retinoids, Everolimus, Azathioprine, 6-mercaptopurine.
Antisense oligonucleotides used in HCC	ISIS5132. ISIS2513

Table 1. Growth factors, proteasome-inhibitors, immunomodulators and antisense oligomers in HCC

3. Approaches

A selection of agents currently in the development and/or testing stages for the clinical application in targeted HCC treatment is summarized in the following section.

3.1. Therapies against EGFR

There are two classes of anti-EGFR agents found to have antitumor activity against HCC. One of them belongs to monoclonal antibodies (as an example cetuximab) which competitively inhibit extracellular endogenous ligand binding. The other class belongs to chemicals such as gefitinib, erlotinib which inhibit the intracellular tyrosine kinase domain. EGF, TGF-α, heparin binding-EGF and EGFR have been shown to involve in the pathogenesis of HCC. Thus, EGFR signalling pathways have become a potential investigating area of research to identify the target (s) to inhibit proliferation of HCC and metastasis. Gefitinib, erlotinib, cetuximab were tested in patients with advanced HCC (Thomas et al. 2007; Philip et al. 2005; Asnacios et al. 2008; Wu et al. 2011, Levêque 2011) and were reported to possess signals of activity in controlling the progress of HCC in a variable extent.

3.2. Targeting approaches towards VEGF and VEGFR

HCCs rely on the formation of new blood vessels for growth, and VEGF is critical in this process (Zhu et al. 2011). HCCs are with high vascular architecture and VEGF is a key factor in tumor angiogenesis (Bergers and Hanahan, 2008; Garrett et al. 2008; Hironaka et al. 2009). Therefore, the inhibition of angiogenesis is a potential and promising therapeutic approach in HCC. Anti-VEGF therapy with sorafenib was the first systemic therapy against VEGF to demonstrate improved survival in patients with advanced-stage HCC (Cheng et al. 2009; Zhu et al. 2011, Miller et al. 2009; Zhu 2008, Llovet et al. 2008a). Sorafenib was also tested in advanced stage liver cirrhosis patients with unresectable HCC (Pinter et al. 2009). Bevacizumab alone or in combination with other agents showed promise in patients with advanced HCC (Siegel et al. 2008; Thomas et al. 2009; Thomas et al. 2008; Kaseb et al. 2012). However, the common bevacizumab-related side effects were hypertension, bleeding, and proteinuria (Thomas et al. 2009; Siegel et al. 2008a; Kopetz et al. 2009). Besides, inhibition of the tyrosine kinase activity of VEGFR has been tried as an effective measure to inhibit angeogenesis in HCC (Bhide et al. 2010). PTK787/ ZK222584 (vatalanib) is an oral angiogenesis inhibitor that targets tyrosine kinase activity of VEGFR (Gauler et al. 2012). Pan-VEGFR tyrosine kinase activity inhibitor with activity against PDGFRs also carries a new hope.

3.3. Multi-kinase inhibitor

Like all other cancers diverse signaling pathways in HCC are very complex. One of the key pathways regulating cellular proliferation is the mitogen activated protein Kinase (MAPK) pathway. Other pathways involved in the development of HCC include the PI3K/Akt/mTOR, hepatocyte growth factor (HGF)/c-MET, insulin-like growth factor (IGF) and its receptor (IGFR) pathways, and the Wnt-β catenin pathway (Cavard et al. 2008;Chen et al. 2009; Desbois-Mouthon et al. 2009; Takigawa and Nouso 2008; Zhang et al. 2008). The Raf family of kinases are central to this pathway where the transduction of extracellular growth signals from the cell surface to the nucleus occurs via the ras-raf-MEK-ERK signaling cascade. The several experiments have shown that Raf, MEK, MAP Kinase are downstream effector molecules of Ras and their sequential order in the pathway. The Raf serine/threonine kinases are the principal effectors of Ras in this mitogen activated protein Kinase (MAPK) signaling pathway. As serine/threonine kinases, Raf proteins phosphorylate and activate serine and threonine residues on subsequent downstream effector proteins of Ras. Therefore, molecularly targeted agents that interact with multiple signaling pathways/effectors appear to be very promising in the treatment of patients with HCC (Cervello et al. 2012; Cheng et al. 2009). The novel bi-aryl urea sorafenib, an orally available multi-kinase inhibitor, targets kinases of wild-type B-Raf, mutant V559EB-Raf and cRaf, thereby blocking tumor growth (Spangenberg et al. 2008). There are three ras protooncogenes that encode 21 Kd proteins – H-Ras (Harvey murine sarcoma virus), N-Ras (neuroblastoma cell line) and two alternatively spliced K-Ras, K-Ras 4A, and K-Ras 4B; These isoforms are capable of differentially activating various critical effectors, thereby exerting distinct biologic effects. Sorafenib, an inhibitor of receptor tyrosine kinases was found to stabilize the advanced unresectable HCC patients by regulating angiogenesis, and was approved by regulatory agencies in 2007. It has a role on human VEGF receptors-2 and -3 (VEGFR-2/-3) and PDGF-βR. However, sorafenib has been also suggested to provide antitumor action in HCC by inhibition of the Raf/MEK/ERK pathway (Llovet and Bruix, 2008 and 2009). Multikinase inhibitor sunitinib is a small molecule that inhibits members of the split-kinase domain family of receptor tyrosine kinase including VEGFR types 1 and 2 (Llovet et al. 2008a). Antiangiogenic effects of sunitinib have been suggested through VEGFR and PDGFR.

However, a randomized phase 3 study in HCC failed to show a significant survival benefit as compared to sorafenib and study stopped in 2011.

3.4. mTOR inhibitors

mTOR inhibitors are potential anti-HCC agents for future (Zhou et al. 2009). Promising mTOR inhibitors are rapamycin and its analogues such as sirolimus, temsirolimus (CCI-779), everolimus (RAD001) and AP23573 (Nocera et al 2008; Rizell et al. 2008). Rapamycin and its analogues such as temsirolimus (the cell cycle inhibitor) and everolimus and AP23573 (an orally bioavailable derivative of rapamycin) modulate angiogennesis to improve survival of patients in advanced HCC (Heuer 2009, Huynh et al. 2008). RAD001, an orally-administered, novel mTOR inhibitor was evaluated in a phase I study (Huynh et al. 2008 and 2008a; Chen et al 2009). Treatment of patients with the combination of rapamycin/ rapamycin-analogue(s) with conventional anticancer drug(s) such as doxorubicin, vinblastine has been found to improve survival in advanced HCC patients (Spangenberg et al. 2008).

3.5. Proteasome inhibition

HCC is highly ubiquitinated. The ubiquitination is important to the development and progression of HCC. Proteasome inhibitor such as bortezomib blocks multi-ubiquitinated protein degradation by reversible and competitive inhibition of the active site threonine residue of the 26S proteasome (Cao and Mao, 2011; Boozari et al. 2009). Antineoplastic activity of bortezomib approved for the treatment of mantle cell lymphoma has already been shown to stabilize advanced HCC in patients (Höpfner et al 2008).

3.6. Immunomodulatory agents

An immunomodulator is a substance which has an effect on the immune system. An immunomodulator may be at the same time an immunosuppressant or an immunostimulant and can act on different targets within the immune system. Cell signalling process regulates immune system consisting of immunomodulatory endogenic chemicals and cells. Immunomodulators interfere with the signalling process by shifting the homeostasis of the immune system to reduce or eliminate disease symptoms. Thus these compounds are the obvious choice for therapeutic intervention of HCC. Thymostimulin (a standardized low molecular protein fraction containing thymosin alpha 1 and thymic humoral factor) has been shown to produce cytotoxic immune reaction against HCC. Phase II trials using thymostimulin in patients with advanced and metastasised HCC have shown to control metastatic HCC without predominant side-effects (Dollinger et al. 2010). However, thymostimulin administration in some patients was found to accumulate ascites and cause renal failure (Dollinger et al. 2010).

3.7. Antisense therapy

Antisense oligonucleotides offer one approach to target genes involved in cancer progression. They are typically less than 50 nucleotides long and are specifically designed to hybridize to corresponding gene/ mRNA by Watson-Crick binding. They inhibit mRNA function in several

http://dx.doi.org/10.5772/56867

ways, including modulation of splicing and inhibition of protein translation by disruption of ribosome assembly. Single stranded synthetic nucleic acid (oligonucleotide) when hybridize with DNA or RNA alters transcription or prevents translation thus, preventing or modifying protein production. Because of the volume of information nowadays available on gene sequencing, there has been burst of exploration of capacity for oligomers to inhibit gene/ protein expression. Thus, antisense therapies focus on controlling the production of the proteins on a genetic level. A strand of mRNA is transcribed from DNA, and is a copy of the "coding" or "sense" strand of the gene. The main form of therapy uses the complementary or antisense strand to hybridize the sense strand or mRNA and thus it prevents production of the protein by blocking or altering transcription or translation (Figure 1). With the backbone chemical modifications (in phosphate linkage), antisense oligonucleotides increase resistance to nuclease digestion, prolong their biological half-lives and significantly suppress target-gene expression. Antisense oligonucleotides have been studied for several years as treatments for many diseases and genetic disorders. The therapy is based on the principles of genetic expression. The most widely used modified oligomers in antisense therapies is phosphorothioate oligonucleotides, which have much greater resistance to digestion by nucleases. Phosphorothioate oligonucleotides are rapidly and extensively absorbed and distributed from blood.

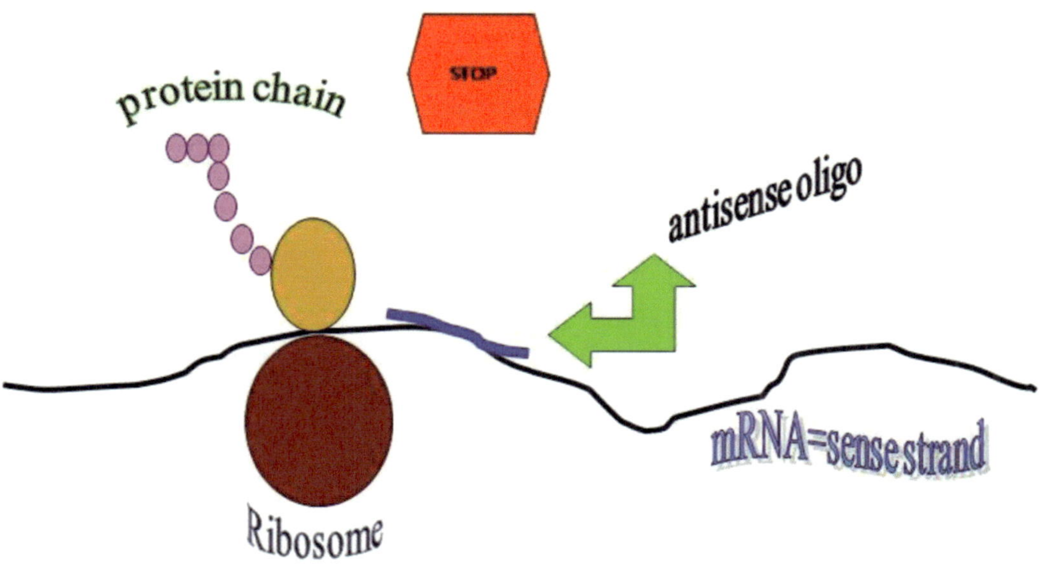

Figure 1. Antisense oligomer-mRNA duplex inhibiting to synthesize peptide chain

The first antisense treatment to get FDA approval to date has been Formivirsen (Vitravene), which is a treatment for cytomegalovirus (CMV) retinitis in people with acquired immunodeficiency disease (AIDS) (Rahman et al. 2008). Several antisense oligonucleotides were shown to target various oncogenes, to overcome tumour escape and to improve therapeutic activity.

Several studies have shown the anticancer potential of antisense oligonucleotides (Das et al. 2010; Rayburn and Zhang, 2008) and many of them are in clinical trial. They have less cytotoxic side-effects than conventional chemotherapy agents. Systemic treatment with fomivirsen is a milestone in the field of antisense treatment with antisense oligonucleotides. This has led the way for development of antisense oligonucleotides for various new potential targets for the treatment of cancer, including HCC.

4. Conclusion

Several experimental evidences have established that targeted inhibition of genes/ proteins involved in controlling HCC growth combined with cytostatic anticancer treatments is a promising approach for HCC therapy. Blocking of single gene/ protein has been found to control neoplastic cellular proliferation *in vitro* effectively. However, considering the multitude of molecular entities and signalling pathways that regulate the proliferation and the life/death decision in cancer cells, inhibition of a single target gene may not be sufficient to suppress tumor growth. The preclinical/ clinical trials of several potential compounds targeting liver cancer-relevant genes/ proteins may address more specific and adequate future therapies for HCC.

Acknowledgements

Authors are indebted to the grants from Department of Science Technology (Govt. of India) (DST/Inspire Fellowship/ 2010/ 87) and Indian Council of Medical Research (58/7/2009-BMS) for funding the related projects and findings of which have helped us partially to write this work.

Author details

Mukherjee Biswajit*, Hossain Chowdhury Mobaswar , Bhattacharya Sanchari and Shampa Ghosh

*Address all correspondence to: biswajit55@yahoo.com

Department of Pharmaceutical Technology, Jadavpur University, Kolkata, India

References

[1] Andreana L, Isgr Ó G, Pleguezuelo M. Surveillance and diagnosis of hepatocellular carcinoma in patients with cirrhosis. World J Hepatol 2009; 1 (1) 48–61.

[2] Arii S, Sata M, Sakamoto M, Shimada M, Kumada T, Shiina S. Management of hepatocellular carcinoma Report of Consensus Meeting in the 45th Annual Meeting of the Japan Society of Hepatology. Hepatol Res 2010; 40 (7) 667–685.

[3] Asnacios A, Fartoux L, Romano O, Tesmoingt C, Louafi SS, Mansoubakht T. Gemcitabine plus oxaliplatin Gemox combined with cetuximab in patients with progressive advanced stage hepatocellular carcinoma: results of a multicenter phase 2 studies. Cancer 2008; 112 (12) 2733–2739.

[4] Bartolomeo N, Trerotoli P, Serio G. Progression of liver cirrhosis to HCC: an application of hidden Markov model. BMC Med Res Methodol 2011; 11 (38) 1–8.

[5] Bergers G, Hanahan D. Modes of resistance to anti-angiogenic therapy. Nat Rev Cancer 2008; 8 (8) 592–603.

[6] Besaratinia A, Kim SI, Hainaut P, Pfeifer GP. In vitro recapitulating of TP53 mutagenesis in hepatocellular carcinoma associated with dietary aflatoxin B1 exposure. Gastroenterology 2009; 137 (3) 1127–1137.

[7] Bhide RS, Lombardo LJ, Hunt JT. The antiangiogenic activity in xenograft models of brivanib alaninate a dual inhibitor of VEGFR-2 and FGFR-1 kinases. Mol Cancer Ther 2010; 9 (2) 369–378.

[8] Böhm F, Köhler UA, Speicher T, Werner S. Regulation of liver regeneration by growth factors and cytokines. EMBO Mol Med 2010; 2 (8) 294–305.

[9] Boozari B, Wirth T, Woller N, Manns MP, Kubicka S, Kühnel F. Efficacy of HCC treatment with proteasome inhibitor Bortezomib is increased by oncolytic virotherapy mediated downregulation of Mcl-1 and Bip. Z Gastroenterol 2009; 47 3–4.

[10] Bruix J, Sherman M. Management of hepatocellular carcinoma: an update. Hepatology 2011; 53 (3) 1020–1022.

[11] Calvisi DF, Pinna F, Ladu S, Pellegrino R, Simile MM, Frau M. Forkhead box M1B is a determinant of rat susceptibility to hepatocarcinogenesis and sustains ERK activity in human HCC. Gut 2009; 58 (5) 679–87.

[12] Cammà C, Di Marco V, Cabibbo G. Survival of patients with hepatocellular carcinoma in cirrhosis: a comparison of BCLC CLIP and GRETCH staging systems. Aliment Pharmacol Ther 2008; 28 (1) 62–75.

[13] Cao B, Mao X. The ubiquitin-proteasomal system is critical for multiple myeloma: implications in drug discovery. Am J Blood Res 2011; 1 (1) 46–56.

[14] Cao CQ, Yan TD, Bester L, Liauw W, Morris DL. Radioembolization with yttrium microspheres for neuroendocrine tumour liver metastases. Brit J Surg 2010; 97 (4) 537–543.

[15] Carr BI, Kondragunta V, Buch SC, Branch RA. Therapeutic equivalence in survival for hepatic arterial chemoembolization and yttrium 90 microsphere treatments in un-

resectable hepatocellular carcinoma: a two-cohort study. Cancer 2010; 116 (5) 1305–1314.

[16] Cavard C, Colnot S, Audard V. Wnt/β-catenin pathway in hepatocellular carcinoma pathogenesis and liver physiology. Future Oncol 2008; 4 (5) 647–660.

[17] Cervello M, McCubrey JA, Cusimano A, Lampiasi N, Azzolina A, Montalto G. Targeted therapy for hepatocellular carcinoma: novel agents on the horizon. Oncotarget 2012; 3 (3) 236–260.

[18] Cha CH, Saif MW, Yamane BH, Weber SM. Hepatocellular carcinoma: current management. Curr Prob Surg 2010; 47 (1) 10–67.

[19] Chagas AL, Kikuchi LOO, Oliveira CPMS. Does hepatocellular carcinoma in non-alcoholic steatohepatitis exist in cirrhotic and non-cirrhotic patients? Braz J Med Biol Res 2009; 42 (10) 958–962.

[20] Chen JS, Wang Q, Fu XH. Involvement of PI3K/PTEN/AKT/mTOR pathway in invasion and metastasis in hepatocellular carcinoma: association with MMP-9. Hepatol Res 2009; 39 (2) 177–186.

[21] Cheng AL, Kang YK, Chen Z, Tsao CJ, Queen S, King JS. Efficacy and safety of sorafenib in patients in the Asia-Pacific region with advanced hepatocellular carcinoma: a phase III randomised double-blind placebo-controlled trial. Lancet Oncol 2009; 10 (1) 25–34.

[22] Chung H, Kudo M, Takahashi S. Comparison of three current staging systems for hepatocellular carcinoma: Japan integrated staging score new Barcelona Clinic Liver Cancer staging classification and Tokyo score. J Gastroen Hepatol 2008; 23 (3) 445–452.

[23] Das T, Patra F, Mukherjee B. Effect of antisense oligomer in controlling c-raf1 overexpression during diethylnitrosamine-induced hepatocarcinogenesis in rats. Cancer Chemother Pharmacol 2010; 65 (2) 309–318.

[24] Desbois-Mouthon C, Baron A, Blivet-Van Eggelpoël MJ. Insulin-like growth factor-1 receptor inhibition induces a resistance mechanism via the epidermal growth factor receptor/ HER3/AKT signaling pathway: rational basis for cotargeting insulin-like growth factor-1 receptor and epidermal growth factor receptor in hepatocellular carcinoma. Clin Cancer Res 2009; 15 (17) 5445–5456.

[25] Dollinger MM, Lautenschlaeger C, Lesske J, Tannapfel A, Wagner AD, Schoppmeyer K. Thymostimulin versus placebo for palliative treatment of locally advanced or metastasised hepatocellular carcinoma: a phase III clinical trial. AIO Hepatobiliary Study Group BMC Cancer 2010; 24 (10) 457–467.

[26] Forner A, Reig ME, de Lope CR, Bruix J. Current strategy for staging and treatment: the BCLC update and future prospects. Semin Liv Dis 2010; 30 (1) 61–74.

[27] Frau M, Biasi F, Feo F, Pascale RM. Prognostic markers and putative therapeutic targets for hepatocellular carcinoma. Mol Aspects Med 2010; 31 (2) 179–193.

[28] Friedman SL. Hepatic stellate cells: protean multifunctional and enigmatic cells of the liver. Physiol Rev 2008; 88 (1) 125–172.

[29] Garrett C, Siu L, El-Khoueiry A. A phase I study of brivanib alaninate BMS-582664 an oral dual inhibitor of VEGFR and FGFR tyrosine kinases in combination with full-dose cetuximab in patients with advanced gastrointestinal malignancies who failed prior therapy. J Clin Oncol 2008; 26 suppl:abstr 4111.

[30] Gauler TC, Besse B, Mauguen A, Meric JB, Gounant V. Phase II trial of PTK787/ZK 222584 vatalanib administered orally once-daily or in two divided daily doses as second-line monotherapy in relapsed or progressing patients with stage IIIB/IV non-small-cell lung cancer NSCLC. Ann Oncol 2012; 23 (3) 678–687.

[31] Gomaa AI, Khan SA, Toledano MB, Waked I,Taylor-Robinson SD. Hepatocellular carcinoma: epidemiology risk factors and pathogenesis. World J Gastroentrol 2008; 14 (27) 4300–4308.

[32] Gomaa AI, Khan SA, Leen ELS, Waked I, Taylor-Robinson SD. Diagnosis of hepatocellular carcinoma. World J Gastroentrol 2009; 15 (11) 1301–1314.

[33] Gouas DA, Shi H, Hautefeuille AH. Effects of the TP53 pR249S mutant on proliferation and clonogenic properties in human hepatocellular carcinoma cell lines: Interaction with hepatitis B virus X protein. Carcinogenesis 2010; 31 (8) 1475–1482.

[34] Hadziyannis SJ. Natural history of chronic hepatitis B in Euro-Mediterranean and African countries. J Hepatol 2011; 55 (1) 183–191.

[35] Heuer M, Benko T, Cicinnati VR, Kaiser GM, Sotiropoulos GC, Baba HA. Effect of low-dose rapamycin on tumor growth in two human hepatocellular cancer cell lines. Transplant Proc 2009; 41 (1) 359–365.

[36] Hironaka S, Onozawa Y, Aramaki T. Phase 1 study of brivanib alaninate a novel FGF and VEGF receptor inhibitor. Japanese Society for Clinical Oncology JSCO Annual Conference Yokohama October 2009; 22– 24 abstr OS036-3.

[37] Höpfner M, Schuppan D, Scherübl H. Growth factor receptors and related signalling pathways as targets for novel treatment strategies of hepatocellular cancer. World J Gastroenterol 2008; 14 (1) 1–14.

[38] Hoshida Y, Villanueva A, Kobayashi M, Peix J, Chiang DY, Camargo A. Gene expression in fixed tissues and outcome in hepatocellular carcinoma. N Engl J Med 2008; 359 (19) 1995–2004.

[39] Hoshida Y, Villanueva A, Llovet JM. Molecular profiling to predict hepatocellular carcinoma outcome. Expert Rev Gastroenterol Hepatol 2009; 3 (2) 101–103.

[40] Huynh H, Chow KP, Soo KC, Toh HC, Choo SP, Foo KF. Rad001 (Everolimus) inhibits tumor growth in xenograft models of human hepatocellular carcinoma. J Cell Mol Med 2009; 13 (7) 1371–1380.

[41] Huynh H, Ngo VC, Fargnoli J. Brivanib alaninate a dual inhibitor of vascular endothelial growth factor receptor and fibroblast growth factor receptor tyrosine kinases induces growth inhibition in mouse models of human hepatocellular carcinoma. Clin Cancer Res 2008a; 14 (19) 6146–6153.

[42] Iavarone M, Colombo M. HBV-related HCC clinical issues and therapy. Digest Liver Dis 2011; 43 supplement 1 S32–S39.

[43] Kaseb AO, Garrett-Mayer E, Morris JS, Xiao L, Lin E, Onicescu G. Efficacy of Bevacizumab plus Erlotinib for advanced hepatocellular carcinoma and predictors of outcome: final results of a phase II trial. Oncology 2012; 82 (2) 67–74.

[44] Kew MC. Epidemiology of chronic hepatitis B virus infection hepatocellular carcinoma and hepatitis B virus-induced hepatocellular carcinoma. Pathol Biol 2010; 58 (4) 273–277.

[45] Kopetz S, Hoff PM, Eng MJ. Angiogenic cytokines are increased prior to disease progression in metastatic colorectal cancer patients treated with bevacizumab. ASCO Gastrointestinal Cancers Symposium San Francisco January 15–17 2009; abstr 292.

[46] Lachenmayer A, Alsinet C, Chang CY, Llovet JM. Molecular approaches to treatment of hepatocellular carcinoma. Digest Liver Dis 2010; 42(3) 264–272.

[47] Levêque D. Pharmacokinetics of gefitinib and erlotinib. Lancet Oncol 2011; 12 (12) 1093.

[48] Lim SG, Mohammed R, Yuen MF, Kao JH. Prevention of hepatocellular carcinoma in hepatitis B virus infection. J Gastroenterol Hepatol 2009; 24 (8) 1352–1357.

[49] Llovet JM, Bruix J. Molecular targeted therapies in hepatocellular carcinoma. Hepatology 2008; 48 (4) 1312–1327.

[50] Llovet JM, Bruix J. Testing molecular therapies in hepatocellular carcinoma: the need for randomized phase II trials. J Clin Oncol 2009; 27 833–835.

[51] Llovet JM, Ricci S, Mazzaferro V, Hilgard P, Gane E, Blanc JF. Sorafenib in advanced hepatocellular carcinoma. N Engl J Med 2008a; 359 (4) 378–390.

[52] Masuzaki R, Yoshida H, Tateishi R, Shiina S, Omata M. Hepatocellular carcinoma in viral hepatitis: improving standard therapy. Best Pract Res 2008; 22 (6) 1137–1151.

[53] Miller AA, Murry DJ, Owzar K, Hollis DR, Kennedy EB, Abou-Alfa G. Phase I and pharmacokinetic study of sorafenib in patients with hepatic or renal dysfunction: CALGB 60301. J Clin Oncol 2009; 27 (11) 1800–1805.

[54] Nocera A, Andorno E, Tagliamacco A, Morelli N, Bottino G, Ravazzoni F. Sirolimus therapy in liver transplant patients: an initial experience at a single center. Transplant Proc 2008; 40 (6) 1950–1952.

[55] Orlando A, Leandro G, Olivo M, Andriulli A, Cottone M. Radiofrequency thermal ablation vs percutaneous ethanol injection for small hepatocellular carcinoma in cirrhosis: meta-analysis of randomized controlled trials. Am J Gastroenterol 2009; 104 (2) 514–524.

[56] Philip P, Mahoney M, Allmer C, Thomas J, Pitot H, Kim G. Phase II study of Erlotinib (OSI-774) in patients with advanced hepatocellular cancer. J Clin Oncol 2005; 23 (27) 6657–6663.

[57] Pinter M, Sieghart W, Graziadei I, Vogel W, Maieron A, Konigsberg R. Sorafenib in unresectable hepatocellular carcinoma from mild to advanced stage liver cirrhosis. Oncologist 2009 ; 14 (1) 70–76.

[58] Rahman SMA, Seki S, Obika S, Yoshikawa H, Miyashita K, Imanishi T. Design synthesis and Properties of 2', 4'-BNA^{NC}: a bridged nucleic acid analogue. J Am Chem Sc 2008; 130 (14) 4886–4896.

[59] Raphael SW, Yangde Z, Xiang CY. Hepatocellular carcinoma: focus on different aspects of management. ISRN Oncology 2012; 2012 1–12.

[60] Rayburn ER, Zhang R. Antisense RNAi and gene silencing strategies for therapy: mission possible or impossible? Drug Discov Today 2008; 13 (11-12) 513–521.

[61] Rizell M, Andersson M, Cahlin C, Hafstrom L, Olausson M, Lindner P. Effects of the mTOR inhibitor sirolimus in patients with hepatocellular and cholangiocellular cancer. Int J Clin Oncol 2008; 13 (1) 66–70.

[62] Roncalli M, Park YN, di Tommaso L. Histopathological classification of hepatocellular carcinoma. Digest Liver Dis 2010; 42 (3) 228–234.

[63] Rosen HR. Clinical practice chronic hepatitis C infection. N Engl J of Med 2011; 364 (25) 2429–2438.

[64] Shariff MIF, Cox IJ, Gomaa AI, Khan SA, Gedroyc W, Taylor-Robinson SD. Hepatocellular carcinoma: current trends in worldwide epidemiology risk factors diagnosis and therapeutics. Expert Rev Gastroenterol Hepatol 2009; 3 (4) 353–367.

[65] Sherman M. Epidemiology of hepatocellular carcinoma. Oncology 2010; 78 (1) 7–10.

[66] Sherman M. Hepatocellular carcinoma: screening and staging. Clin Liver Dis 2011; 15 (2) 323–334.

[67] Siegel AB, Cohen EI, Ocean A, Lehrer D, Goldenberg A, Knox JJ. Phase II trial evaluating the clinical and biologic effects of bevacizumab in unresectable hepatocellular carcinoma. J Clin Oncol 2008; 24 (26) 2992–2998.

[68] Siegel AB, McBride RB, El-Serag HB, Hershman DL, Brown Jr RS, Renz JF. Racial disparities in utilization of liver transplantation for hepatocellular carcinoma in the United States 1998-2002. Am J Gastroenterol 2008a; 103 (7) 120–127.

[69] Simile MM, Frau M, Pascale RM, Feo F. New putative prognostic markers and therapeutic targets for the molecular approach to treatment of hepatocellular carcinoma. J Exp Integr Med 2011; 1 85–97.

[70] Sonja K, Olsen RS, Brown JR, Siegel AB. Review: Hepatocellular carcinoma: review of current treatment with a focus on targeted molecular therapies. Therap Adv Gastroenterol 2010; 3 (1) 55–56.

[71] Spangenberg HC, Thimme R, Blum HE. Evolving therapies in the treatment of hepatocellular carcinoma. Biologics 2008; 2 (3) 453–462.

[72] Takigawa Y, Brown AM. Wnt signaling in liver cancer. Curr Drug Targets 2008; 9 (11) 1013–1024.

[73] Thomas MB, Chadha R, Glover K, Wang X, Morris J, Brown T. Phase 2 study of erlotinib in patients with unresectable hepatocellular carcinoma. Cancer 2007; 110 (5) 1059–1067.

[74] Thomas MB, O'Beirne JP, Furuse J, Chan ATC, Abou-Alfa G Johnson P. Systemic therapy for hepatocellular carcinoma: cytotoxic chemotherapy targeted therapy and immunotherapy. Ann Surg Oncol 2008; 15 (4) 1008–1014.

[75] Thomas MB, Morris JS, Chadha R, Iwasaki M, Kaur H, Lin E. Phase II trial of the combination of bevacizumab and erlotinib in patients who have advanced hepatocellular carcinoma. J Clin Oncol 2009; 27 (6) 843–850.

[76] Woo HG, Park ES, Cheon JH, Kim JH, Lee JS, Park BJ. Gene Expression-based recurrence prediction of hepatitis B virus-related human hepatocellular carcinoma. Clin Cancer Res 2008; 14 (7) 2056–2064.

[77] Wu JY, Wu SG, Yang CH, Chang YL, Chang YC, Hsu YC, Shih JY, Yang PC. Comparison of gefitinib and erlotinib in advanced NSCLC and the effect of EGFR mutations. Lung cancer 2011; 72 (2) 205–212.

[78] Yang JD, Roberts LR. Epidemiology and management of hepatocellular carcinoma infectious disease. Clin N Am 2010; 24 (4) 899–919.

[79] Zhang XF, Yu L, Lu Y. Wnt/β-catenin signaling pathway and its role in hepatocellular carcinoma. Front Med China 2008; 2 (3) 216–228.

[80] Zhou L, Huang Y, Li J , Wang Z. The mTOR pathway is associated with the poor prognosis of human hepatocellular carcinoma. Med Oncol 2009; 27(2) 255–261.

[81] Zhu AX, Duda DG, Sahani DV, Jain RK. HCC and angiogenesis: possible targets and future directions. Nat Rev Clin Oncol 2011; 8 (5) 292–302.

[82] Zhu AX. Development of sorafenib and other molecularly targeted agents in hepatocellular carcinoma. Cancer 2007; 112 (2) 250–259.

Chapter 7

Early Chronic Inflammation and Subsequent Somatic Mutations Shift Phospho-Smad3 Signaling from Tumor-Suppression to Fibro-Carcinogenesis in Human Chronic Liver Diseases

Miki Murata, Katsunori Yoshida and
Koichi Matsuzaki

Additional information is available at the end of the chapter

http://dx.doi.org/10.5772/56739

1. Introduction

Hepatocellular carcinoma (HCC) is the fifth most common cancer and the third leading cause of cancer death worldwide [1]. HCC is strongly associated with chronic hepatitis B virus (HBV) or hepatitis C virus (HCV) infection, which are implicated in about 80% of HCCs in certain geographic area [2]. Risk of HCC is increased 5- to 15-fold in chronic HBV carriers [1] and 11.5- to 17-fold in HCV-infected patients [3]. In addition, epidemiological studies have shown that chronic inflammation of the liver predisposes individuals to HCC. Most HCCs are associated with severe fibrosis or cirrhosis caused by unresolved inflammation. Both HBV and HCV show a wide spectrum of clinical manifestations, ranging from a healthy carrier state to chronic hepatitis, cirrhosis and HCC. Notably, HCC occurs less often in chronic viral hepatitis without cirrhosis. As liver fibrosis progresses from chronic hepatitis to cirrhosis, HCC occurrence increases [4]. Thus, unresolved inflammation with long-term viral infection leads to HCC associated with cirrhosis. Approaches to understanding how human HCC develops in chronic inflammatory liver diseases should therefor focus on molecular mechanisms shared between liver fibrosis and carcinogenesis (fibro-carcinogenesis).

Transforming growth factor (TGF)-β is a key regulator of many important biologic processes. TGF-β can inhibit epithelial cell growth, physiologically acting as a tumor suppressor, but it also can promote neoplasia. TGF-β has been shown to play both tumor-suppressive and tumor promoting roles [5-7]. As disease progresses toward malignancy, cancer cells gain advantage by selective reduction of the tumor-suppressive activity of TGF-β together with augmentation of TGF-β oncogenic activity [6]. In concert with mitogens, TGF-β induces accumulation of extracellular matrix (ECM), while mitogenic signaling antagonizes cytostatic TGF-β function [8,9]. These results indicate that perturbation of TGF-β signaling by mitogens can promote hepatic fibro-carcinogenesis.

The TGF-β superfamily includes many multifunctional cytokines including TGF-β, activin, and others [6,10]. Progress over the past 10 years has disclosed important details of how the TGF-β family elicits its responses [11-14]. Smads, central mediators conveying signals from receptors for TGF-β superfamily members to the nucleus, are modular proteins with conserved Mad-homology (MH)1, intermediate linker, and MH2 domains [13]. In cell-signaling pathways, various transcription factors are phosphorylated at multiple sites by upstream kinases. Catalytically active TGF-β type I receptor (TβRI) phosphorylates COOH-tail serine residues of receptor-activated Smads (R-Smads), which include Smad2 and the highly similar protein Smad3 [12]. Mitogenic signals alternatively cause phosphorylation of R-Smad at specific sites in their middle linker regions [15-20]. After a phosphorylated R-Smad rapidly oligomerizes with Smad4, this complex translocates to the nucleus, where it regulates transcription of target genes.

Monitoring phosphorylation status of signaling molecules is a key step in dissecting their pathways. In Smad signaling, phosphorylation of not only the COOH-tail but also the linker regions of R-Smads are likely to be important in regulating Smad activity under physiologic and pathologic conditions [21]. Understanding of molecular mechanisms underlying hepatitis virus-induced fibro-carcinogenesis can help to guide early management and improve therapy for patients with chronic liver diseases. This review describes current knowledge of the molecular pathogenesis of human fibro-carcinogenesis, especially concerning Smad3 phosphorylation profiles. We further consider how enhanced understanding of phospho-Smad3 signaling could lead to more effective prevention of human fibro-carcinogenesis.

2. Smad3 phosphoisoforms

The canonical TGF-β pathway involves Smad2 and Smad3 signaling through direct serine phosphorylation of COOH termini by TβRI upon TGF-β binding (Figure 1A), [10,13]. TβRI-mediated phosphorylation of Smad2 and Smad3 induces their association with the shared partner Smad4, followed by translocation into the nucleus where these complexes activate transcription of specific genes [10-14]. Smad2 and Smad3 proteins contain a conserved Mad-homology (MH)1 domain that binds DNA, and a conserved MH2 domain that binds to receptors, Smad4, and transcription co-activators.

More divergent linker regions separate the two domains [13]. The linker domain undergoes regulatory phosphorylation by Ras/mitogen-activated protein kinase (MAPK) pathways including extracellular signal-regulated kinase (ERK), c-Jun N-terminal kinase (JNK), p38 MAPK, and cyclin-dependent kinase (CDK)-2/4, as well as glycogen synthase kinase 3-β, Ca (2+)-calmodulin-dependent protein kinase II, and G protein-coupled receptor kinase-2 (Figure

http://dx.doi.org/10.5772/56739

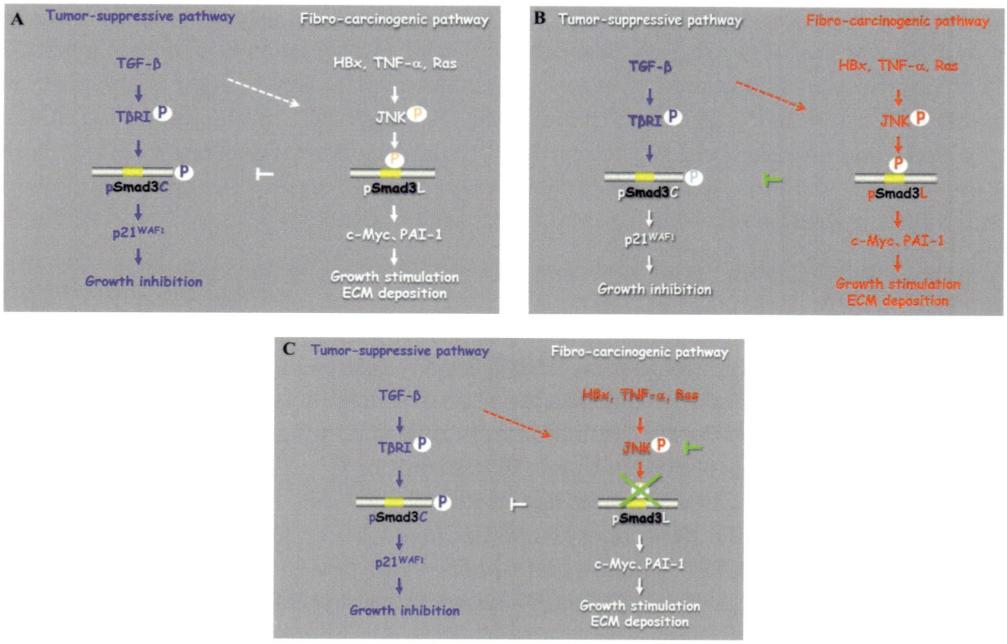

Figure 1. Reversible phospho-Smad3 signaling between tumor-suppression and fibro-carcinogenesis A) TGF-β treatment activates TβRI, further leading to direct phosphorylation of Smad3C, which inhibits normally hepatocytic growth by up-regulating $p21^{WAF1}$ transcription. B) Mitogens drastically alter phospho-Smad3 signaling via the JNK pathway, increasing basal nuclear fibro-carcinogenic pSmad3L activity while shutting down TGF-β-dependent cytostatic pSmad3C. Although TGF-β signal weakly phosphorylates Smad3L in normal hepatocytes (dotted line), hepatitis viral components including HBx, pro-inflammatory cytokines including TNF-α, and somatic mutations such as Ras additively transmit fibro-carcinogenic signal through the JNK-dependent pSmad3L pathway to participate in hepatocytic growth and ECM deposition, possibly by stimulating transcription of *c-Myc* and *PAI-1* genes. Linker phosphorylation of Smad3 indirectly prevents COOH-tail phosphorylation, pSmad3C-mediated $p21^{WAF1}$ transcriptions and cytostatic function. C) Either various JNK inhibitors or a Smad3 mutation causing lack of JNK phosphorylation sites in the linker region can eliminate fibro-carcinogenic pSmad3L signaling, restoring or maintaining the tumor-suppressive pSmad3C signaling characteristic of mature hepatocytes.

1B), [15-26]. TGF-β alternatively elicits signaling responses through non-Smad pathways representing important effectors for TGF-β activated kinase (TAK) 1 in response to pro-inflammatory cytokines. TAK1 activates JNK and p38 MAPK signaling through mitogen-activated kinase kinase (MKK) 4/7 and MKK3/6 [27,28]. JNK and p38 MAPK have been linked to modification of TGF-β signaling by pro-inflammatory cytokines through their regulation of distinct processes such as cytoskeleton organization, cell growth, survival, migration and invasion [29]. Imbalances between signaling through non-Smad and Smad pathways may occur during fibro-carcinogenesis, with interaction between these pathways mediating pro-fibrogenic and pro-tumorigenic effects of TGF-β [30]

Findings in mice with targeted deletion of Smad3 and JNK1 indicate that both Smad3 and JNK1 pathways promote hepatic fibro-carcinogesis. When acute liver injury was induced by administration of CCl_4, *Smad3*$^{-/-}$ mice showed approximately half as much of the induction of collagen type I mRNA as seen in wild-type mice [31]. *JNK1*$^{-/-}$ mice resisted not only liver fibrosis but also HCC development. Remarkable collagen deposition in wild-type and *JNK2*$^{-/-}$ was less evident in *JNK1*$^{-/-}$ mice, suggesting importance of JNK1 in development of liver fibrosis [32]. *JNK1*$^{-/-}$ mice exhibited impaired liver carcinogenesis with reduced tumor mass, size, and number [33]. Importantly, *JNK1*$^{-/-}$ mice displayed decreased HCC proliferation in a carcinogenic model and decreased hepatocytic growth in a model of liver regeneration. In both cases, the impaired proliferation was caused by increased expression of p21^{WAF1}, a cell-cycle inhibitor, and reduced expression of c-Myc, a negative regulator of p21^{WAF1}.

Mitogens simultaneously activate linker-phosphorylated R-Smad and non-Smad signaling, with both usually operating in parallel. Biologic significance of linker-phosphorylated R-Smad pathways is therefore difficult to assess in isolation. Here we will review recent work in this area with a particular focus on how mitogens modulate TGF-β signaling through Smad3 linker phosphorylation, using hepatic fibro-carcinogenesis as an example. Antibodies (Abs) reactive with structurally related phosphorylated peptides are emerging as valuable tools for determining phosphorylation sites *in vivo* and for investigating distinct signals via phosphorylated domains. Domain-specific phospho-Smad3 Abs have allowed us to reveal that TβRI and JNK differentially phosphorylate Smad3 to create 2 phosphorylated forms (phosphoisoforms): COOH-terminally phosphorylated Smad3 (pSmad3C) and linker phosphorylated Smad3 (pSmad3L) [34-37]. Linker phosphorylation can modify COOH-terminally phosphorylated R-Smad signaling [15-17,19-24]. Differential localization of kinases and phosphatases in the cytoplasm or nucleus raises the intriguing possibility of differences in temporal dynamics between cytoplasmic and nuclear R-Smad phosphoisoforms, adding to the repertoire of signaling responses that determine cell-fate decisions [8,9]. Immunohistochemical and immunofluorescence analyses using specific Abs in human tissues can examine the clinical significance of context-dependent and cell type-specific signaling mediated by R-Smad phosphoisoforms by comparison of their tissue and cellular localization in pathologic specimens.

3. Tumor-suppressive (cytostatic) TGF-β signaling: the pSmad3C pathway

TGF-β inhibits proliferation of normal hepatocytes, a crucial function in hepatic homeostasis [38]. In the context of cell cycle control, the most important targets of action by TGF-β are the genes encoding two CDK inhibitors (*p21*^{WAF1} and *p15*^{INK4B}) and *c-Myc* [39]. The pSmad3C signal induces expression of these CDK inhibitors and represses expression of c-Myc, shutting down cell cycle progression in the early to mid G_1 phase of the cell cycle (Figure 1A). Development of HCC is ordinarily blocked through actions of the pSmad3C pathway, which causes normal hepatocytes to cease growth and enter apoptosis after hepatocytic proliferation.

4. Carcinogenic (mitogenic) JNK signaling: the pSmad3L pathway

Mitogens strongly activate the JNK pathway, as TGF-β does more weakly (Figure 1B) [40]. Ras/MAPK signaling has been shown to induce phosphorylation of Smad2 and Smad3 at their linker regions [15]. Smad2 phosphorylation at the linker region inhibits nuclear accumulation of Smad2 without interfering with TGF-β-induced phosphorylation of its COOH-tail [19,41-50]. In contrast, linker phosphorylation does not retain Smad3 in the cytoplasm, permitting further consequences of Ras/JNK signaling. Mechanisms underlying this difference between the two R-Smads are not known, but phosphorylation sites of Smad3 at clusters of 3 serine residues in its linker region (Ser^{204}, Ser^{208}, and Ser^{213}) somewhat differ in sequence location from the corresponding linker phosphorylation sites of Smad2 (Ser^{245}, Ser^{250}, and Ser^{255}).

Several lines of evidence indicate that JNK transmits carcinogenic (mitogenic) signal via the pSmad3L pathway. First, JNK can directly phosphorylate Smad3 linker sites *in vitro*, while JNK inhibitors block Smad3 linker phosphorylation *in vivo* [16,19]. Second, mitogens translocate pSmad3L into the nucleus [16,19,20]. Third, nuclear pSmad3L forms a hetero-complex with Smad4 [16,23]. Fourth, nuclear pSmad3L binds to the Smad-binding element in the promoter with high affinity and specificity [23,51-53]. Finally, mitogens induce growth of normal epithelial cells by up-regulating c-Myc, and such mitogenic effects are blocked in Smad3 mutants lacking linker phosphorylation sites and by JNK inhibitors [19,54]. These results strongly support the notion that JNK specifically signals via Smad3 [55].

5. Reversible shifts in phospho-Smad3 signaling between tumor-suppression and carcinogenesis

JNK/pSmad3L and TβRI/pSmad3C signals oppose each other; most importantly, the balance between carcinogenesis and tumor-suppression can shift (Figure 1C). Linker phosphorylation of Smad3 blocks COOH-tail phosphorylation induced by TβRI [16,19,24,54,56]. Mitogenic signaling accelerates nuclear transport of pSmad3L from the cytoplasm, while preventing Smad3C phosphorylation, pSmad3C-mediated transcription, and anti-proliferative effects of TGF-β [16,19]. Smad3 mutants lacking linker phosphorylation sites, as well as JNK inhibitors, can restore growth inhibitory and transcriptional responses to TGF-β in Ras-transformed cells and pre-neoplastic hepatocytes, both *in vitro* and *in vivo* [19,54,56]. Our model implies that the JNK pathway directly or indirectly modulates pSmad3C- and pSmad3L-mediated signaling to regulate target genes, resulting in an antagonistic relationship between carcinogenesis and tumor-suppression. Thus, effectiveness of tumor-suppressive TGF-β signaling can depend on extent of Smad3 phosphorylation at the linker region.

6. Homeostatic termination of mitogenic JNK/pSmad3L/c-Myc signaling after liver regeneration by hepatocytic TβRI/pSmad3C/$p21^{WAF1}$ signaling

Carcinogenesis is currently thought to occur as a sequence of steps termed initiation, promotion, and progression. Each step is characterized by disruption of normal cellular control mechanisms. Thus, development of HCC involves sequential alterations of physiological mechanisms regulating hepatocytic growth. Before consideration of molecular mechanisms of hepatocarcinogenesis, examination of the physiologic role of phospho-Smad3 signaling in liver regeneration is instructive. A unique feature of adult mammalian liver is its ability to accurately regenerate lost mass, which occurs following surgical resection or diffuse liver injury [57]. Although precise identities of cytokines and molecular mechanisms involved in liver regeneration are largely unknown, TGF-β and tumor necrosis factor (TNF)-α apparently act as positive and negative regulators of hepatocytic growth, respectively (Figure 1 A and 1B).

Hepatocytes undergo transition from a resting to a proliferative state after acute liver injury or partial hepatectomy [57]. Loss of parenchyma rapidly induces a wave of hepatocytic proliferation capable of restoring the total mass of the liver to normal. Several converging lines of evidence have established that pro-inflammatory cytokines such as TNF-α and interleukin (IL)-6 are important components of the mitogenic pathways leading to regeneration after acute liver injury [58]. Treatment of hepatocytes with antibodies against TNF-α resulted in decreased DNA synthesis and JNK activity [38]. DNA synthesis during liver regeneration was severely impaired in mice with a TNF-α type I receptor deficiency [59]. After acute liver injury, TGF-β increases in damaged livers within a time frame similar to that of increases in pro-inflammatory cytokines [60-62]. This raises the problem of how hepatocytes manage to proliferate in response to a mitogenic pro-inflammatory cytokine signal despite elevated TGF-β concentration. During liver regeneration, hepatocytes acquire temporary resistance to cytostatic effect of TGF-β, allowing them to proliferate [61-63]. The phosphorylation pattern of Smad3 in regenerative hepatocytes after acute liver injury suggested important participation of phospho-Smad3 in hepatocytic growth regulation. In actively growing hepatocytes, intracellular phosphorylation at Smad3L was found to be high [54,56,64]. Translocated to the nucleus, inflammatory cytokine-induced pSmad3L stimulated c-Myc transcription [54,64,65], which increased proliferation of hepatocytes and opposed the cytostatic action of the pSmad3C/ $p21^{WAF1}$ pathway (Figure 1B). Accordingly, pSmad3C/$p21^{WAF1}$ was undetectable in regenerative hepatocytic nuclei; escape from TGF-β-induced cytostasis was crucial in a subset of progenitor cells devoted to ensuring epithelial renewal. Thus, pSmad3L signaling can permit liver regeneration in response to mitogenic pro-inflammatory cytokines even though TGF-β concentration is elevated after acute liver injury.

Liver regeneration is tightly controlled by a delicate balance between hepatocytic growth and inhibition. Anti-mitotic effects of TGF-β contribute to the termination of hepatocyte proliferation observed following the wave of DNA synthesis in the regenerating liver. Post regeneration, return of TGF-β sensitivity thus limits hepatocyte proliferation and terminates liver regeneration [61,63]. After TNF-α and pSmad3L decreased, hepatocytic proliferation ceased, as decreases in pSmad3L allowed increased sensitivity to phosphorylation at Smad3C by TβRI (Figure 1C). TGF-β-dependent pSmad3C appears to limit the proliferative response of regenerating hepatocytes through inhibition of the G1 to S phase transition in the cell-cycle. Such signaling represents a highly effective defense mechanism against development of HCC, since nonproliferating hepatocytes containing pSmad3C that might have sustained any mutations are destined to die [66].

7. Liver fibrosis as the largest single risk factor for HCC occurrence

Liver fibrosis usually precedes the multistage process of HCC development. Liver fibrosis is strongly associated with HCC, with 80 to 90% of HCCs arising in cirrhotic livers [67]. In hepatitis B infection is a risk factor for HCC, along with age, gender, viral DNA load, and viral core promoter mutation [68]. Fibrosis has also been identified as risk factor in hepatitis C infection, where cancer risk is directly related to fibrosis severity [69]. Similarly, HCC development is linked to alcoholic cirrhosis [70], nonalcoholic steatohepatitis (NASH) [70], and hemochromatosis [71], with a yearly HCC incidence of 1.7% in alcoholic cirrhosis [70] and 2.6% in NASH cirrhosis [72].

8. Involvement of both myofibroblasts and hepatocytes in liver fibrosis

Hepatic fibrosis is characterized by accumulation of excess ECM proteins, regardless of underlying etiology. Amount of matrix deposition reflects a balance between matrix synthesis and degradation [73,74]. When synthesis of ECM exceeds degradation, pathologic accumulation of ECM leads to liver fibrosis. Reversibility of experimental hepatic fibrosis and a striking decrease in collagenolytic activity observed in liver fibrosis models suggest crucial importance of impaired matrix degradation in hepatic fibrogenesis [75]. The plasminogen activator/plasmin system, which is situated upstream of the fibrolysis system, can directly degrade matrix components, and indirectly inhibit ECM deposition [76]. Plasminogen activator inhibitor-1 (PAI-1), the major physiologic inhibitor of plasminogen activator, is a potent promoter of fibrosis. Introduction of a PAI-1 small interfering RNA attenuates deposition of ECM and hydroxyproline content in experimental hepatic fibrosis [77].

Liver fibrosis is one of the most common pathologic processes occurring in response to increased inflammatry factors. A complex interplay among different hepatic cell types takes place in injured livers. Hepatocytes are the targets for most hepatotoxic agents, including hepatitis viruses, alcohol metabolites, and chemical toxins [78]. Damaged hepatocytes induce recruitment of white blood cells by local inflammatory cells. Apoptosis of damaged hepatocytes stimulates fibrogenesis by Kupffer cells. Activated Kupffer cells secrete pro-inflammatory cytokines including TNF-α and IL, as well as TGF-β. Intensive studies have shown that hepatic stellate cells (HSC) are the major cell type responsible for matrix production in damaged liver tissues [75]. HSC, characterized by retinoid droplets in the cytoplasm, are present in the space of Disse [79].

Standardized methods of obtaining HSC from livers have been developed [80]. Long-term culture of HSC on plastic substrates is widely accepted as a model of liver fibrosis [79]. HSC spontaneously transdifferentiate to a myofibroblast (MFB) phenotype on plastic dishes, and this response reproduces the features of activation *in vivo*. MFB usually retain fibrogenic TGF-β signaling component, but have lost the capacity to respond to TGF-β with growth arrest [81]. Such a state of altered TGF-β responsiveness is also observed in pre-neoplastic hepatocytes, which typically exhibit a limited growth inhibitory response to TGF-β, instead responding to TGF-β with pro-fibrogenic behavior [9].

Hepatic fibrosis results from a wound-healing response to repeated injury in chronic liver diseases [82], in which HSC undergo dramatic phenotypic activation, with acquisition of fibrogenic properties. Patients develop liver fibrosis as a result of chronic liver damage, characterized by ECM accumulation that distorts hepatic architecture by forming a fibrous scar [79]. Ultimately, nodules of regenerating hepatocytes become enclosed by scar tissue, an event defining cirrhosis. Excess deposition of ECM of which type I collagen predominates disrupts the normal architecture of the liver, resulting in pathologic damage with pathophysiologic consequences.

A new concept has been proposed that epithelial cells undergo a phenotypical change termed epithelial-mesenchymal transition (EMT), acquiring a fibroblastic phenotype. EMT facilitates metastasis and cancer development [83]. Pioneering studies on EMT in organ fibrosis were carried out in kidney, ocular lens, and lung [84,85]. Involvement of EMT also has been proposed in liver fibrosis. Zeisberg et al. demonstrated that hepatocytes acquire expression of fibroblast-specific protein 1 in response to CCl_4 injury *in vivo* or TGF-β *in vitro* [86].

9. Fibrogenic pSmad3L signaling shared between MFB and pre-neoplastic hepatocytes

As a result of chronic liver damage, HSC undergo progressive activation to become MFB-like cells. During transdifferentiation in culture, pSmad3C-mediated signal decreases while the pSmad3L pathway predominates [23]. These observations complement the finding of pSmad3L rather than pSmad3C in nuclei of α-smooth muscle actin (SMA)-immunoreactive MFB in portal tracts of chronically HCV-infected liver specimens [64]. The presence of α-SMA is associated with transdifferentiation of HSC into scar-forming MFB, an event considered pivotal in the fibrogenic response [75].

Plasma TGF-β, TNF-α, and PAI-1 concentrations are usually elevated in patients with chronic liver diseases [87-89]. Since pSmad3L can transmit a fibrogenic signal by stimulating PAI-1 transcription (Figure 1B) [23], we investigated the pSmad3L pathway in human chronic liver disease. The results indicated nuclear localization of pSmad3L in PAI-1-immunoreactive MFBs and hepatocytes in chronic hepatitis specimens [64]. Thus, hepatocytes are regulated by the same pSmad3L pathway as are MFBs. Hepatocytes in HCV-infected livers, particularly those adjacent to inflamed portal tracts, exhibited phosphorylation at Smad3L [64]. Extent of phosphorylation at Smad3L was less in hepatocytes distant from portal tracts, in sharp contrast to pSmad3C, which was predominantly located in hepatocytic nuclei distant from portal tracts [64]. Extent of hepatocytic pSmad3L/PAI-1 increased in proportion to fibrotic stage in chronic liver diseases [56,74]. TGF-β and pro-inflammatory cytokines are released from infiltrating Kupffer cells in portal tracts to activate JNK [90,91]. Considering these findings together with a previous observation showing transcriptional activation of the *PAI-1* gene by JNK [92], TGF-β and TNF-α can mediate JNK/pSmad3L signaling that in turn induces PAI-1 expression and promotes ECM deposition in both hepatocytes and MFB. Thus, hepatocytes affected by chronic inflammation undergo transition from the tumor-suppressive pSmad3C pathway, characteristic of mature hepatocytes, to the JNK/pSmad3L/PAI-1 pathway, which favors a state of flux characterized by MFB.

Our findings support many important papers reporting that hepatocytes can promote fibrogenesis via TGF-β/Smad signaling. Dooley et al. reported that overexpression of inhibitory Smad7 in hepatocytes attenuated TGF-β-mediated fibrogenesis by blocking Smad signaling [93]. Since the large latent TGF-β complex consisting of TGF-β, the N-terminal part of its precursor, and the latent TGF-β binding protein exists in not only HSC but also hepatocytes, the complex can transmit a pro-fibrogenic signal [94], although intracellular functions of the TGF-β complex are poorly understood. TGF-β down-stream mediator connective tissue growth factor (CTGF) also involves hepatic fibro-carcinogenesis [95]. CTGF expression increases in fibrotic livers and various tumor tissues [96]. More importantly, *in vivo* knockdown of CTGF by small interfering RNA leads to substantial attenuation of experimental liver fibrosis. Differential regulation of CTGF expression in hepatocytes and HSC by Smad2 signaling may contribute to hepatic fibro-carcinogenesis [97]. Interestingly, a methylxanthine, caffeine, inhibits synthesis of CTGF in hepatocytes and HSC, primarily by inducing degradation of Smad2 [96].

10. Additive promotion of human carcinogenesis by persistent hepatitis viral infection and chronic inflammation

Various experiments support the notion that a single promoting agent is insufficient for development of cancer. Hepatocarcinogenesis is multi-factorial, involving collaboration between 2 or more promoting agents in HCC occurrence [98]. Among tumor-promoting agents, hepatitis viruses and chronic inflammation directly participate in HCC pathogenesis, which frequently occurs during long-standing hepatitis viral infection.

Many clinical observations suggest that persistent hepatitis viral infection and chronic inflammation additively influence development of human HCC. For example, alcohol consumption is a recognized major cause of liver disease, and plays an important role in progression to HCC. However, alcoholic hepatitis progresses less frequently to HCC than HBV- or HCV- related hepatitis. In addition, patients with both viral infection and alcohol consumption have a higher risk of developing HCC than those with alcohol consumption alone [3,99,100]. Autoimmune hepatitis (AIH) and primary billiary cirrhosis (PBC) are chronic inflammatory disorders that proceed to cirrhosis. However, HCC only rarely arises from AIH or PBC, particularly in the absence of HBV or HCV infection [101,102]. Conversely, asymptomatic HBV or HCV carriers maintaining normal alanine aminotransferase (ALT) levels despite intensive viral replication less frequently develop HCC than patients with chronic hepatitis B. The annual risk of HCC occurrence in HBV healthy carriers is 0.26% to 0.6%, while risk increases to 1% in patients with chronic active hepatitis B [103]. Moreover, HBV can act synergistically with HCV. Patients co-infected with HBV and HCV have a 2- to 6-fold higher risk of HCC occurrence than those with either infection alone [104,105]. Accordingly, we will consider how the oncogenic JNK/pSmad3L pathway induces development of HCC, with particular attention to potential synergy between hepatitis viruses and inflammation in formation of pre-neoplastic hepatocytes.

11. Hepatitis virus components can activate oncogenic JNK/pSmad3L pathway

One of the earliest evidence linking HBV to development of HCC was obtained in the woodchuck hepatitis virus model, in which 100% of rodents infected with woodchuck hepatitis virus developed HCC [106]. Because HBV contains partially double stranded-DNA, it can directly cause HCC by integrating its DNA into the host genome. HBV genomic integration is present in over 85% to 90% of HBV-related HCC, usually even before development of HCC [107]. Integration of HBV DNA is not restricted to HCC but also is found in non-tumor tissue in patients with chronically HBV infection [108,109]. HBV integration induces a wide range of genetic alterations within the host genome, including chromosomal deletions, translocations, production of fusion transcripts, amplification of cellular DNA, and generalized genomic instability [110,111]. Many integration events occur near or within fragile sites or other cancer-associated regions of the human genome that are prone to instability in tumor development and progression. Genetic instability associated with integration may alter expression of oncogenes, tumor suppressor genes, and microRNAs [111]. A recent large-scale analysis of HBV DNA integration sites in cellular DNA found a preference for sites regulating cell signaling, proliferation, and viability [112]. A large proportion of HCC have integrated HBV sequences encoding HBV X (HBx) and/or truncated envelope pre-S2/S proteins.

The HBx protein encoded by the X gene has been long suspected as a viral oncoprotein participating in hepatocarcinogenesis. This protein is involved in liver cell transformation because of its pleiotropic activities on cell cycle regulation, cell signaling pathways and DNA repair [113-115]. Numerous attempts have been made to examine the oncogenic potential of HBx in cell culture. However, its transforming ability was barely measurable evident only when cells were immortalized by other oncogenes, such as SV40 T-antigen [116,117] or TGF-α [118]. Furthermore, most transgenic mice harboring the HBx gene did not develop serious liver diseases or tumors [119]. Only in a certain transgenic lineage of CD-1 strain, HBx weakly promoted carcinogenesis, where HBx was highly expressed [120]. A second mouse lineage with lower HBx expression developed liver tumors at the same rate as normal CD-1 mice [121]. HBx was shown to potentiate c-Myc-induced liver carcinogenesis in transgenic mice [122]. Thus, HBx does not have strong transforming activity, but HBx overexpression in a certain genetic background might induce tumor formation in a multistage transformation, most likely in collaboration with other cellular oncogenic pathways.

HBx is mainly located in the cytoplasm and exhibits pleiotropic effects that modulate cell responses to oncogenic signaling pathways [114]. HBx protein do not bind directly to DNA, but rather acts on cellular promoters. Such protein-protein interaction can modulate cytoplasmic pathways [113,114,123]. For example, HBx protein was found to activate the JNK-dependent pathway and up-regulate oncogenic c-Myc gene expression [124].

To investigate whether HBx alters phospho-Smad3 signaling in hepatocytes, we stably transfected immortalized rat hepatocytes using a construct of HBx with a mammalian expression vector, resulting in high HBx-expressing cells [56]. High expression of HBx protein in hepatocytes tended to shut down pSmad3C-mediated signaling and favored acquisition of constitutively active JNK-mediated pSmad3L signaling, which fostered hepatocytic growth by up-regulating c-Myc (Figure 1B).

In transgenic models, HBx played an important role in hepatocarcinogenesis via the pSmad3L/c-Myc pathway [56]. HBx transgenic mouse livers progressed through hyperplasia to HCC. HBx, pSmad3L, and c-Myc were not detected in normal mouse livers. Beginning at the age of 2 months, HBx transgenic mouse liver showed centrilobular foci of cellular alteration with cytoplasmic vacuolation surrounding central veins where Bromodeoxyuridine (BrdU) was uptaken into the hepatocytes [121]. Smad3L was phosphorylated in hepatocytic nuclei of the centrilobular region, where HBx and c-Myc were expressed. Hepatocytic HBx, pSmad3L, and c-Myc increased as mouse liver progressed through hyperplasia to HCC.

Positivity of hepatocytic nuclei for pSmad3L in early chronic hepatitis B specimens increases with amount of HBV-DNA [56]. Taken together with results of *in vitro* experiments using HBx-expressing hepatocytes and HBx transgenic livers, these human findings indicate that HBx oncoprotein participates directly in hepatocarcinogenesis by shifting hepatocytic phospho-Smad3 signaling from the tumor-suppressive pSmad3C/p21^{WAF1} pathway to the oncogenic JNK/pSmad3L/c-Myc pathway (Figure 1B), [56].

Unlike HBV, HCV is a positive-single-strand RNA virus, apparently incapable of integration into the host's genome. The HCV genome has a long open reading frame, which encodes a polyprotein precursor [125,126]. This polyprotein is cleaved by both host and viral proteases to generate 4 structural proteins (C, E1, E2, and P7) and 6 nonstructural proteins (xlink, NS3, NS4A, NS4B, NS5A, and NS5B) [127,128]. The HCV components modulate a number of cellular regulatory functions by targeting a wide spectrum of cellular signaling pathways [129-136]. HCV core expression has been shown to induce activation of the JNK pathway in regulation of vascular endothelial growth factor [136]. NS5A acts as a positive regulator of the JNK signaling pathway by interacting with tumor necrosis factor receptor-associated factor 2, which may play a key role in HCV pathogenesis [137]. In an HCV infection model, Lin *et al.* demonstrated that HCV directly induced TGF-β release from hepatocytes in reactive oxygen species (ROS)-dependent and JNK-dependent manner [138]. Moreover, recent studies using transgenic mouse models indicate that HCV directly involves hepatocarcinogenesis. Three different HCV core transgenic lines develop liver steatosis and HCC [139-141]. Accordingly, future studies are expected to prove that the HCV components can activate the oncogenic JNK/pSmad3L pathway.

12. Activation of the oncogenic JNK/pSmad3L pathway by chronic inflammation

Inflammatory microenvironments are present in human hepatocarcinogenesis before malignant change occurs. A hepatitis virus infection triggers chronic inflammation, increasing the risk of HCC development. Several studies have discussed how chronic inflammation affects the proliferation and survival of hepatocytes [142,143]. TNF-α, IL-1β and IL-6 are multifunctional pro-inflammatory cytokines largely responsible for the hepatic response to chronic inflammation [144-146]. Serum concentrations of these cytokines are increased in chronic liver inflammation including hepatitis viral infection and steatohepatitis [147]. JNK is a key signal transducer for inflammatory cytokines and has emerged as an important endogenous tumor promoter [148,149].

TGF-β is also released by infiltrating Kupffer cells, the liver's resident macrophages, in portal tracts during chronic inflammation [150]. These findings suggest that elevated pro-inflammatory cytokines might alter hepatocytic TGF-β signaling in inflammatory microenvironments. We investigated this hypothesis using rat cultured hepatocytes [64]. Pretreatment of hepatocytes with SP600125, a JNK inhibitor, reduced the subsequent increase in pSmad3L, c-Myc transcription, and hepatocytic growth triggered by pro-inflammatory cytokine stimulation (Figure 1C), suggesting a direct role of the JNK/pSmad3L/c-Myc pathway in facilitating hepatocytic growth in response to cytokine stimulation (Figure 1B).

Experimental models of HCC including inflammation can elucidate how chronic inflammation contributes to hepatocarcinogenesis. In a rat model involving diethylnitrosamine (DEN)-induced carcinogenesis, chronic inflammation liver accompanies abnormalities that progress to HCC [151]. This DEN-induced rat HCC is histologically and genetically similar to human HCC, and also is associated with chronic inflammation [152]. In this chemical model, JNK act participates importantly in hepatocarcinogenesis via pSmad3L/c-Myc signaling. In DEN-treated livers, the JNK/pSmad3L/c-Myc pathway was activated in early pre-neoplastic hepatocytes (Figure 1B), [54]. Moreover, a JNK inhibitor SP600125 suppressed HCC development in DEN-treated rat livers by restoring carcinogenic pSmad3L/c-Myc to the basal pSmad3C/p21^{WAF1} pathway in the pre-neoplastic hepatocytes (Figure 1C), [54].

In human chronic hepatitis C specimens, mainly in groups of hepatocytes adjoining inflammatory cells in portal tracts, Smad3 was found to be phosphorylated at the linker region [64]. Furthermore, positivity of hepatocytic nuclei for pSmad3L/c-Myc in chronic hepatitis C specimens showed a significant relationship with necrosis and inflammatory activity [64]. Taken together with the results of *in vitro* experiments and DEN-treated rat livers, the human findings indicate that chronic inflammation directly participates in hepatocarcinogenesis by shifting hepatocytic phospho-Smad3 signaling from the tumor-suppressive pSmad3C/p21^{WAF1} pathway to the oncogenic JNK/pSmad3L/c-Myc pathway [54,64].

Many tumor-enhancing effects of pro-inflammatory cytokines on hepatocytes are exerted at the level of tumor promotion [58]. TNF-α promotes HCC occurrence in mice lacking the P-glycoprotein Mdr2 [153]. HCC follows cholestatic inflammation in these mice. Incidence of HCC can be enhanced by another member of the TNF family, lymphotoxin β [154]. Tumor-promoting cytokines produced by Kupffer cells activate several transcription factors, including NF-kB, STAT3, and AP-1, in pre-malignant hepatocytes [155]. The activated transcription factors stimulate transcription of their target genes involved in hepatocytic proliferation and survival, representing a major tumor-promoting mechanism. Similarly to these transcription factors, tumor-promoting actions of hepatocytic Smad3 in human chronic liver disease rarely result from direct mutations [156]. Instead, pSmad3L depends on mitogenic pro-inflammatory cytokine signals produced by neighboring Kupffer cells.

13. Constitutive phosphorylation at Smad3L in pre-neoplastic hepatocytes in cirrhotic human liver

The mechanism regulating regeneration, which avoids accumulation of deleterious mutations in genes that promote cell growth and division, must be disrupted before hepatocytes can throw off normal restraints and behave as an asocial HCC. Constitutive phosphorylation at Smad3L is observed in pre-malignant hepatocytes in cirrhosis [56,64]. Constitutively active pSmad3L stimulates hepatocytes to proliferate continuously in human livers that normally experience little proliferation because hepatocytic regeneration is tightly regulated by cytostatic pSmad3C signaling. Since JNK is constitutively activated in pre-neoplastic hepatocytes in cirrhotic human liver [157], constitutive Smad3L phosphorylation in pre-malignant lesions can be a direct consequence of proto-oncogene-mediated JNK signaling. Somatic mutations in pre-neoplastic hepatocytes include changes in the *Ras* pathway that favor progression from cirrhosis toward HCC [158]. In pre-neoplastic hepatocyte nuclei, pSmad3L/c-Myc can accumulate when somatic mutations constitutively activate the JNK pathway to phosphorylate Smad3 at the linker region (Figure 1B). Then, the proliferative effect mediated via the pSmad3L/c-Myc pathway constitutively keeps on suppresses the growth-inhibitory pSmad3C/p21^{WAF1} pathway in the nuclei of pre-neoplastic hepatocytes.

Pre-neoplastic hepatocytes and HCC show reduction of anti-mitogenic responses to TGF-β [20,37]. Escaping the cytostatic action of pSmad3C is a critical step for progression to full malignancy in cancers, which must overcome multiple fail-safe genetic controls [39,159,160]. The TGF-β/pSmad3C pathway is required for maintenance of genomic stability, induction of replicative senescence, and suppression of telomerase [161-163]. Selection for genetic instability occurs in clones of aberrant cells able to produce tumors, since genetic instability greatly accelerates accumulation of further genetic and epigenetic changes required for tumor progression. In this regard, the TGF-β/pSmad3C pathway contributes to tumor suppression along with its cytostatic effect.

14. Chronic inflammation together with hepatitis virus effects in shifting phospho-Smad3 signaling into oncogene-dependent fibro-carcinogenic signaling

In the pathogenesis of HCC, continuous viral infection and chronic inflammation have a prominent role. On the other hand, detailed analysis of HCC development in experimental animals and correlation of these results with HCC in humans has identified a variety of genomic and molecular alterations in fully developed HCC [164]and to a lesser extent in morphologically defined pre-neoplastic precursor lesions [165]. Thus, a series of mutations may accumulate in individual hepatocytes over time. Finally, hepatocytes come to carry somatic mutations that lead to focal uncontrolled hepatocytic growth and eventual malignant cell transformation, in some cases, HCC [166].

Chronic inflammation associated with hepatitis virus infection may be the primary initial requirement in multistep hepatocarcinogenesis. If pSmad3L-positive and pSmad3C-negative hepatocytes survive in the course of chronic hepatitis, such hepatocytes and their descendants can accumulate, and acquire various mutated alleles. Mutations may involve genes in *Ras* pathway [158]that impel pre-neoplastic hepatocytes with constitutive phosphorylation at Smad3L toward a neoplastic growth [8]. Tumor promotion results in further selective clonal expansion of initiated cells, thereby enhancing the likelihood of additional genetic damage as a consequence of endogenous mutations. During tumor progression, premalignant cells continue to develop progressive phenotypic changes and genomic instability, developing into overt HCC.

15. The JNK/pSmad3L pathway as a therapeutic target to avert HCC development

Clinical analyses of pSmad3L and pSmad3C in human tumor formation have provided substantial mechanistic insights. For example, specimens from patients with chronic hepatitis B who develop HCC show abundant Smad3L but limited Smad3C phosphorylation in hepatocytic nuclei, while other patients with abundant hepatocytic pSmad3C but limited pSmad3L do not develop HCC [56]. The same relationships are observed in human HCV-related hepatocarcinogenesis [64]. These clinical observations support roles for pSmad3C as a tumor-suppressor and pSmad3L as a promoter during human carcinogenesis.

HCC is a highly chemoresistant cancer with no effective systemic cytotoxic chemotherapy [167]. Despite surgical or locoregional therapies, the prognosis remains poor because of high likelihood of tumor recurrence or progression and there are no well-established effective adjuvant therapies [168]. Molecular events that affect carcinogenesis need to be identified and targeted to validate new treatment approaches and expand available therapeutics to include chemoprevention to other therapeutics. Since JNK acts as an important regulator of Smad3 signaling that increases the basal amount of hepatocytic pSmad3L available for cell growth

http://dx.doi.org/10.5772/56739

while inactivating the TGF-β-dependent cytostatic actions of pSmad3C (Figure 1B), pharmacologic interference with JNK/pSmad3L signaling could interrupt carcinogenesis. A key therapeutic aim in chronic liver disorders is restoration of lost tumor-suppressive function observed in normal hepatocytes, at the expense of effects promoting hepatic carcinogenesis [169]. To accomplish this difficult aim, Nagata *et al*. (2009) administered a JNK inhibitor SP600125 to rats and were able to suppress chemical carcinogenesis by shifting hepatocytic Smad3 signaling from the carcinogenic pSmad3L pathway to the tumor-suppressive pSmad3C pathway (Figure 1C), [54]. These studies provide evidence that JNK/pSmad3L is an important target for development of chemopreventive and therapeutic measures to reduce emergence of HCC in the context of chronic liver injury and to slow progression of existing tumors. We must also consider whether long-term use of any drug inhibiting C-terminal phosphorylation of R-Smads might cause cancer development [7].

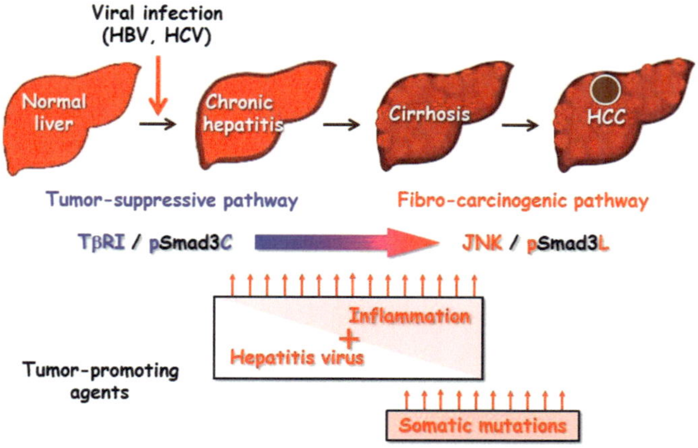

Figure 2. After hepatitis virus infection, early chronic inflammation and subsequent somatic mutations shift hepatocytic phospho-Smad3 signaling from the tumor-suppressive TβRI/pSmad3C made to the fibro-carcinogenic JNK/pSmad3L mode characteristic of MFB, accelerating liver fibrosis while increasing risk of HCC. Both hepatitis virus infection and chronic inflammation represent early fibro-carcinogenic steps representing non-mutagenic tumor-promoting stimuli. In advanced liver fibrosis, mitogenic genetic or epigenetic alterations can drive multistep fibro-carcinogenesis via the pSmad3L pathway. Escaping the cytostatic action of pSmad3C is a critical step for progression to full malignancy in cancers, which must overcome multiple fail-safe genetic controls.

16. Conclusion and perspectives

Human fibro-carcinogenesis is a complex multistep process, which involves dysregulation of physiological signal transduction pathways. To maintain hepatic homeostasis, hepatocytic TβRI/pSmad3C/p21^{WAF1} terminates mitogenic JNK/pSmad3L/c-Myc signaling after liver regeneration. During progression of chronic liver diseases, however, early pro-inflammatory cytokines together with hepatitis viruses and subsequent somatic mutations switch hepatocytic phospho-Smad3 signaling from the tumor-suppressive TβRI/pSmad3C to the fibro-carcinogenic JNK/pSmad3L mode characteristic of MFB, which accelerates liver fibrosis while increasing risk of HCC (Figure 2). Our model is likely to represent a crucial molecular mechanism by which most HCCs arise in from fibrosis or cirrhosis caused by chronic inflammation associated with persistent hepatitis virus infection [164]. Thus, Smad phosphoisoforms function as an important orchestrator of a human chronic inflammation-fibrosis-HCC axis [9,170].

Recent studies in animal models using conditional transgenic expression have suggested an intriguing reversibility of malignant transformation at specific time points if the primary inciting cause of the neoplasia is eliminated [171,172]. However, the fibro-carcinogenic stage in human chronic liver at which the process becomes irreversible. Chronic hepatitis B and C can be cured if patients are treated with antiviral therapy that arrests chronic inflammation by eradicating hepatic HBV and HCV populations. Continued histologic improvement and reversal of fibrosis by antiviral therapy can lead to reduction of HCC development [173,174], but prevention appears most effective when therapy is given before development of cirrhosis. Chronic hepatitis is clearly dependent on continued promoter stimulation - involving in this case the presence of hepatitis viruses and chronic inflammation. However, many patients with cirrhosis have evolved beyond dependence on inflammation because hepatocytes have acquired genetic and epigenetic carcinogenic properties. We are carrying out several trials to determine whether or not antiviral therapy can decrease liver fibrosis and lower HCC incidence. The trials will bear upon important questions regarding relative participation in fibro-carcinogenesis of inflammation-dependent and oncogene-dependent Smad3 phosphoisoform signaling in HBV- and HCV-related chronic liver disorders. In the trials, pathologic analyses using domain-specific phospho-Smad3 Abs, together with clinical data, will be used to evaluate the benefit from antiviral therapy, which decreases stimulation of the inflammation-dependent Smad phosphorisoform pathway. After antiviral therapy, hepatocytic pSmad3L and pSmad3C assessment in liver specimens should prove clinically useful for predicting progression of fibrosis and risk of HCC.

Author details

Miki Murata*, Katsunori Yoshida and Koichi Matsuzaki

*Address all correspondence to: muratami@takii.kmu.ac.jp

Departments of Gastroenterology and Hepatology, Kansai Medical University, Osaka, Japan

References

[1] El-Serag HB, Rudolph KL. Hepatocellular carcinoma: epidemiology and molecular carcinogenesis. Gastroenterology 2007;132(7) 2557-2576.

[2] McGlynn KA, London WT. Epidemiology and natural history of hepatocellular carcinoma. Best Pract Res Clin Gastroenterol 2005;19(1) 3-23.

[3] Donato F, Tagger A, Gelatti U, Parrinello G, Boffetta P, Albertini A, Decarli A, Trevisi P, Ribero ML, Martelli C, Porru S, Nardi G. Alcohol and hepatocellular carcinoma: the effect of lifetime intake and hepatitis virus infections in men and women. Am J Epidemiol 2002;155(4) 323-331.

[4] Tsukuma H, Hiyama T, Tanaka S, Nakao M, Yabuuchi T, Kitamura T, Nakanishi K, Fujimoto I, Inoue A, Yamazaki H, Kawashima T. Risk factors for hepatocellular carcinoma among patients with chronic liver disease. N Engl J Med 1993;328(25) 1797-1801.

[5] Moses HL, Yang EY, and Pietenpol JA. TGF-β stimulation and inhibition of cell proliferation: new mechanistic insights. Cell 1990;63(2) 245-247.

[6] Roberts AB, Sporn MB. The transforming growth factor-βs. In: Sporn MB, Roberts AB. (eds.) Peptide Growth Factors and Their Receptors. Springer, Berlin; 1990. p 419-472.

[7] Bellam N, Pasche B. TGF-β signaling alterations and colon cancer. Cancer Treat Res 2010;155:85-103.

[8] Matsuzaki K. Smad phosphoisoform signaling specificity: the right place at the right time. Carcinogenesis 2011;32(11) 1578-1588.

[9] Matsuzaki K. Smad phosphoisoform signals in acute and chronic liver injury: similarities and differences between epithelial and mesenchymal cells. Cell Tissue Res 2012;347(1) 225-243.

[10] Derynck R, Miyazono K. The TGF-β signaling. Cold Spring Harbor Laboratory Press, NewYork; 2008.

[11] Heldin CH, Miyazono K, ten Dijke P. TGF-β signaling from cell membrane to nucleus through SMAD proteins. Nature 1997;390(6659) 465-471.

[12] Wrana JL. Regulation of Smad activity. Cell 2000;100(2) 189-192.

[13] Shi Y, Massagué J. Mechanisms of TGF-β signaling from cell membrane to the nucleus. Cell 2003;113(6) 685-700.

[14] Guo X, Wang XF. Signaling cross-talk between TGF-β/BMP and other pathways. Cell Res 2009;19(1) 71-88.

[15] Kretzschmar M, Doody J, Timokhina I, Massagué J. A mechanism of repression of TGF-β/Smad signaling by oncogenic Ras. Genes Dev 1999;13(7) 804-816.

[16] Mori S, Matsuzaki K, Yoshida K, Furukawa F, Tahashi Y, Yamagata H, Sekimoto G, Seki T, Matsui H, Nishizawa M, Fujisawa J, Okazaki K. TGF-β and HGF transmit the

signals through JNK-dependent Smad2/3 phosphorylation at the linker regions. Oncogene 2004;23(44) 7416-7429.

[17] Matsuura I, Denissova NG, Wang G, He D, Long J, Liu F. Cyclin-dependent kinases regulate the antiproliferative function of Smads. Nature 2004;430(6996) 226-231.

[18] Kamaraju AK, Roberts AB. Role of Rho/ROCK and p38 MAP kinase pathways in transforming growth factor-β-mediated Smad-dependent growth inhibition of human breast carcinoma cells in vivo. J Biol Chem 2005;280(2) 1024-1036.

[19] Sekimoto G, Matsuzaki K, Yoshida K, Mori S, Murata M, Seki T, Matsui H, Fujisawa J, Okazaki K. Reversible Smad-dependent signaling between tumor suppression and oncogenesis. Reversible Smad-dependent signaling between tumor suppression and oncogenesis. Cancer Res 2007;67(11) 5090-5096.

[20] Matsuzaki K, Kitano C, Murata M, Sekimoto G, Yoshida K, Uemura Y, Seki T, Taketani S, Fujisawa J, Okazaki K. Smad2 and Smad3 phosphorylated at both linker and COOH-terminal regions transmit malignant TGF-β signal in later stages of human colorectal cancer. Cancer Res 2009;69(13) 5321-5330.

[21] Liu F. Smad3 phosphorylation by cyclin-dependent kinases. Cytokine Growth Factor Rev 2006;17(1-2) 9-17.

[22] Wicks SJ, Lui S, Abdel-Wahab N, Mason RM, Chantry A. Inactivation of Smad-transforming growth factor β signaling by Ca(2+)-calmodulin-dependent protein kinase II. Mol Cell Biol 2000;20(21) 8103-8111.

[23] Furukawa F, Matsuzaki K, Mori S, Tahashi Y, Yoshida K, Sugano Y, Yamagata H, Matsushita M, Seki T, Inagaki Y, Nishizawa M, Fujisawa J, Inoue K. p38 MAPK mediates fibrogenic signal through Smad3 phosphorylation in rat myofibroblasts. Hepatology 2003;38(4) 879-889.

[24] Ho J, Cocolakis E, Dumas VM, Posner BI, Laporte SA, Lebrun JJ. The G protein-coupled receptor kinase-2 is a TGF-β-inducible antagonist of TGF-β signal transduction. EMBO J 2005;24(18) 3247-3258.

[25] Millet C, Yamashita M, Heller M, Yu LR, Veenstra TD, Zhang YE. A negative feedback control of transforming growth factor-β signaling by glycogen synthase kinase 3-mediated Smad3 linker phosphorylation at Ser-204. J Biol Chem 2009;284(30) 19808-19816.

[26] Alarcón C, Zaromytidou AI, Xi Q, Gao S, Yu J, Fujisawa S, Barlas A, Miller AN, Manova-Todorova K, Macias MJ, Sapkota G, Pan D, Massagué J. Nuclear CDKs drive Smad transcriptional activation and turnover in BMP and TGF-β pathways. Cell 2009;139(4) 757-769.

[27] Akira S, Takeda K. Toll-like receptor signalling. Nat Rev Immunol 2004;4(7) 499-511.

[28] Shim JH, Xiao C, Paschal AE, Bailey ST, Rao P, Hayden MS, Lee KY, Bussey C, Steckel M,Tanaka N, Yamada G, Akira S, Matsumoto K, Ghosh S. TAK1, but not TAB1 or

TAB2, plays an essential role in multiple signaling pathways in vivo. Genes Dev 2005;19(22) 2668-2681.

[29] Xu J, Lamouille S, Derynck R. TGF-β-induced epithelial to mesenchymal transition. Cell Res 2009;19(2) 156-172.

[30] Derynck R, Akhurst RJ. Differentiation plasticity regulated by TGF-β family proteins in development and disease. Nat Cell Biol 2007;9(9) 1000-1004.

[31] Schnabl B, Kweon YO, Frederick JP, Wang XF, Rippe RA, Brenner DA. The role of Smad3 in mediating mouse hepatic stellate cell activation. Hepatology 2001;34(1) 89-100.

[32] Kodama Y, Kisseleva T, Iwaisako K, Miura K, Taura K, De Minicis S, Osterreicher CH, Schnabl B, Seki E, Brenner DA. c-Jun N-terminal kinase-1 from hematopoietic cells mediates progression from hepatic steatosis to steatohepatitis and fibrosis in mice. Gastroenterology 2009;137(4) 1467-1477.

[33] Hui L, Zatloukal K, Scheuch H, Stepniak E, Wagner EF. Proliferation of human HCC cells and chemically induced mouse liver cancers requires JNK1-dependent p21 downregulation. J Clin Invest 2008;118(12) 3943-3953.

[34] Matsuzaki K. Smad3 phosphoisoform-mediated signaling during sporadic human colorectal carcinogenesis. Histol Histopathol 2006;21(6) 645-662.

[35] Sapkota G, Knockaert M, Alarcón C, Montalvo E, Brivanlou AH, Massagué J. Dephosphorylation of the linker regions of Smad1 and Smad2/3 by small C-terminal domain phosphatases has distinct outcomes for bone morphogenetic protein and transforming growth factor-β pathways. J Biol Chem 2006;281(52) 40412-40419.

[36] Wrighton KH, Lin X, Feng X-H. Phospho-control of TGF-β superfamily signaling. Cell Res 2009;19(1) 8-20.

[37] Matsuzaki K. Modulation of TGF-β signaling during progression of chronic liver diseases. Front Biosci 2009;14: 2923-2934.

[38] Fausto N, Campbell JS, Riehle KJ. Liver regeneration. Hepatology 2006;43(2 Suppl 1) S45-53.

[39] Massagué J. TGF-β in Cancer. Cell 2008;134(2) 215-230.

[40] Derynck R, Zhang YE. Smad-dependent and Smad-independent pathways in TGF-β family signaling. Nature 2003;425(6958) 577-584.

[41] Caestecker MP de, Parks WT, Frank CJ, Castagnino P, Bottaro DP, Roberts AB, Lechleider RJ. Smad2 transduces common signals from receptor serine-threonine and tyrosine kinases. Genes Dev 1998;12(11) 1587-1592.

[42] Lehmann K, Janda E, Pierreux CE, Rytomaa M, Schulze A, McMahon M, Hill CS, Beug H, Downward J. Raf induces TGF-β production while blocking its apoptotic but

not invasive responses: a mechanism leading to increased malignancy in epithelial cells. Genes Dev 2000;14(20) 2610-2622.

[43] Yue J, Mulder KM. Requirement of Ras/MAPK pathway activation by transforming growth factor beta for transforming growth factor beta 1 production in a Smad-dependent pathway. J Biol Chem 2000;275(40) 30765-30773.

[44] Oft M, Akhurst RJ, Balmain A. Metastasis is driven by sequential elevation of H-ras and Smad2 levels. Nat Cell Biol 2002;4(7) 487-494.

[45] Funaba M, Zimmerman CM, Mathews LS. Modulation of Smad2-mediated signaling by extracellular signal-regulated kinase. J Biol Chem 2002;277(44) 41361-41368.

[46] Janda E, Lehmann K, Killisch I, Jechlinger M, Herzig M, Downward J, Beug H, Günter S. Ras and TGF-β cooperatively regulate epithelial cell plasticity and metastasis: dissection of Ras signaling pathways. J Cell Biol 2002;156(2) 299-313.

[47] Suzuki K, Wilkes MC, Garamszegi N, Edens M, Leof EB. Transforming growth factor β signaling via Ras in mesenchymal cells requires p21-activated kinase 2 for extracellular signal-regulated kinase-dependent transcriptional responses. Cancer Res 2007;67(8) 3673-3682.

[48] Li F, Zeng B, Chai Y, Cai P, Fan C, Cheng T. The linker region of Smad2 mediates TGF-beta-dependent ERK2-induced collagen synthesis. Biochem Biophys Res Commun 2009;386(2) 289-293.

[49] Burch ML, Yang SN, Ballinger ML, Getachew R, Osman N, Little PJ. TGF-β stimulates biglycan synthesis via p38 and ERK phosphorylation of the linker region of Smad2. Cell Mol Life Sci 2010;67(12) 2077-2090.

[50] Jiang W, Zhang Y, Wu H, Zhang X, Gan H, Sun J, Chen Q, Guo M, Zhang Z. Role of cross-talk between the Smad2 and MAPK pathways in TGF-β1-induced collagen IV expression in mesangial cells. Int J Mol Med 2010;26(4) 571-576.

[51] Wang G, Long J, Matsuura I, He D, Liu F. The Smad3 linker region contains a transcriptional activation domain. Biochem J 2005;386(Pt 1) 29-34.

[52] Prokova V, Mavridou S, Papakosta P, Kardassis D. Characterization of a novel transcriptionally active domain in the transforming growth factor beta-regulated Smad3 protein. Nucleic Acids Res 2005;33(12) 3708-3721.

[53] Vasilaki E, Siderakis M, Papakosta P, Skourti-Stathaki K, Mavridou S, Kardassis D. Novel regulation of Smad3 oligomerization and DNA binding by its linker domain. Biochemistry 2009;48(35) 8366-8378.

[54] Nagata H, Hatano E, Tada M, Murata M, Kitamura K, Asechi H, Narita M, Yanagida A, Tamaki N, Yagi S, Ikai I, Matsuzaki K, Uemoto S. Inhibition of c-Jun NH2-terminal kinase switches Smad3 signaling from oncogenesis to tumor-suppression in rat hepatocellular carcinoma. Hepatology 2009;49(6) 1944-1953.

[55] Engel ME, McDonnell MA, Law BK, Moses HL. Interdependent SMAD and JNK signaling in transforming growth factor-β-mediated transcription. J Biol Chem 1999;274(52) 37413-37420.

[56] Murata M, Matsuzaki K, Yoshida K, Sekimoto G, Tahashi Y, Mori S, Uemura Y, Sakaida N, Fujisawa J, Seki T, Kobayashi K, Yokote K, Koike K, Okazaki K. Hepatitis B virus X protein shifts human hepatic transforming growth factor (TGF)-beta signaling from tumor suppression to oncogenesis in early chronic hepatitis B. Hepatology 2009;49(4) 1203-1217.

[57] Michalopoulos GK. Liver regeneration. J Cell Physiol 2007;213(2) 286-300.

[58] Grivennikov SI, Greten FR, Karin M. Immunity, inflammation, and cancer. Cell 2010;140(6) 883-899.

[59] Yamada Y, Kirillova I, Peschon JJ, Fausto N. Initiation of liver growth by tumor necrosis factor: deficient liver regeneration in mice lacking type I tumor necrosis factor receptor. Proc Natl Acad Sci U S A 1997;94(4) 1441-1446.

[60] Tilg H, Kaser A, Moschen AR. How to modulate inflammatory cytokines in liver diseases. Liver Int 2006;26(9) 1029-1039.

[61] Date M, Matsuzaki K, Matsushita M, Sakitani K, Shibano K, Okajima A, Yamamoto C, Ogata N,Okumura T, Seki T, Kubota Y, Kan M, McKeehan WL, Inoue K. Differential expression of transforming growth factor-β and its receptors in hepatocytes and nonparenchymal cells of rat liver after CCl4 administration. J Hepatol 1998;28(4) 572-581.

[62] Date M, Matsuzaki K, Matsushita M, Tahashi Y, Sakitani K, Inoue K. Differential regulation of activin A for hepatocyte growth and fibronectin synthesis in rat liver injury. J Hepatol 2000;32(2) 251-260.

[63] Date M, Matsuzaki K, Matsushita M, Tahashi Y, Furukawa F, Inoue K. Modulation of transforming growth factor β function in hepatocytes and hepatic stellate cells in rat liver injury. Gut 2000;46(5) 719-724.

[64] Matsuzaki K, Murata M, Yoshida K, Sekimoto G, Uemura Y, Sakaida N, Kaibori M, Kamiyama Y, Nishizawa M, Fujisawa J, Okazaki K, Seki T. Chronic inflammation associated with hepatitis C viral infection perturbs hepatic TGF-β signaling, promoting cirrhosis and hepatocellular carcinoma. Hepatology 2007;46(1) 48-57.

[65] Kawamata S, Matsuzaki K, Murata M, Seki T, Matsuoka K, Iwao Y, Hibi T, Okazaki K. Oncogenic Smad3 signaling induced by chronic inflammation is an early event in ulcerative colitis-associated carcinogenesis. Inflamm Bowel Dis 2011;17(3) 683-695.

[66] Yang YA, Zhang GM, Feigenbaum L, Zhang YE. Smad3 reduces susceptibility to hepatocarcinoma by sensitizing hepatocytes to apoptosis thorough downregulation of Bcl-2. Cancer Cell 2006;9(6) 445-457.

[67] Caldwell S, Park SH. The epidemiology of hepatocellular cancer: from the perspectives of public health problem to tumor biology. J Gastroenterol 2009;44 (Suppl 19) S96-101.

[68] Seitz and Stickel. Risk factors and mechanisms of hepatocarcinogenesis with special emphasis on alcohol and oxidative stress. Biol Chem 2006;387(4) 349-360.

[69] Yuen MF, Tanaka Y, Fong DY, Fung J, Wong DK, Yuen JC, But DY, Chan AO, Wong BC, Mizokami M, Lai CL. Independent risk factors and predictive score for the development of hepatocellular carcinoma in chronic hepatitis B. J Hepatol 2009;50(1) 80-88.

[70] Fattovich G, Stroffolini T, Zagni I, Donato F. Hepatocellular carcinoma in cirrhosis: incidence and risk factors. Gastroenterology 2004;127(Suppl 1) S35-50.

[71] Kris VK. Iron, hemochromatosis and hepatocellular carcinoma. Gastroenterology 2004;127(5 Suppl 1) S79-86.

[72] Ascha MS, Hanouneh IA, Lopez R, Tamimi TA, Feldstein AF, Zein NN. The incidence and risk factors of hepatocellular carcinoma in patients with nonalcoholic steatohepatitis. Hepatology 2010;51(6) 1972-1978.

[73] Arthur MJ. Fibrogenesis II. Metalloproteinases and their inhibitors in liver fibrosis. Am J Physiol Gastrointest Liver Physiol 2000;279(2) G245-249.

[74] Popov Y, Schuppan D. Targeting liver fibrosis: strategies for development and validation of antifibrotic therapies. Hepatology 2009;50(4) 1294-1306.

[75] Pinzani M, Macias-Barragan J. Update on the pathophysiology of liver fibrosis. Expert Rev Gastroenterol Hepatol 2010;4(4) 459-472.

[76] Eddy AA. Serine proteases, inhibitors and receptors in renal fibrosis. Thromb Haemost 2009;101(4) 656-664.

[77] Hu PF, Chen H, Zhong W, Lin Y, Zhang X, Chen YX, Xie WF. Adenovirus-mediated transfer of siRNA against PAI-1 mRNA ameliorates hepatic fibrosis in rats. J Hepatol 2009;51(1) 102-113.

[78] Taub R. Liver regeneration: from myth to mechanism. Nat Rev Mol Cell Biol 2004;5(10) 836-847.

[79] Friedman SL. Evolving challenges in hepatic fibrosis. Nat Rev Gastroenterol Hepatol 2010;7(8) 425-436.

[80] Kawada N. The hepatic perisinusoidal stellate cell. Histol Histopathol 1997;12(4) 1069-1080.

[81] Inagaki Y, Okazaki I. Emerging insights into transforming growth factor β Smad signal in hepatic fibrogenesis. Gut 2007;56(2) 284-292.

[82] Bataller R, Brenner DA. Liver fibrosis. J Clin Invest 2005;115(2) 209-218.

[83] Weinberg RA.The Biology of Cancer. Garlang Science, New York; 2007

[84] Iwano M, Plieth D, Danoff TM, Xue C, Okada H, Neilson EG. Evidence that fibroblasts derive from epithelium during tissue fibrosis. J Clin Invest 2002;110(3) 341-350.

[85] Saika S, Kono-Saika S, Ohnishi Y, Sato M, Muragaki Y, Ooshima A, Flanders KC, Yoo J, Anzano M, Liu CY, Kao WW, Roberts AB. Smad3 signaling is required for epithelial-mesenchymal transition of lens epithelium after injury. Am J Pathol 2004;164(2) 651-663.

[86] Zeisberg M, Yang C, Martino M, Duncan MB, Rieder F, Tanjore H, Kalluri R. Fibroblasts derive from hepatocytes in liver fibrosis via epithelial to mesenchymal transition. J Biol Chem 2007;282(32) 23337-23347.

[87] Shirai Y, Kawata S, Tamura S, Ito N, Tsushima H, Takaishi K, Kiso S, Matsuzawa Y. Plasma transforming growth factor-β1 in patients with hepatocellular carcinoma: comparison with chronic liver diseases. Cancer 1994;73(9) 2275-2279.

[88] Tilg H. Cytokines and liver diseases. Can J Gastroenterol 2001;15(10) 661-668.

[89] Sugano Y, Matsuzaki K, Tahashi Y, Furukawa F, Mori S, Yamagata H, Yoshida K, Matsushita M, Nishizawa M, Fujisawa J, Inoue K. Distortion of autocrine transforming growth factor β signal accelerates malignant potential by enhancing cell growth as well as PAI-1 and VEGF production in human hepatocellular carcinoma cells. Oncogene 2003;22(15) 2309-2321.

[90] Yoshida K, Matsuzaki K, Mori S, Tahashi Y, Yamagata H, Furukawa F, Seki T, Nishizawa M, Fujisawa J, Okazaki K. Transforming growth factor-β and platelet-derived growth factor signal via c-Jun N-terminal kinase-dependent Smad2/3 phosphorylation in rat hepatic stellate cells after acute liver injury. Am J Pathol 2005;166(4) 1029-1039.

[91] Kluwe J, Pradere JP, Gwak GY, Mencin A, De Minicis S, Osterreicher CH, Colmenero J, Bataller R, Schwabe RF. Modulation of hepatic fibrosis by c-Jun-N-terminal kinase inhibition. Gastroenterology 2010;138(1) 347-359.

[92] Nagamine Y. Transcriptional regulation of the plasminogen activator inhibitor type 1-with an emphasis on negative regulation. Thromb Haemost 2008;100(6) 1007-1013.

[93] Dooley S, Hamzavi J, Ciuclan L, Godoy P, Ilkavets I, Ehnert S, Ueberham E, Gebhardt R, Kanzler S, Geier A, Breitkopf K, Weng H, Mertens PR. Hepatocyte-specific Smad7 expression attenuates TGF-β-mediated fibrogenesis and protects against liver damage. Gastroenterology 2008;135(2) 642-659.

[94] Roth-Eichhorn S, Kühl K, Gressner AM. Subcellular localization of (latent) transforming growth factor beta and the latent TGF-beta binding protein in rat hepatocytes and hepatic stellate cells. Hepatology 1998;28(6) 1588-1596.

[95] Weng HL, Ciuclan L, Liu Y, Hamzavi J, Godoy P, Gaitantzi H, Kanzler S, Heuchel R, Ueberham U, Gebhardt R, Breitkopf K, Dooley S. Profibrogenic transforming growth

factor-beta/activin receptor-like kinase 5 signaling via connective tissue growth factor expression in hepatocytes. Hepatology 2007;46(4) 1257-1270.

[96] Gressner OA. Less Smad2 is good for you! A scientific update on coffee's liver benefits. Hepatology 2009;50(3) 970-978.

[97] Gressner OA, Lahme B, Demirci I, Gressner AM, Weiskirchen R. Differential effects of TGF-beta on connective tissue growth factor (CTGF/CCN2) expression in hepatic stellate cells and hepatocytes. J Hepatol 2007;47(5) 699-710.

[98] Aravalli RN, Steer CJ, Cressman EN. Molecular mechanisms of hepatocellular carcinoma. Hepatology 2008;48(6) 2047-2063.

[99] Bréchot C, Nalpas B, Courouc é AM, Duhamel G, Callard P, Carnot F, Tiollais P, Berthelot P. Evidence that hepatitis B virus has a role in liver-cell carcinoma in alcoholic liver disease. N Engl J Med 1982;306(23) 1384-1387.

[100] Hassan MM, Hwang LY, Hatten CJ, Swaim M, Li D, Abbruzzese JL, Beasley P, Patt YZ. Risk factors for hepatocellular carcinoma: synergism of alcohol with viral hepatitis and diabetes mellitus. Hepatology 2002;36(5) 1206-1213.

[101] Park SZ, Nagorney DM, Czaja AJ. Hepatocellular carcinoma in autoimmune hepatitis. Dig Dis Sci 2000;45(10) 1944-1948.

[102] Shibuya A, Tanaka K, Miyakawa H, Shibata M, Takatori M, Sekiyama K, Hashimoto N, Amaki S, Komatsu T, Morizane T. Hepatocellular carcinoma and survival in patients with primary biliary cirrhosis. Hepatology 2002;35(5) 1172-1178.

[103] But DY, Lai CL, Yuen MF. Natural history of hepatitis-related hepatocellular carcinoma. World J Gastroenterol 2008;14(11) 1652-1656.

[104] Tsai JF, Jeng JE, Ho MS, Chang WY, Hsieh MY, Lin ZY, Tsai JH. Effect of hepatitis C and B virus infection on risk of hepatocellular carcinoma: a prospective study. Br J Cancer 1997;76(7) 968-974.

[105] Chiaramonte M, Stroffolini T, Vian A, Stazi MA, Floreani A, Lorenzoni U, Lobello S, Farinati F, Naccarato R. Rate of incidence of hepatocellular carcinoma in patients with compensated viral cirrhosis. Cancer 1999;85(10) 2132-2137.

[106] Buendia MA. Mammalian hepatitis B viruses and primary liver cancer. Semin Cancer Biol 1992;3(5) 309-320.

[107] Jiang Z, Jhunjhunwala S, Liu J, Haverty PM, Kennemer MI, Guan Y, Lee W, Carnevali P, Stinson J, Johnson S, Diao J, Yeung S, Jubb A, Ye W, Wu TD, Kapadia SB, de Sauvage FJ, Gentleman RC, Stern HM, Seshagiri S, Pant KP, Modrusan Z, Ballinger DG, Zhang Z. The effects of hepatitis B virus integration into the genomes of hepatocellular carcinoma patients. Genome research 2010;22(4) 593-601.

[108] Bréchot C, Pourcel C, Louise A, Rain B, Tiollais P. Presence of integrated hepatitis B virus DNA sequences in cellular DNA of human hepatocellular carcinoma. Nature 1980;286(5772) 533-535.

[109] Shafritz DA, Shouval D, Sherman HI, Hadziyannis SJ, Kew MC. Integration of hepatitis B virus DNA into the genome of liver cells in chronic liver disease and hepatocellular carcinoma studies in percutaneous liver biopsies and post-mortem tissue specimens. N Engl J Med 1981;305(18) 1067-1073.

[110] Guerrero RB, Roberts LR. The role of hepatitis B virus integrations in the pathogenesis of human hepatocellular carcinoma. J Hepatol 2005;42(5) 760-777.

[111] Feitelson MA, Lee J. Hepatitis B virus integration, fragile sites, and hepatocarcinogenesis. Cancer Lett 2007;252(2) 157-170.

[112] Murakami Y, Saigo K, Takashima H, Minami M, Okanoue T, Bréchot C. Large scaled analysis of hepatitis B virus (HBV) DNA integration in HBV related hepatocellular carcinomas. Gut 2005;54(8) 1162-1168.

[113] Andrisani OM, Barnabas S. The transcriptional function of the hepatitis B virus X protein and its role in hepatocarcinogenesis. Int J Oncol 1999;15(2) 373-379.

[114] Bouchard MJ, Schneider RJ. The enigmatic X gene of hepatitis B virus. J Virol 2004;78(23) 12725-12734.

[115] Tang H, Oishi N, Kaneko S, Murakami S. Molecular functions and biological roles of hepatitis B virus x protein. Cancer Sci 2006;97(10) 977-983.

[116] Seifer M, Höhne M, Schaefer S, Gerlich WH. In vitro tumorigenicity of hepatitis B virus DNA and HBx protein. J Hepatol 1991;13(Suppl 4) S61-65.

[117] Gottlob K, Pagano S, Levrero M, Graessmann A. Hepatitis B virus X protein transcription activation domains are neither required nor sufficient for cell transformation. Cancer Res 1998;58(16) 3566-3570.

[118] Oguey D, Dumenco LL, Pierce RH, Fausto N. Analysis of the tumorigenicity of the X gene of hepatitis B virus in a nontransformed hepatocyte cell line and the effects of cotransfection with a murine p53 mutant equivalent to human codon 249. Hepatology 1996;24(5) 1024-1033.

[119] Reifenberg K, Löhler J, Pudollek HP, Schmitteckert E, Spindler G, Köck J, Schlicht HJ. Long-term expression of the hepatitis B virus core-e- and X-proteins does not cause pathologic changes in transgenic mice. J Hepatol 1997;26(1) 119-130.

[120] Kim CM, Koike K, Saito I, Miyamura T, Jay G. HBx gene of hepatitis B virus induces liver cancer in transgenic mice. Nature 1991;351(6324) 317-320.

[121] Koike K, Moriya K, Iino S, Yotsuyanagi H, Endo Y, Miyamura T. High-level expression of hepatitis B virus HBx gene and hepatocarcinogenesis in transgenic mice. Hepatology 1994;19(4) 810-819.

[122] Terradillos O, Billet O, Renard CA, Levy R, Molina T, Briand P, Buendia MA. The hepatitis B virus X gene potentiates c-myc-induced liver oncogenesis in transgenic mice. Oncogene 1997;14(4) 395-404.

[123] Pang R, Tse E, Poon RT. Molecular pathways in hepatocellular carcinoma. Cancer Lett 2006;240(2) 157-169.

[124] Feitelson MA. c-myc overexpression in hepatocarcinogenesis. Hum Pathol 2004;35(11) 1299-1302.

[125] Choo QL, Richman KH, Han JH, Berger K, Lee C, Dong C, Gallegos C, Coit D, Medina-Selby R, Barr PJ. Genetic organization and diversity of the hepatitis C virus. Proc Natl Acad Sci U S A 1991;88(6) 2451-2455.

[126] Takamizawa A, Mori C, Fuke I, Manabe S, Murakami S, Fujita J, Onishi E, Andoh T, Yoshida I & Okayama H. Structure and organization of the hepatitis C virus genome isolated from human carriers. J Virol 1991;65(3) 1105-1113.

[127] Lin C, Lindenbach BD, Pragai BM, McCourt DW, Rice CM. Processing in the hepatitis C virus E2-xlink region: identification of p7 and two distinct E2-specific products with different C termini. J Virol 1994;68(8) 5063-5073.

[128] Reed KE, Rice CM. Overview of hepatitis C virus genome structure, polyprotein processing, and protein properties. Curr Top Microbiol Immunol 2000;242:55-84.

[129] Hayashi J, Aoki H, Kajino K, Moriyama M, Arakawa Y, Hino O. Hepatitis C virus core protein activates the MAPK/ERK cascade synergistically with tumor promoter TPA, but not with epidermal growth factor or transforming growth factor alpha. Hepatology 2000;32(5) 958-961.

[130] Erhardt A, Hassan M, Heintges T, Haussinger D. Hepatitis C virus core protein induces cell proliferation and activates ERK, JNK, and p38 MAP kinases together with the MAP kinase phosphatase MKP-1 in a HepG2 Tet-Off cell line. Virology 2002;292(2) 272-284.

[131] He Y, Nakao H, Tan SL, Polyak SJ, Neddermann P, Vijaysri S, Jacobs BL, Katze MG. Subversion of cell signaling pathways by hepatitis C virus nonstructural 5A protein via interaction with Grb2 and P85 phosphatidylinositol 3-kinase. J Virol 2002;76(18) 9207-9217.

[132] Qadri I, Iwahashi M, Capasso JM, Hopken MW, Flores S, Schaack J, Simon FR. Induced oxidative stress and activated expression of manganese superoxide dismutase during hepatitis C virus replication: role of JNK, p38 MAPK and AP-1. Biochem J 2004;378(Pt 3) 919-928.

[133] Zhao LJ, Wang L, Ren H, Cao J, Li L, Ke JS, Qi ZT. Hepatitis C virus E2 protein promotes human hepatoma cell proliferation through the MAPK/ERK signaling pathway via cellular receptors. Exp Cell Res 2005;305(1) 23-32.

[134] Hassan M, Ghozlan H, Abdel-Kader O. Activation of c-Jun NH2-terminal kinase (JNK) signaling pathway is essential for the stimulation of hepatitis C virus (HCV) nonstructural protein 3 (NS3)- mediated cell growth. Virology 2005;333(2) 324-336.

[135] Choi SH, Hwang SB. Modulation of the transforming growth factor-beta signal transduction pathway by hepatitis C virus nonstructural 5A protein. J Biol Chem 2006;281(11) 7468-7478.

[136] Hassan M, Selimovic D, Ghozlan H, Abdel-kader O. Hepatitis C virus core protein triggers hepatic angiogenesis by a mechanism including multiple pathways. Hepatology 2009;49(5) 1469-1482.

[137] Park KJ, Choi SH, Choi DH, Park JM, Yie SW, Lee SY, Hwang SB. 1Hepatitis C virus NS5A protein modulates c-Jun N-terminal kinase through interaction with tumor necrosis factor receptor-associated factor 2. J Biol Chem 2003;278(33) 30711-30718.

[138] Lin W, Tsai WL, Shao RX, Wu G, Peng LF, Barlow LL, Chung WJ, Zhang L, Zhao H, Jang JY, Chung RT. Hepatitis C virus regulates transforming growth factor beta1 production through the generation of reactive oxygen species in a nuclear factor kappaB-dependent manner. Gastroenterology 2010;138(7) 2509-2518.

[139] Moriya K, Yotsuyanagi H, Shintani Y, Fujie H, Ishibashi K, Matsuura Y, Miyamura T, Koike K. Hepatitis C virus core protein induces hepatic steatosis in transgenic mice. J Gen Virol 1997;78 (Pt 7) 1527-1531.

[140] Moriya K, Fujie H, Shintani Y, Yotsuyanagi H, Tsutsumi T, Ishibashi K, Matsuura Y, Kimura S, Miyamura T, Koike K. Hepatitis C virus core protein induces hepatocellular carcinoma in transgenic mice. Nat Med 1998;4(9) 1065-1067.

[141] Lerat H, Honda M, Beard MR, Loesch K, Sun J, Yang Y, Okuda M, Gosert R, Xiao SY, Weinman SA, Lemon SM. Steatosis and liver cancer in transgenic mice expressing the structural and nonstructural proteins of hepatitis C virus. Gastroenterology 2002;122(2) 352-365.

[142] Balkwill F, Charles KA, Mantovani A. Smoldering and polarized inflammation in the initiation and promotion of malignant disease. Cancer Cell 2005;7(3) 211-217.

[143] Coussens LM, Werb Z. Inflammation and cancer. Nature 2002;420(6917) 860-867.

[144] Grivennikov S, Karin M. Autocrine IL-6 signaling: a key event in tumorigenesis? Cancer Cell 2008;13(1) 7-9.

[145] Szlosarek PW, Balkwill FR. Tumour necrosis factor alpha: a potential target for the therapy of solid tumours. Lancet Oncol 2003;4(9) 565-573.

[146] Voronov E, Shouval DS, Krelin Y, Cagnano E, Benharroch D, Iwakura Y, Dinarello CA, Apte RN. IL-1 is required for tumor invasiveness and angiogenesis. Proc Natl Acad Sci U S A 2003;100(5) 2645-2650.

[147] Jonsson JR, Barrie HD, O'Rourke P, Clouston AD, Powell EE. Obesity and steatosis influence serum and hepatic inflammatory markers in chronic hepatitis C. Hepatology 2008;48(1) 80-87.

[148] Karin M. The regulation of AP-1 activity by mitogen-activated protein kinases. J Biol Chem 1995;270(28) 16483-16486.

[149] Davis RJ. Signal transduction by the JNK group of MAP kinases. Cell 2000;103(2) 239-252.

[150] Mantovani A, Allavena P, Sica A, Balkwill F. Cancer-related inflammation. Nature 2008;454(7203) 436-444.

[151] Tada M, Hatano E, Taura K, Nitta T, Koizumi N, Ikai I, et al. High volume hydrodynamic injection of plasmid DNA via the hepatic artery results in a high level of gene expression in rat hepatocellular carcinoma induced by diethylnitrosamine. J Gene Med 2006;8(8) 1018-1026.

[152] Schiffer E, Housset C, Cacheux W, Wendum D, Desbois-Mouthon C, Rey C, Clergue F, Poupon R, Barbu V, Rosmorduc O. Gefitinib, an EGFR inhibitor, prevents hepatocellular carcinoma development in the rat liver with cirrhosis. Hepatology 2005;41(2) 307-314.

[153] Pikarsky E, Porat RM, Stein I, Abramovitch R, Amit S, Kasem S, Gutkovich-Pyest E, Urieli-Shoval S, Galun E, Ben-Neriah Y. NF-κB functions as a tumour promoter in inflammation-associated cancer. Nature 2004;431(7007) 461-466.

[154] Haybaeck J, Zeller N, Wolf MJ, Weber A, Wagner U, Kurrer MO, Bremer J, Iezzi G, Graf R, Clavien PA, Thimme R, Blum H, Nedospasov SA, Zatloukal K, Ramzan M, Ciesek S, Pietschmann T, Marche PN, Karin M, Kopf M, Browning JL, Aguzzi A, Heikenwalder M. A lymphotoxin-driven pathway to hepatocellular carcinoma. Cancer Cell 2009;16(4) 295-308.

[155] He G, Karin M. NF-κB and STAT3 - key players in liver inflammation and cancer. Cell Res 2011;21(1) 159-168.

[156] Roberts AB, Tian F, Byfield SD, Stuelten C, Ooshima A, Saika S, Flanders KC. Smad3 is key to TGF-β-mediated epithelial-to-mesenchymal transition, fibrosis, tumor suppression and metastasis. Cytokine Growth Factor Rev 2006;17(1-2) 19-27.

[157] Sugioka Y, Watanabe T, Inagaki Y, Kushida M, Niioka M, Endo H, Higashiyama R, Okazaki I. c-Jun NH2-terminal kinase pathway is involved in constitutive matrix metalloproteinase-1 expression in a hepatocellular carcinoma-derived cell line. Int J Cancer 2004; 109(6) 867-874.

[158] Guichard C, Amaddeo G, Imbeaud S, Ladeiro Y, Pelletier L, Maad IB, Calderaro J, Bioulac-Sage P, Letexier M, Degos F, Clément B, Balabaud C, Chevet E, Laurent A, Couchy G, Letouzé E, Calvo F, Zucman-Rossi J. Integrated analysis of somatic muta-

tions and focal copy-number changes identifies key genes and pathways in hepatocellular carcinoma. Nat Genet 2012;44(6) 694-698.

[159] Wakefield LM, Roberts AB. TGF-β signaling: positive and negative effects on tumorigenesis. Curr Opin Genet Dev 2002;12(1) 22-29.

[160] Pardali K, Moustakas A. Actions of TGF-β as tumor suppressor and pro-metastatic factor in human cancer. Biochim Biophys Acta 2007;1775(1) 21-62.

[161] Glick AB, Weinberg WC, Wu IH, Quan W, Yuspa SH. Transforming growth factor β1 suppresses genomic instability independent of a G1 arrest, p53, and Rb. Cancer Res 1996;56(16) 3645-3650.

[162] Tremain R, Marko M, Kinnimulki V, Ueno H, Bottinger E, Glick A. Defects in TGF-β signaling overcome senescence of mouse keratinocytes expressing v-Ha-ras. Oncogene. 2000;19(13) 1698-1709.

[163] Yang H, Kyo S, Takatura M, Sun L. Autocrine transforming growth factor beta suppresses telomerase activity and transcription of human telomerase reverse transcriptase in human cancer cells. Cell Growth Differ 2001;12(2) 119-127.

[164] Thorgeirsson SS, Grisham JW. Molecular pathogenesis of human hepatocellular carcinoma. Nat Genet 2002;31(4) 339-346.

[165] Llovet JM, Burroughs A, Bruix J. Hepatocellular carcinoma. Lancet 2003;362(9399) 1907-1917.

[166] Kew MC, Yu MC, Kedda MA, Coppin A, Sarkin A, Hodkinson J. The relative roles of hepatitis B and C viruses in the etiology of hepatocellular carcinoma in Southern African Blacks. Gastroenterology 1997;112(1) 184-187.

[167] Lopez PM, Villanueva A, Llovet JM. Systematic review: evidence-based management of hepatocellular carcinoma–an updated analysis of randomized controlled trials. Aliment Pharmacol Ther 2006;23(11) 1535-1547.

[168] Poon RT, Fan ST, Lo CM, Ng IO, Liu CL, Lam CM, Wong J. Improving survival results after resection of hepatocellular carcinoma: a prospective study of 377 patients over 10 years. Ann Surg 2001;234(1) 63-70.

[169] Felsher DW. Reversibility of oncogene-induced cancer. Curr Opin Genet Dev 2004;14(1) 37-42.

[170] Elsharkawy AM, Mann DA. Nuclear factor-kappaB and the hepatic inflammation-fibrosis-cancer axis. Hepatology 2007;46(2) 590-597.

[171] Ewald D, Li M, Efrat S, Auer G, Wall RJ, Furth PA, Hennighausen. Time-sensitive reversal of hyperplasia in transgenic mice expressing SV40 T antigen. Science 1996;273(5280) 1384-1386.

[172] Felsher DW, Bishop JM. Reversible tumorigenesis by MYC in hematopoietic lineages. Mol Cell 1999;4(2) 199-207.

[173] Yoshida H, Shiratori Y, Moriyama M, Arakawa Y, Ide T, Sata M, Inoue O, Yano M, Tanaka M, Fujiyama S, Nishiguchi S, Kuroki T, Imazeki F, Yokosuka O, Kinoyama S, Yamada G, Omata M. Interferon therapy reduces the risk for hepatocellular carcinoma: national surveillance program of cirrhotic and noncirrhotic patients with chronic hepatitis C in Japan. IHIT Study Group. Inhibition of Hepatocarcinogenesis by Interferon Therapy. Ann Intern Med 1999;131(3) 174-181.

[174] Shiratori Y, Imazeki F, Moriyama M, Yano M, Arakawa Y, Yokosuka O, Kuroki T, Nishiguchi S, Sata M, Yamada G, Fujiyama S, Yoshida H, Omata M. Histologic improvement of fibrosis in patients with hepatitis C who have sustained response to interferon therapy. Ann Intern Med 2000;132(7) 517-524.

Surgical Treatment Strategies and Prognosis of Hepatocellular Carcinoma

Alessandro Uzzau, Maria Laura Pertoldeo,
Vittorio Cherchi, Serena Bertozzi,
Claudio Avellini and Giorgio Soardo

Additional information is available at the end of the chapter

http://dx.doi.org/10.5772/55890

1. Introduction

Hepatocellular carcinoma (HCC is the fifth most common cause of mortality worldwide and the third cancer related cause and is responsible for about 1 million deaths yearly [1]. The age-adjusted worldwide incidence is 5.5-14.9 per 100.000 population. In some areas of the world, such as sub-Saharan Africa and Southeast Asia, HCC represents the first cause of cancer death with an incidence of 52 per 100.000. Furthermore, in Europe and USA, HCC incidence has progressively raised in the past decade representing a burden problem.

HCC is one of the few cancers for which a number of risk factors are known in great detail [2, 3]. HCC is almost always (80%) associated with cirrhosis, at least in developed countries, and chronic hepatitis C and B infection, alcoholic cirrhosis and haemocromatosis are some of the established risk factors [4]. The metabolic syndrome related to hypertension, central obesity, diabetes and obesity has been identified as a new risk factor. As a result, screening programs have developed, with the use of ultrasound and α-fetoprotein (AFP), with a hope to increase the chances of diagnosing small HCC and unltimately increase the rate of curability.

Definitive diagnosis relies on the demonstration of a typical vascular pattern per liver imaging techniques (triple-phase CT-scan or MRI) of tumors larger than 2 cm with arterial hypervascularity and venous wash- out. Nodules, smaller than 2 cm, should be rechecked every six months or, if highly suspect, subjected to needle biopsy. It's likely that the study of tumor-specific tissue markers with prognostic value could introduce a systematic use of needle biopsy.

Over the past 20 years, surgical treatment of hepatocellular carcinoma has seen an immense boost and improvement, with good survival outcomes and reduced morbidity and mortality.

Liver resection (LR) and orthotopic liver transplantation (OLT) and ablative therapies are now considered the only potentially curative treatments for this cancer. LR has achieved improvement in survival within the past decade as a result of advances in diagnosis, surgical management of HCC and perioperative care. However, the long-term prognosis remains poor, and the 5-year overall survival rate ranges between 33% and 44%, with a 5-year cumulative recurrence rate of 80% to 100%.

OLT could be viewed as the optimal treatment for HCC that is accompanied by advanced cirrhosis because of the widest possible resection margins for tumour and for a definitive cure of cirrhosis and its related complications. OLT for HCC performed within well-defined oncologic criteria (Milan criteria "reference") has shown long-term results comparable with those of transplantation for non-HCC patients. However, the critical shortage of available donated organs, together with the increasing number of patients awaiting transplantation, makes this therapeutic option available to only a small percentage of patients. Owing to the limited organ supply, many liver transplant centers usually make a selection to resect patients with compensated liver cirrhosis, defined as Child–Pugh A chronic liver disease and resectable tumor and to reserve transplantation for those with impaired liver function (Child-Pugh class B-C) and small oligonodular HCC considered within the currently accepted criteria for transplantation.

Radiofrequency and microwave ablation are relatively new percutaneous techniques in clinical use for HCC, that can produce tumour necrosis. Complete response rates are high in large series if tumour is less that 3 cm in diameter.

This chapter will consider the main surgical techniques for the treatment of HCC in the light of the major guidelines currently available and of personal experience.

Also, we will review HCC prognostic factors, and the particular situation of "large" HCC and the strategy for liver tumours located at the hepato-caval confluence.

2. Surgical approach to HCC

Until two decades ago, prognosis of HCC was considered inevitably poor. Survival values of 54%, 40% and 28% at 1, 3 and 5 years in a group of patients with unresectable HCC were reported [5]. Since then, the therapeutic approach and the prognosis have been significantly modified [6], overall survival rates at 5 yearsreached values of 35-70% for liver resection [7, 8] and 40-75% for liver transplantation, depending on the stratification system of patients [9, 10]. This mainly related to better allocation of patients to current available treatments (OLT, LR, local therapies), enhancement of post-operative care, and treating patients at centers with a high-volume of hepatic surgeries. With regard to LR there has been an improved balance between extent of resection and parenchymal volume spared, a systematic use of intraoperative ultrasound examination (IOUS), and meticulous care to minimize blood loss by mean of intermittent clamping of the portal triad [11], selective clamping, and use of innovative hemostatic tools for dissection as ultrasound dissectors, harmonic scalpel, and argon-beamers.

Side by side, some new techniques, such as portal vein embolization to induce hypertrophy of the remnant liver, and intraoperative radiofrequency (RFA) or microwave (MWA) ablation have allowed it to expand and optimize the surgical offer. HCC occurs in over 80% of cases of cirrhosis. Furthermore, both tumor and cirrhosis contribute to the risk of mortality, and cirrhosis represents a limit for hepatic resection due to the risk of liver failure.

For HCC arising in the setting of healthy liver, it is undisputed that resection represents the first line of treatment; parenchymal resections extended up to 60% of the organ fall within an acceptable risk of post-operative liver failure and mortality.

Conversely, for HCC accompanied by cirrhosis, surgical outcome and prognosis are dependent on the degree of cirrhosis, independent of the tumor stage. In general, considering only the size of the tumor, three categories of HCC could be defined: (<3 cm), -(3-5 cm), a (5-10 cm) and (> 10 cm). The outcome after resection is good in the setting of smaller tumorsand the results after transplantation are optimal for single tumor<5cm or up to 3 tumors, <3cm each (Milan criteria). Furthermore tumor ablation by percutaneous alcohol treatment or RF ablation is optimal for tumors in the first category, and in select cases in the second, not applicable for tumors >5 cm. These results depend on the fact that, with an increase in the tumor size there increases the likelihood of vascular infiltration, poor tumor grading 3-4, satellites nodules, and/or multinodularity which represent (in particular the first two) a strong negative prognostic factors. If it is true that the best results in terms of survival are obtained for single lesion, there is now agreement that multiple nodules, up to 3, and no larger than 3cm can be addressed to transplantation with results similar to those of single tumor < 3 cm. Percutaneous ablative therapies or multiple resections, or resections supplemented by intraoperative ablation also offer discrete survival results in selected cases. The presence of a peritumoral capsule (in the so-called expansive capsulated HCC) represents another favorable prognostic element, while vascular infiltration, both microscopic and macroscopic, even more drastically reduces survival expectancy, because it determines an additional risk of early recurrence. Improved knowledge of the weight of these prognostic factors has led to the development of pathological classification systems very useful for evaluating the prognosis in non-surgical cases. AJCC / UICC pathological classification [12] devotes particular concern to the presence of macroscopic vascular infiltration or infiltration of large venous branches seen on imaging scans, but not to the size of the lesion, which is useful for prognostic purposes. The classification of the American Liver Tumor Study Group [13] also used by the United Network of Organ Sharing (United Network for Organ Sharing - UNOS 2012) [14] takes into account the size and nodularity of HCC tumors and is used to evaluate patients before resection or transplantation.

Finally, another HCC tumor parameter, which is critical to treatment decisionsis of the tumor location within the liver and its relationship with vascular structures. This technical aspect isespecially relevant to small tumors that are centrally located, or close to the main portal branches or to the hepato caval confluence, which should be considered for percutaneous therapy or transplantation, given the difficulty of extensive resection in this setting. In addition, other aspects related to the underlying liver disease must be addressed, such as the presence of portal hypertension (with pressures > 10mmHg), or platelets <100,000 that are associated with poor survival outcome following surgery, and increased bilirubin levels.

3. Liver resection and assessment of liver function

Problems to be faced in order to formulate a correct indication to resection are linked to 1) general conditions of the patient, in particular the presence of co-morbidities, 2) stage of the tumor, and 3) presence of advanced cirrhosis and hepatic function status which represent a limiting condition to hepatic resection and a real risk of postoperative liver failure, this being the major cause of mortality.

Liver function in cirrhotic liver is evaluated using different models, none of which is more useful than others in predicting of residual liver function after resection. Child-Turcotte-Pugh (CTP) [15] is the functional classification still widely used in most Western Centers: patients who fall within class A can be submitted to resection, even extended, with a low risk of liver failure, patients in class B are better candidates for non-surgical procedures (such as RFA, or transarterial chemoembolization), while those belonging to class C can only aspire to a transplant (Table 1) if within Milan criteria and good surgical candidates. However, the accuracy of CTP in predicting survival and treatment outcome has been questioned. Furthermore, this classification based only on few functional aspect of the liver is of limited utility in a decisional algorithm that must take into account also pathological aspects of the tumor.

For this reason, attempts have been made to integrate functional aspects of cirrhotic liver and tumor features. An example of these attempts is the Okuda classification (Table 2) [16] which combines tumor burden expressed as a percentage value of liver measure (< 50% or > 50%), with other functional and clinical variables: bilirubin and albumin levels, and the presence of ascites. Okuda's classification is certainly useful for predicting the risk of post-operative complications but not the results of long-term survival. In untreated patients with HCC on cirrhosis, this classification has proved to be highly predictive of survival.

Point	Bilirubin (mg/dL)	**Prothrombin time**	Albumin (g/dL)	**Ascites**	**Encefphalopathy (grade)**
1	< 2	"/> 70%	"/> 3.5	None	None
2	2-3	40-70%	2.8-3.5	Slight	1-2
3	"/>3	< 40 %	< 2.8	Moderate	3-4
Stage	Score				
A	5-6				
B	7-9				
C	≥ 10				

Table 1. Child-Pugh-Turcotte Score

In many Centers, especially Asians, CPT score is supplemented with the indiocyanin green clearance test (ICG) [17, 18]. Indocyanine Green dye is exclusively cleared from the blood by

Criterion	Cut-off	
	+	-
Tumor size (*)	"/> 50%	< 50%
Ascites	Clinically detectable	Absence
Albumin	< 3g/dL	"/> 3 g/dL
Bilirubin	"/> 3 mg/dL	< 3mg/dL
Stage I	No positives	
Stage II	One or two positives	
Stage III	Three or four positives	

Table 2. Okuda staging system. (*) Largest cross-sectional area of tumor to largest cross-sectional area of liver

the liver. A value of ICG at 15 minutes ≤ 14% is considered as predictive of a good functional reserve that allows resection of more than two segments according to Couinaud classification, both in patients in class A as well as for those in CPT class B [17, 19, 20]. Compared to only CPT score, ICG15r offers a prediction of the extent of liver resection [11] (Figure 1).

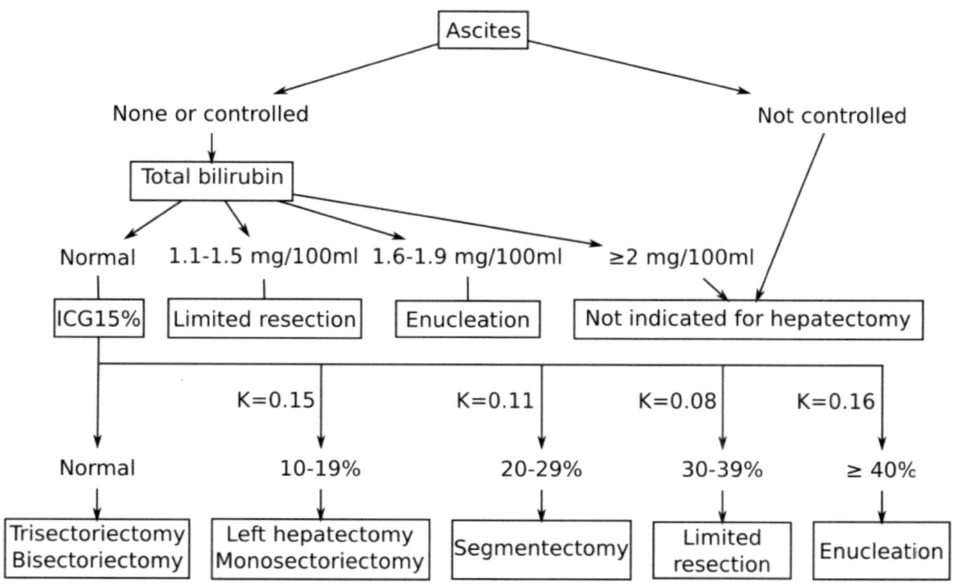

Figure 1. Possible extent of liver resection based on ICGr15 test.

It should be noted that these methods of evaluating liver function do not directly consider the presence and degree of portal hypertension, which instead is withheld as an high risk factor of post-operative morbidity in most Western Centers. Guidelines of the 'European Association of the Study of the Liver (EASL 2005) in fact, strongly recommend to preclude resection to patients with portal hypertension (PHT) with hepatic venous portal gradient (HVPG) > 10mmHg [5, 21, 22]. According to EASL guidelines, direct measurement of veno-portal gradient is more appropriate than an indirect assessment for the presence of esophageal varices, splenomegaly, and thrombocytopenia [23]. Recently hepatic elastography, which is a measure of the parenchymal "stiffness" would seem to linearly correlate with the values of HVPG, and may be considered as a simple alternative to the direct measurement [24, 25].

Notably, in late 1990s, another classification was proposed, named Barcelona Clinic Liver Cancer (BCLC) staging; which takes into account both variables linked to the tumor, and patient's conditions (CTP), to be also used as a treatment alloction system (Table 3) [5].

BCLC stratifies patients depending on the size and features of the tumor in four categories or stages: early stage (quite broad: single tumor up to 5 cm in diameter or up to three HCC with a diameter of <3 cm), intermediate stage, advanced and terminal stages. For each category, after considering the performance status, values of bilirubin and presence or absence of portal hypertension, each patient is assigned to a specific treatment modality (resection, transplantation, percutaneous treatment (PEI, RF, MW) which should offer the expectation of survival and treatment outcome.

Stadio	Tumor features	Clinical features
Stage A (EC early)		
A1 PST 0	Single tumor	Portal hypertension absent, normal bilirubin levels
A2 PST 0	Single tumor	Portal hypertension present, normal bilirubin levels
A3 PST 0	Single tumor	Portal hypertension present, abnormal bilirubin levels
A4 PST 0	3 nodules less than 3 cm	Child Pugh A-B
B (EC intermediate) PST 0	Multinodular	Child Pugh A-B
C (EC advanced) PST 1-2	Vascular infiltration and extrahepatic extension	Child Pugh A-B
D (EC end stage) PST 3-4	Any	Child Pugh C

Table 3. BCLC staging system (Barcelona Clinic Liver Cancer). PST: performance Status Test.

Notably, the American Association for the Study of the Liver guidelines (AASLD) [26], adopted BCLC HCC staging. The Asia-Pacific Association for the Study of the Liver (APASL) [27] maintained a bolder position: it does not evaluate a "functional reserve", and even puts a limit in the presence of portal hypertension, reflecting different development experience in Eastern Centers. The gap between the two guidelines is expanded even more if it considers the tumor burden, in fact AASLD guidelines recommend liver resection only in the presence of a single HCC, while APASL guidelines allows resection if HCC is confined to the liver, if the portal trunk is patent and the resection technically feasible, verbatim "Liver resection is a first-line curative treatment of solitary or multi-focal HCC confined to the liver, anatomically resectable, and with satisfactory liver function". This recommendation is obviously very different from that of the AASLD, verbatim "Patients who have a single lesion can be offered surgical resection if they are non-cirrhotic or have cirrhosis but still have preserved liver function, normal bilirubin and hepatic vein pressure < 10 mm Hg".

Thus, HCC staging and treatment allocation reflect a certain methodological variability [28] determined by ethical and social influences, and different practical needs of the different health care systems worldwide, which ultimately produce center-specific selection criteria.

4. Indication to liver resection

Resection for HCC is placed on the basis of two preliminary "technical" considerations:

1. Amount of liver function reserve and value of residual liver volume (RLV).
2. Anatomical location and extent of the tumor.

Single HCC below 5 cm, or multifocal HCC (not more than three tumors) without vascular invasion and with limited dimensions (<3 cm each), offer very good survival results that reach 50% at 5 years [29–31], and up to 70% at 5 years in a category of patients with normal bilirubin values and absence of portal hypertension [5]. In view of these results, there is a rather frequent disease relapse, estimated in terms of 50% at 3 years, 70% at 5 years and > 80% at 10 years [29–32]. Since these hopeful survival results (in particular for single HCC < 3 cm) were consistent with those of percutaneous ablation therapies, and slightly lower than those of transplantation, the choice of the procedure essentially depends on the experiences of the treating center [26].

The best results in terms of survival and low disease recurrence are offered by transplant specially in cases with established cirrhosis, even if, on a basis of "intention-to-treat" comparison the difference tends to be closer [33]. However, the option of liver transplantation is clearly limited by the shortage of organs supply. In 2010, based on the Organ Procurement and estimated Transplantation Network (OPTN), average waiting list time ranged from 140 days for American Indians up to 651 days for Hispanics [34]. Depending on the wait time period and the selection criteria used, the dropout rate for patients with HCC awaiting LT ranged between 12% and 38% [10, 35–37], and was essentially linked to tumor progression. Therefore, for early stage HCC transplantation should be reserved for those patients with poor liver function (eg CPT class C), and/or with evidence of portal hypertension. Since the report from Mazzaferro on the results of liver transplantation in a very well defined category of HCC, with actuarial 4-year overall survival of 85% and disease-free survival of 92%, subsequently confirmed by others, the "Milan criteria" [9] has marked an important turning point towards a more homogeneous transplant indication. Subsequently, other centers [38] have attempted to expand these criteria with fairly consistent results. However, the favorable results of transplantation for HCC within the Milan criteria must be considered very carefully, because it may be influenced from a selection bias. In fact, stratifying patients for factors other than size (for example for the presence of vascular invasion), survival curves between OLT and LR showed a similar trend [39]. Many high volume centers for HCC treatment reported that patients eligible for OLT (within the Milan criteria), but subjected to liver resection showed 5-year actuarial survival rate of about 60-70%, [6, 8, 40–45], in particular in a subgroup of patients without vascular invasion [39, 42–48].

Taking into account these observations, it seems appropriate to offer hepatic resection to patients with preserved liver functions who may be also eligible for transplantation, thanks to the rapidity of care, the greater simplicity of resection compared to transplant, and the lower rate of post-operative morbidity and mortality. Furthermore, it must be considered that transplant exposes patients to the risk of toxicity and potentially fatal infections related to immunosuppressive therapy, and predispose to the development of "de novo tumors".

In contrast, as previously mentioned, resection is associated with a higher recurrence rate (50-70% at 5 years) given the persistent background defect of the underlying liver disease that led to HCC development in the first place. Liver recurrence could be managed surgically (with a re-resection) in selected cases, or through the use of percutaneous ablative therapies, or by mean of "salvage transplant". Recurrences rates are lower if tumors are within the Milan criteria could benefit after orthotopic liver transplant as well as from split liver transplantation (SLT), the latter, using of a portion of liver from a living or dead donor, allows a more rapid access to liver transplantation. Two recent studies showed 5-year survival, morbidity and recurrence rate after salvage transplant to be similar to OLT performed as first choice [41, 49].

Recurrence is influenced in part by HCC pathological criteroa such as satellites nodules, vascular invasion, and poor histologic grading G3-G4. Translational research aimed at identifying molecular characteristics of HCC predictive of high risk of recurrence will be promising to avance this area of clinical challenge. Thus far, different chemoterapeutic agents have been tested in the adjuvant setting to reduce the recurrence rate. However, the small numbers of patients and the confounding variables did not lead to conclusive results.

The evidence gained to date for reducing the risk of recurrence has been linked to the surgical technique details. In particular, during the exploratory time, intraoperative ultrasonography should be systematically used for the correct evaluation of the position of the lesion, for the exclusion of further lesions not identified at pre-operative imaging, and yet for a correct evaluation of the vascular anatomy (Figure 2). It is estimated that 22 to 35% of the planned resections could change as a result of the IOUS examination.

HCC tend to permeate portals pedicles causing "anatomical" metastases or tumor thrombi that in turn are responsible of liver metastases (Figure 3). For this reason, many surgeons prefer to perform anatomical segmental or sub-segmental resections rather than atypical or wedge resections to ensure the inclusion of any microscopic satellite nodules, and tumor segmental embolization [50]. The advantage of anatomic resections remains valid, even in cases of multifocal lesions, as an alternative to extended resections such as hepatectomy or extended hepatectomy, given the advantage of preserving the hepatic functional reserve [51]. In the case of small centrally located HCC, and/or HCC proximal to major vascular pedicles, extensive resections are required [52], but alternatively bi- or three-segmentectomy whenever feasible,

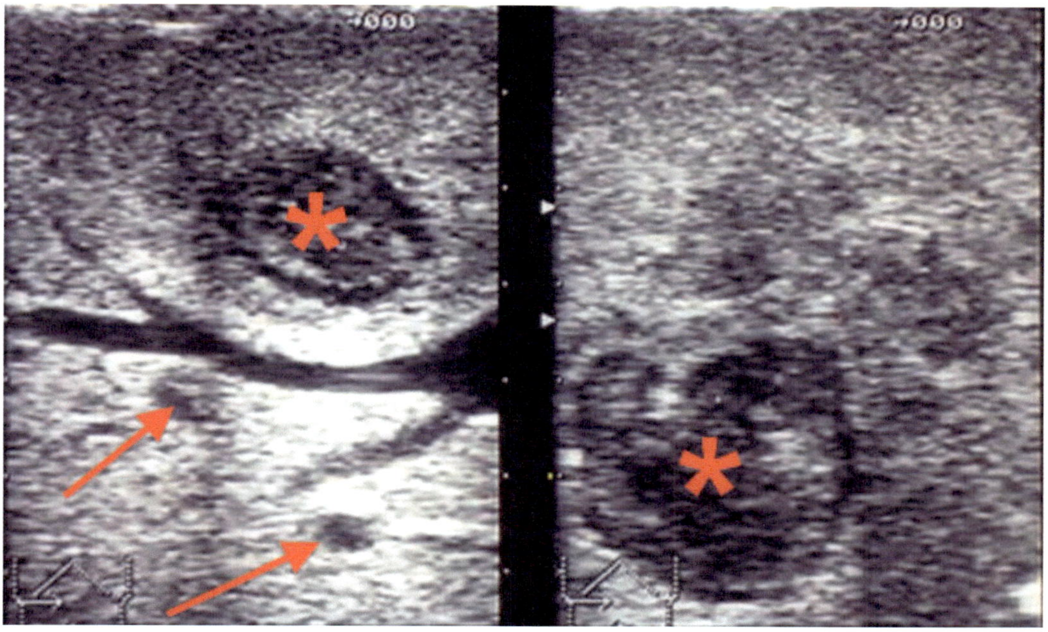

Figure 2. Intraoperative ultrasound examination showing a small HCC of 2 cm (star mark) located in the eighth segment and two minimal HCC (5 and 4 mm) (arrows) in the contiguous seventh segment. The planned resect on of the eight segment was changed to a bisegmentectomy of 7+8.

offers the same oncologic advantage, and at the same time allows a second surgical approach in case of relapse. Central resection (segments 5, 8, and 4), anterior-central resection (segments 4b and 5), posterior-central resection (segments 4° and 8), and lateral-superior bisegmentectomy (segments 7 and 8), and inferior-right bisegmentectomy (segments 6 and 5) represent an economic alternatives to standard right hepatectomy.

The segmental nature of the liver has been reported by Bismuth [53] who described eight segments, each of which is provided by an independent artero-portal and biliary pedicle. Segments are easily identified by anatomical landmarks, or through the intraoperative ultrasonography study of the portal branches distribution. A clear segmental demarcation could be obtained through by ultrasound-guided direct puncture and flushing of the portal branch with intravenous dye (methylene blue) tattooing the liver surface corresponding to the perfused district; using small bilumen-catheters equipped with inflatable balloon, and the Seldinger technique it is possible to simultaneously tattooing the liver surface (Figure 4) and occluding the vascular lumen in order to stop blood flow to the segment, minimizing blood loss, and theoretically reducing the risk of retrograde embolization from the tumor.

In general HCC ≤ 3cm can be treated with a segmentectomy, or with sub-segmentectomy, HCC 3-5 cm with segmentectomy eventually extended to contiguous subsegments, HCC> 5 cm may require more extensive resections in order to provide a free margin from neoplasm of at least 1 cm (Figure 5).

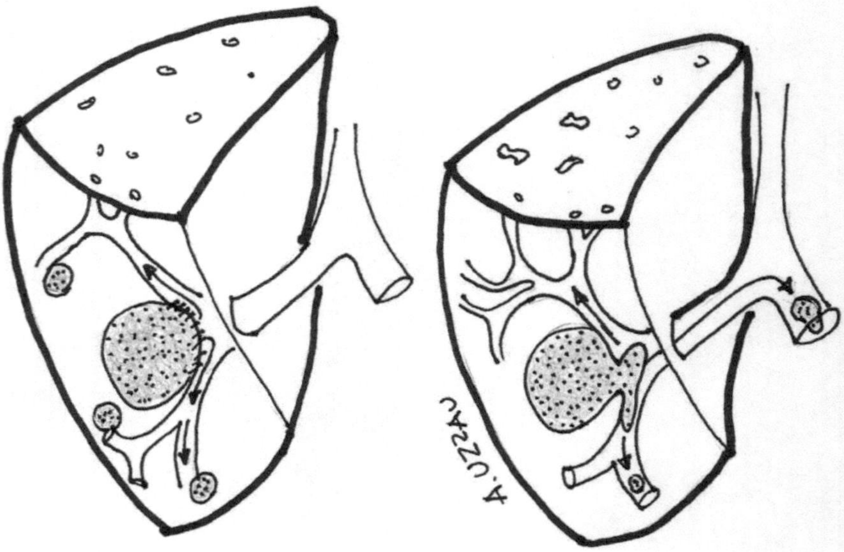

Figure 3. Modality of intrahepatic spreading of HCC. Tumor infiltrating sub-segmentary portal branches and delivering tumor cells to the perifery (intra-segmental diffusion) (left). Tumor thrombus has invaded a portal pedicle and becomes a source of dissemination at distance (intra- extra-segmental diffusion) (right).

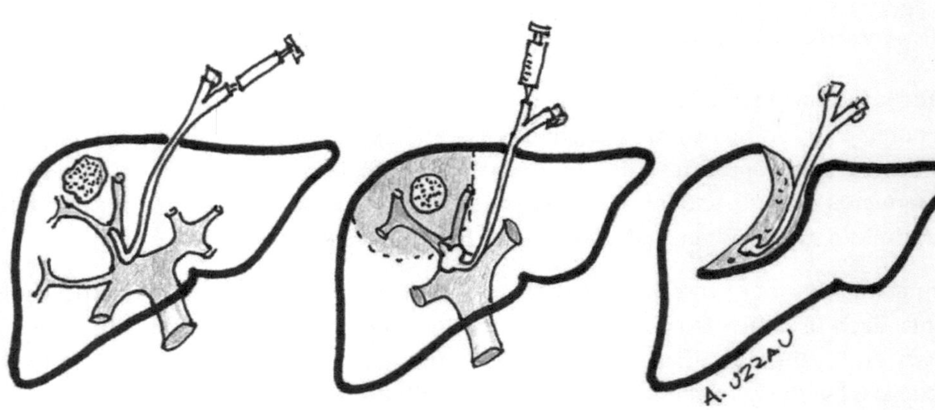

Figure 4. Technic of tattooing liver segment. Staining a segment through a bilumen catheter introduced according to Seldinger technique, after direct puncture under US guidance of a segmental portal pedicle (left). Blood flow occlusion inflating the balloon (optional) (center). Division of the parenchyma in segmental ischemic condition (left).

With regard to the definition of the so-called "high-risk HCC", it is still controversial. The high-risk HCC could be defined as:

1. "large", those > 5 cm in diameter (Figure 6). Large HCC increases the risk of vascular infiltration, worsening the prognosis. Even 10 years ago, 5-year survival after resection was no more than 33%. Today survival rate for large HCC without vascular infiltration are reported to be about 70% at 5 years [54] and 45% for so-called "giant HCC" (> 10cm) [55].

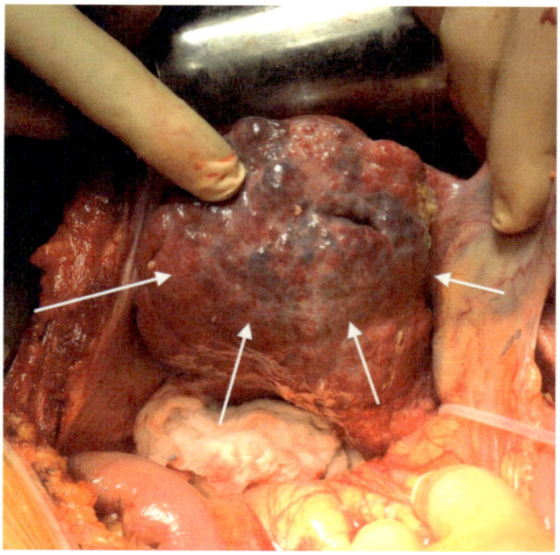

Figure 5. Tattooing of sub-segment of the fifth segment for a small HCC deeply located.

2. "multifocal tumors". Multifocality was considered for a long time as a contraindication to surgical approach, since it is associated with a poor prognosis. The only feasible treatment within the limits of small dimensions (3 nodules < 3cm each) is liver transplantation. However, many patients do not fall within the selection criteria and about 20% of those selected experience progression and dropout from the waiting list. Thus, surgical resection for patients with preserved liver functions may be the only curative option for multifocal HCC. Global survivals from 29.9% to 58% are reported at present, depending on the selection criteria [56, 57].

3. "macroscopic portal/hepatic vein involvement". This condition indicates the worst prognosis with a life expectancy of a few months in the absence of treatment.

In general, resectability for high-risk HCC is considered in absence of extrahepatic disease (lymph node metastasis or extrahepatic hematogenous spread and contiguous organs involvement), and in presence of preserved liver function. Due to the size, number, location and vascular involvement of the tumor, major resections or multiple resections are required, and are often associated with vascular reconstruction procedures. Limits to indication are the percentage value of the estimated remnant liver, and feasibility of vascular reconstruction. This configure a complex liver surgery that exposes at significatively higher morbidity/mortality risk and different survival rates depending on specific Centers selection and influenced by three main prognostic factors: grading, vascular infiltration, and size of the tumor. However, if resection is technically feasible, long-term survival for these patients is better than second-line therapy as trans-arterial chemo-embolization (TACE) [58, 59].

For multifocal and bilobar HCC although there are no randomized trials,there is anevidence of cohort studies that rported successful resection in select cases [60, 61]. Resection can be

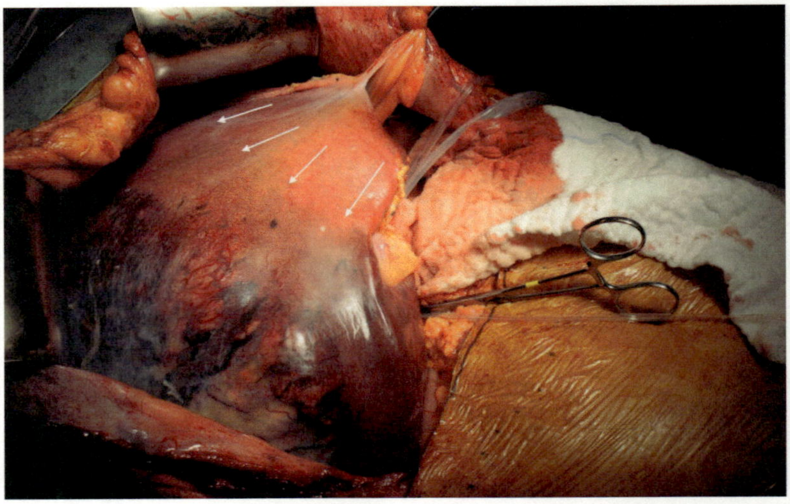

Figure 6. A case of very large, or so-called "giant HCC" which measured > 30 cm in diameter and weighted 5 Kg, involving the entire right hepatic lobe. The tumor did not involve the portal trunk and the left lobe was hypertrophic. Note the ischemic demarcation line (arrows) after selective right pedicle clamping.

combined with intraoperative ablation (RFA) expanding the rate of curability. Overall 5 years survival between 39% and 58% for large, multifocal and vascular infiltrating HCC [57, 58, 62–65] compared with the results of TACE overall survival of 24-63% at 2 years, and lowest rate of survival at 5 years [66–68].

Recently, Delis [69] compared a group of 59 patients within the UCSF (abbreviation needs to be defined..) liver transplant criteria (single tumor ≤6.5 cm, or three or fewer tumors of which the largest ≤4.5 cm and the sum of the tumor diameter ≤8 cm) [38] and another group of 27 pateints who exceeded these criteria: all patients underwent hepatectomy or extended hepatectomy with no mortality, but with higher rates of complications in the group that exceeded the UCSF criteria. 1, 3 and 5 years disease-free survival were 66%, 37% and 34%, respectively, in the first group and 56%, 29% and 26%, respectively, in the second group ($p < 0.01$), and the rate of recurrence was significantly higher in the second group, 74% vs 69% ($p < 0.002$). Vascular invasion was a strong predictive factor of intrahepatic and distant recurrences. Therefore, major vascular invasion is considered a contraindication to surgery and transplant in many surgical centers. Ikai [62] reports results of 66% and 43% 5-year survival in HCC with and without vascular infiltration, and found better survival values for the cases with tumor invasion of the portal branches of 2nd and 3rd order compared with invasion of the portal trunk or main branches, or contralateral infiltration. The recurrence rate was high (percentage??), but a considerable proportion of cases may be candidates for re-resection or ablative treatments. In the presence of tumor invasion of the portal trunk, 5-year survival of 26.4% is reported (thrombosis with portal infiltration) and 28.5% ($p = .33$) (without portal infiltration) [70]. According to some authors pre-treatment with TACE before resection can increase the global values of 5-year survival up to 42% that is a value significantly higher than 7% observed in non resected patients [71]. Resection and reconstruction of the portal trunk or of the main portal branches represent a very small percentage of the total resections, but they impose considerable technical difficulty because they require mobilization of the portal vein to the pancreas, an accurate posterior skeletonization, and dissection of the contralateral portal pedicle before the venotomy.

In the presence of hepatic veins involvement resection also extended to venous segments is accompanied by global survival at 1 and 3 years of 88% and 50% respectively, with mortality rates of 12% [72]. These are very selective indication procedure, which must be addressed at highly skilled centers in the hepato-biliary-pancreatic surgery.

In conclusion, for high-risk HCC there are no guidelines supported by strong scientific evidence at the moment, but nevertheless, resection is offered more frequently in both Eastern and Western Centers as well as in Academic Centers with a high volume of liver surgery [73–75].

5. Technical details

Major resection, defined as the resection of more than two segments (on liver with chronic disease), does not involve particular risks of liver failure in patients with preserved functional reserve (CTP class A), which can tolerate even more extensive resections, such as right or left hepatectomy. However, except for cases of large HCC where the resected liver accounts for a small proportion of functioning liver parenchyma, in other cases it is appropriate that a greater hepatectomy is replaced by more limited resections, allowing to reduce the risk of postoperative liver failure, and maintaining the chance of a new intervention in case of recurrence.

As aforementioned, the choice of a segmental resection is standard because it reduces the incidence of early complications, such as seromas, abscesses and in particular biliary leak. This aspect should not be underestimated since postoperative infection could lead to increased risk of liver failure.

An adequate knowledge of the vascular anatomy of the liver, the improvement of surgical technique and post-operative care have allowed to extend resections for large tumors, select cases of majorvascular involvement, saving the functioning segments, such as the salvage of segment 6 to preserve the portal postero-inferior pedicle, or reconstructing hepatic vessels in order to avoid vascular congestion of residual segments and/or sectors (Figure 7). Vascular reconstruction can be of direct-type as hepato-caval, or with prosthetic interposition (generally Gore-Tex), or venous segment interposition (portal or gonadal). This procedure can be performed with direct vascular control, or with ex-vivo technique using veno-venous bypass. Vascular reconstructions have the main purpose of avoiding the congestion of segments that have no other way of direct outflow [76]. For these techniques a complete study of vascular distribution preoperatively with CT-angiography and intraoperatively by mean of ultrasonography is mandatory.

Intraoperative bleeding represents a further technical problem., In fact, blood loss affects both the patient outcome in the short term, as well as the long-term survival and relapse. In the case

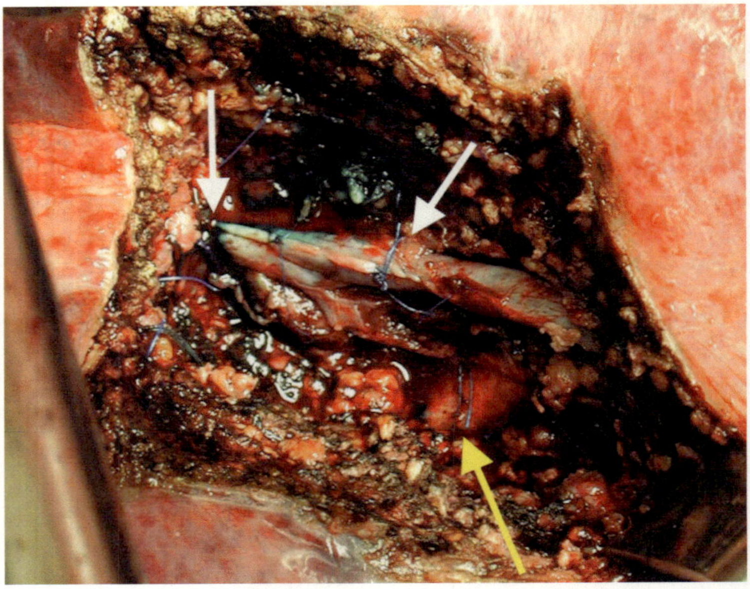

Figure 7. Direct reconstruction of the middle hepatic vein (white arrows) after resection of HCC situated between segment 8 and 4a. The yellow arrow indicates the upper segmental branch for segment 8.

of cirrhotic patients, bleeding is a cofactor of liver failure. Currently in high volume centers for liver surgery, 50-70% of resected patients do not require blood transfusions.

To limit blood loss, Pringle maneuver or clamping the portal triad are the technique most commonly used. Intermittent clamping of the hepatic hilum is preferred in cirrhotic patients compared to continuous clamping aimed to limit ischemia/reperfusion damage. Typically, clamping that determines a state of warm ischemia, is prolonged in cirrhotic up to 15 minutes. In the case of prolonged resection times clamping can be repeated with periods of unclamping (reperfusion) of 5 minutes (intermittent clamping). To limit the risk of ischemia/reperfusion damage many surgeons employ the technique of pre-conditioning, which consists of 10 minutes clamping followed by 10 minutes reperfusion, which precedes the definitive clamping. Pre-conditioning is believed to adapt liver parenchyma to warm ischemia thus reducing the damage of ischemia/reperfusion. In fact, there is much evidence of this advantageous use of the pre-conditioning in animal studies. However, evidence from few clinical studiesdoes not conclude potential definite benefit in humans [77–79].

An elegant and effective alternative to the Pringle maneuver is vascular direct control by means of ligation and division of the portal and arterial branches of the hepatic lobe to be resected if a hepatectomy is planned, or its selective clamping in the course of segmental resections; thus maintaining blood flow to the contralateral lobe. The selective exclusion of blood flow is confirmed by a change in color (ischemic demarcation) on the surface of the liver lobe excluded. Typically, if resections are performed with vascular control outset, the hepatic vein drainage is identified and secured too, thus causing a total parenchymal ischemia. Under certain favorable circumstances of anatomical dissection (easy hilum), inflow vascular control can also be obtained on second order branches (sectorial pedicles) determining a super-selective ischemic control.

Clamping of the hepatic vessels is generally employed during major resections, while it is not necessary if a small segmental resections, or wedge and laparoscopic resection are carried out [80–82].

The interruption of the blood flow from the hepatic pedicle effectively reduces bleeding during transection; however, bleeding could still results from the hepatic veins branches. To limit this further source of bleeding, it is useful to conduct resection under low value of central venous pressure (PVC) at less than 5 mmHg, and to place the patient in 20-25° Trendelemburg decubitus. The value of CVP in fact is reflected both at the level of the hepatic veins as well as at the sinusoidal compartment level, and blood volume lost during resection well correlates with the value of CVP [83–86].

Intraoperative control of bleeding is further optimized by the use of different instruments of parenchymal dissection, all aimed at containing bleeding from venular or sinusoidal origin. Classical hepatic dissection is carried out through parenchymal crushing by means of the Kelly or Klemmer clamps (crushing clamp technique): clamp pressure fractures the parenchyma leaving uncovered blood vessels that, depending on the size, are secured by mean of coagulation device or sutures or clips. Alternatively one can employ tools that divide the parenchyma in a gentler manner, through the ultrasonic dissector (ultrasonic dissection - CUSA-), bipolar current instruments (LigaSure), or radio frequency device (Harmonic Scalpel), to list a few examples. Although simple to use, the usefulness of these instruments is not clearin terms of blood saving or shorter time of resection[87].

Another technical consideration related to expanding the possibility ofresection even in those cases in which the total liver remnant volume is < 30% in healthy liver or < 35-40% in cirrhotic liver is expected, which are the limits generally accepted to contain the risk of postoperative liver failure [88, 89]. It is in fact possible to increase the volume of the hepatic remnant through the mechanism of liver lobe induced hypertrophy occluding the contralateral portal branch, the so-called portal vein embolization (PVE). This procedure is generally carried out under local anesthesia, through the puncture of a portal branch under ultrasound guidance or by fluoroscopy, which is then occluded by different embolizatin materials. This technique determines a volumetric increase of the residual lobe of about 8 to 12% over the time of about 20-30 days. After PVE, the percentage of patients undergoing surgery ranges from 62 to 100% according to recent studies [90, 91].

6. Indication to orthotopic liver transplantation

Since 1968 the "European Liver Transplant Registry" (ELTR) records all data of liver transplants in 145 centers across Europe. These data give an overview on what is the trend of transplants in Europe during each period.

Both the number of centers and the number of liver transplants gradually increased, but after an exponential growth until the 80s, they reached a plateau that was maintained as shown by recent data (ELRT) with about 5800 liver transplants performed per year across Europe. Cirrhosis was the most common indication for liver transplantation (52%) rate, followed by primary tumors of the liver (14%, HCC 12.1%).

Indication for liver transplantation have significantly changed over time. Subsequently, the rate of liver transplantation for increased to 20% in late 1990s. Between 2000-2010, two groups of indications have increased: primary tumors of the liver (16%), especially HCC, and cirrhosis (53%), especially alcohol related (20%).

Transplantation for HCC has thus become a therapeutic approach more commonly used in Europe where it accounted for 25% of all indications for liver transplantation. Improvement of survival of cirrhotic patients given by the pharmacological control of HBV and HCV, has led to an increased rate of survival and lower rate of recurrent HCC. In fact, HCC has gradually become the most common complication in cirrhotic patients. In the last three years the number of patients with HCC in transplant list has grown dramatically: more than 30% in France, 26% in Europe, 34% in the United States [92, 93].

7. The role of liver transplant from living donor

Living donor liver transplantation (LDLT) is a practice used mainly in Asia, where orthotopic organs are not readily available. Its use was later extended to other countries, mostly in Europe and North America to compensate for the shortage of organs and the long time on the waiting list which leads to patients' death, or dropout for medical reasons or progression of cancer beyond acceptable transplant criteria.

The main requirement of the transplant from a living donor is the "donor safety", namely the protection of the donor. Although the risks of this intervention in specialized centers are very low, the incidence of death of the donor ranges from 0.15 to 0.30%, but can reach up to 0.50%. The concept of "double equipoise" was proposed to describe the balance that must be maintained between the benefits related to the survival of the recipient and the risk of morbidity/mortality of the healthy donor. For example, in Europe and North America transplantation for acute liver failure from a living donor is not accepted, as the mortality of the recipient in such cases is higher. Some studies have suggested a higher risk of tumor recurrence related to liver regeneration after transplantation using a hemiliver from living donor compared to cadaveric whole liver. Other studies have shown no significant differences related to the type of graft used, and the only risk factor appeared to be related to the timing of transplantation from a living donor (fast-tracked patients), a short interval between the diagnosis of HCC and transplantation whaich can lead to a greater risk of tumor recurrence in the short term related to the fact that the biological behavior of HCC has not yet fully manifested. For these reasons, it is generally required to have a wiat time ofat least three months between the diagnosis of HCC and transplant before offering a graft from a living donor. The transplant from a living donor is acceptable if the 5-year survival is comparable to that of patients transplanted from cadaveric donor. The use of cadaveric donors in the event of failure of the graft is generally accepted. The need for re-transplantation is still very low however, and the survival after re-OLT is high. In patients transplanted for HCC from a living donor within regionally accepted criteria, re-transplantation for graft failure using a cadaveric liver is also possible and accepted by the scientific community. If the transplant from a living donor had been done over the criteria, re-transplant from a cadaver is not recommended [94–98].

8. Inclusion criteria

Currently, in many countries, the eligibility criteria for transplantation for HCC follow "Milan criteria" [9]:

- the presence of a single tumor of less than or equal to 5 cm in size;
- up to three tumors of size less than or equal to 3 cm;
- absence of extrahepatic or lymph node metastases;
- absence of tumor thrombosis of the portal veins, or hepatic veins per liver imaging.

The tumor should be considered unresectablebased on the location, major vessel involvement, or if the tumor is multifocal or the patient has advanced cirrhosis (Child class B or C) [9, 99].

The expansion of the Milan criteria with the criteria of San Francisco (1 nodule < 6.5 cm in diameter or multiple nodules of 4.5 cm in diameter with the sum of the diameters < 8cm) had mixed results in terms of survival (survival at 5 years of 50%); for patients with HCC outside the limits of the criteria of Milan, the survival tends to decrease mainly in the recurrence of disease. Survival that is reduced to less than 50% at five years after transplantation is considered not acceptable. Given the scarcity of available organs, many countries circumscribe selection of patients exclusively to the Milan criteria. In practice, the problem of the shortage of organs is the principal factor influencing the indications for transplantation. Therefore, it became mandatory to tranplant only patients who can reach an adequate survival.

The "United Network of Organ Sharing or UNOS" has rejected the use of CTP classification to prioritize HCC patients on the waiting list, who may have an increased risk of mortality while on the waiting list. The MELD system became the standard method for assessing the clinical severity of a patient potentially candidate for liver transplantation. It is based on a numerical score that takes into account the levels of serum creatinine, total bilirubin and INR. The score is calculated according to the formula:

9.57*log (creatinin mg/dl) + 11.2*log (INR) +3.78*log (Bilirubin mg/dl) + 6.43

This formula calculates the risk of 3-months mortality. Patients with high scores have priority on the waiting list for transplantation [100].

The limit above which a patient can be enrolled into a waiting list is of MELD 15; whenever the MELD is less than 15 the risk of the transplantation is certainly greater than the risk of mortality by three months in the absence of transplantation. Since patients with HCC often have a MELD < 15 and therefore a lower priority of transplantation, UNOS considered to assign all patients with HCC (T1-T2) a MELD of 22, regardless of the actual state of liver disease. This, however, several others factors are still considered.

In addition to the number and size of lesions (Milan criteria) and serum creatinine, bilirubin and INR (MELD score), great importance is also given to the values of the α-FP. Although there is not a cut-off default, in patients with cirrhosis and HCC, if α-FP levels is increasing by more than 15 microg / L per month, liver transplantation is associated with a 5-year survival of less than 54%. Consequently, α-FP is considered a marker of related HCC aggressiveness and therefore should be considered to select potential candidates [101].

9. Prognosis

The main causes of death after liver transplantation are:

- Perioperative generalized morbidity causes such as multi-organ failure, cerebrovascular, cardiovascular, pulmonary and renal complications (29%).
- Recurrence of the primary disease (20%), especially tumors (11%).
- Sepsis (18%), especially bacterial (9%).
- Technical complications (5%), especially bleeding and vascular disorders (3%).
- Rejection (4%), especially chronic (3%).

Intraoperative death and liver failure represent 3% of all deaths.

Over the past 10 years there is a decrease in mortality in the range of 16%.

Survival after transplantation account for 82% at 1 year, 71% at 5 years, 61% at 10 years, 51% at 15 years and 43% at 20 years.

Survival has improved over the time reaching 85% at one year in 2004, compared to 76% in 1990-1994 to only 33% in 1985 (please list reference(s)..). This improvement over the time is most evident in liver transplantation for liver tumor.

From 1988 to 2009, 5-year survival was statistically higher for patients with cirrhosis (72%) than in patients with primary liver cancer (52%). During the last 10 years, post transplant survival for cirrhosis and liver cancer tended to approach (73 vs. 64%).

Moreover, a recent multicenter study from Europe showed that cumulative 1 and 5 year survival for patients transplanted for HCC on cirrhosis is 86% and 70% respectively in patients within the Milan criteria. Patients beyond the Milan criteriahad an average overall 5-year survival of 61.5% (correct?) [92, 102].

Etiology of liver disease and (n. TX)	Years (1999-2009)			
	1 year actuarial survival (%)		5 years actuarial survival (%)	
	Graft (%)	Pazient (%)	Graft (%)	Pazient (%)
Acute hepatic failure (3449)	70	76	62	69
Colostatic disease (4675)	83	89	74	81
Congenital biliary pathology (2167)	84	90	79	87
Cirrhosis (25424)	81	85	69	73
Primary liver tumors (7640)	81	83	61	64
Metastatic tumors (361)	77	83	50	55
Metabolic diseases (2866)	82	87	72	79
Budd Chiari (400)	76	81	66	73

Table 4. Patients and graft survival over the last 10 years (adat from European studies of liver transplant for HCC (correct?). Modified from [92]

10. Follow-up and treatment of recurrence

The main concern for patients subjected to liver transplant for HCC is recurrence that occurs in 8 to 20% (reference). Recurrence usually occurs within the first two years and is associated with a median survival of less than one year from the time of diagnosis (range 7-18 months). The adoption of α-FP assay and imaging (ultrasound, CT and MRI) every six months in the course of the follow-up has resulted in early detection of recurrence, allowing for a possible treatment to more than 1/3 of the cases.

Recent studies have tried to identify the role of post-transplant adjuvant therapy, but results, while highlighting a benefit in terms of overall survival and disease-free interval, are not conclusive because of their variability in terms of chemotherapeutic regimen, dosage, inclusion criteria and end points.

Sorafenib is a tyrosine kinase multi-targeted inhibitor, approved for treatment of patients with advanced HCC. However, its use post-transplant is not permitted outside of clinical trials. Loco-regional therapies for HCC recurrence (RF, TACE) and resection have been used in patients with limited burden of disease and appear to be useful in selected cases. In conclusion, the HCC recurrence after transplantation provides surgery for resectable lesions or through loco-regional therapies or systemic therapies (including Sorafenib) for unresectable lesions. Liver re-transplantation for HCC recurrence is not established [103–106].

11. Summary

Surgical treatment of HCC has evolved over the last 20 years due to improvements in surgical technique, anesthesiologist care and in particular to more appropriate criteria for carrying out resection or liver transplantation. Using systematic screening of at-risk groups has increased the detection of HCC at an early stage, potentially curable.

Survival rates following HCC surgical treatments, which were disappointing in the past, are very high today exceeding 50% at 5 years, both with resection as well as with transplantation in the category of single and small HCC. The choice between transplant and resection is eventually related to liver function that may be compromised by coexisting cirrhosis, and the availability of grafts that is currently lacking.

The biggest flaw of hepatic resection remains its high rate of relapse of the disease. In part, due to true recurrence, and partly due to the emergence of new HCC. In this situation it is possible to consider a transplant rescue, a second resection or local therapy options if the disease is limited to the liver, or systemic therapies if metastatic.

A most relevant concern remains that of high risk HCC for which transplantation is precluded. In this category of HCC resection with very strict indications can still meet a decent expectation of survival.

Author details

Alessandro Uzzau[1*], Maria Laura Pertoldeo[1], Vittorio Cherchi[1], Serena Bertozzi[1], Claudio Avellini[2] and Giorgio Soardo[1]

*Address all correspondence to: alessandro.uzzau@uniud.it, alessandrouzzau@gmail.com

1 Department of Clinical and Experimental Sciences, University of Udine, Italy

2 Department of Biological and Medical Sciences, University of Udine, Italy

References

[1] Ferlay, J, Shin, H. R, Bray, F, Forman, D, Mathers, C, & Parkin, D. M. Estimates of worldwide burden of cancer in 2008: GLOBOCAN (2008). Int J Cancer. 2010;, 127, 2893-2917.

[2] Colombo, M, & De Franchis, R. Del Ninno E, Sangiovanni A, De Fazio C, Tommasini M, et al. Hepatocellular carcinoma in Italian patients with cirrhosis. N Engl J Med. (1991). , 325, 675-680.

[3] Tsukuma, H, Hiyama, T, Tanaka, S, Nakao, M, Yabuuchi, T, Kitamura, T, et al. Risk factors for hepatocellular carcinoma among patients with chronic liver disease. N Engl J Med. (1993). , 328, 1797-1801.

[4] Schafer, D. F, & Sorrell, M. F. Hepatocellular carcinoma. Lancet. (1999). , 353, 1253-1257.

[5] Llovet, J. M, Bustamante, J, Castells, A, & Vilana, R. Ayuso MdC, Sala M, et al. Natural history of untreated nonsurgical hepatocellular carcinoma: rationale for the design and evaluation of therapeutic trials. Hepatology. (1999). , 29, 62-67.

[6] Fan, S. T. Mau Lo C, Poon RTP, Yeung C, Leung Liu C, Yuen WK, et al. Continuous improvement of survival outcomes of resection of hepatocellular carcinoma: a 20-year experience. Ann Surg. (2011). , 253, 745-758.

[7] Fan, S. T, Lo, C. M, Liu, C. L, Lam, C. M, Yuen, W. K, Yeung, C, et al. Hepatectomy for hepatocellular carcinoma: toward zero hospital deaths. Ann Surg. (1999). , 229, 322-330.

[8] Poon RTP, Fan ST, Lo CM, Liu CL, Wong J. Long-term survival and pattern of recurrence after resection of small hepatocellular carcinoma in patients with preserved liver function: implications for a strategy of salvage transplantation. Ann Surg. (2002). , 235, 373-382.

[9] Mazzaferro, V, Regalia, E, Doci, R, Andreola, S, Pulvirenti, A, Bozzetti, F, et al. Liver transplantation for the treatment of small hepatocellular carcinomas in patients with cirrhosis. N Engl J Med. (1996). , 334, 693-699.

[10] Yao, F. Y, Bass, N. M, Ascher, N. L, & Roberts, J. P. Liver transplantation for hepatocellular carcinoma: lessons from the first year under the Model of End-Stage Liver Disease (MELD) organ allocation policy. Liver Transpl. (2004). , 10, 621-630.

[11] Makuuchi, M, Kosuge, T, Takayama, T, Yamazaki, S, Kakazu, T, Miyagawa, S, et al. Surgery for small liver cancers. Semin Surg Oncol. (1993). , 9, 298-304.

[12] American Joint Committee on CancerAjcc Cancer Staging Handbook: Tnm Classification of Malignant Tumors, chapter Liver (including intrahepatic bile ducts). STAT! Ref electronic medical library. Springer, New York, NY. (2002).

[13] American Liver Tumor Study Grouprandomized prospective multi-institutional trial of orthotopic liver transplantation or partial hepatic resection with or without adjuvant chemotherapy for hepatocellular carcinoma: investigators booklet and protocol. Technical report, National Academies Press, Washington, DC. (1998).

[14] United Network for Organ Sharing (UNOS)Liver Transplant Candidates with hepatocellular carcinoma (HCC). http://optn.transplant.hrsa.gov/PoliciesandBylaws2/policies/pdfs/policy_8.pdf. (accessed August 20, (2012).

[15] Child, C. G, & Turcotte, J. G. Surgery and portal hypertension. Major Probl Clin Surg. (1964). , 1, 1-85.

[16] Okuda, K, Ohtsuki, T, Obata, H, Tomimatsu, M, Okazaki, N, Hasegawa, H, et al. Natural history of hepatocellular carcinoma and prognosis in relation to treatment. Study of 850 patients. Cancer. (1985). , 56, 918-928.

[17] Lau, H, Man, K, Fan, S. T, Yu, W. C, Lo, C. M, & Wong, J. Evaluation of preoperative hepatic function in patients with hepatocellular carcinoma undergoing hepatectomy. Br J Surg. (1997). , 84, 1255-1259.

[18] Clavien, P. A, Petrowsky, H, Deoliveira, M. L, & Graf, R. Strategies for safer liver surgery and partial liver transplantation. N Engl J Med. (2007). , 356, 1545-1559.

[19] Poon, R. T, & Fan, S. T. Assessment of hepatic reserve for indication of hepatic resection: how I do it. J Hepatobiliary Pancreat Surg. (2005). , 12, 31-37.

[20] Imamura, H, Sano, K, Sugawara, Y, Kokudo, N, & Makuuchi, M. Assessment of hepatic reserve for indication of hepatic resection: decision tree incorporating indocyanine green test. J Hepatobiliary Pancreat Surg. (2005). , 12, 16-22.

[21] Bruix, J, & Sherman, M. AAftSoLD Practice Guidelines Committee. Management of hepatocellular carcinoma. Hepatology. (2005). , 42, 1208-1236.

[22] Bruix, J, Castells, A, Bosch, J, Feu, F, Fuster, J, Garcia-pagan, J. C, et al. Surgical resection of hepatocellular carcinoma in cirrhotic patients: prognostic value of preoperative portal pressure. Gastroenterology. (1996). , 111, 1018-1022.

[23] Boleslawski, E, Petrovai, G, Truant, S, Dharancy, S, Duhamel, A, Salleron, J, et al. Hepatic venous pressure gradient in the assessment of portal hypertension before liver resection in patients with cirrhosis. Br J Surg. (2012). , 99, 855-863.

[24] Lemoine, M, Katsahian, S, Ziol, M, Nahon, P, Ganne-carrie, N, Kazemi, F, et al. Liver stiffness measurement as a predictive tool of clinically significant portal hypertension in patients with compensated hepatitis C virus or alcohol-related cirrhosis. Aliment Pharmacol Ther. (2008). , 28, 1102-1110.

[25] Robic, M. A, Procopet, B, Métivier, S, Péron, J. M, Selves, J, Vinel, J. P, et al. Liver stiffness accurately predicts portal hypertension related complications in patients with chronic liver disease: a prospective study. J Hepatol. (2011). , 55, 1017-1024.

[26] Bruix, J, & Sherman, M. AAftSoLD. Management of hepatocellular carcinoma: an update. Hepatology. (2011). , 53, 1020-1022.

[27] Omata, M, Lesmana, L. A, Tateishi, R, Chen, P. J, Lin, S. M, Yoshida, H, et al. Asian Pacific Association for the Study of the Liver consensus recommendations on hepatocellular carcinoma. Hepatol Int. (2010). , 4, 439-474.

[28] Schmidt, S, Follmann, M, Malek, N, Manns, M. P, & Greten, T. F. Critical appraisal of clinical practice guidelines for diagnosis and treatment of hepatocellular carcinoma. J Gastroenterol Hepatol. (2011). , 26, 1779-1786.

[29] Bismuth, H, & Majno, P. E. Hepatobiliary surgery. J Hepatol. (2000). , 32, 208-224.

[30] The Liver Cancer Study Group of JapanPredictive factors for long term prognosis after partial hepatectomy for patients with hepatocellular carcinoma in Japan. Cancer. (1994). , 74, 2772-2780.

[31] Arii, S, Yamaoka, Y, Futagawa, S, Inoue, K, Kobayashi, K, Kojiro, M, et al. Results of surgical and nonsurgical treatment for small-sized hepatocellular carcinomas: a retrospective and nationwide survey in Japan. The Liver Cancer Study Group of Japan. Hepatology. (2000). , 32, 1224-1229.

[32] Cucchetti, A, Piscaglia, F, Cescon, M, Ercolani, G, Terzi, E, Bolondi, L, et al. Conditional survival after hepatic resection for hepatocellular carcinoma in cirrhotic patients. Clin Cancer Res. (2012). , 18, 4397-4405.

[33] Llovet, J. M, Burroughs, A, & Bruix, J. Hepatocellular carcinoma. Lancet. (2003). , 362, 1907-1917.

[34] OPTNOrgan Procurement and Transplantation Network. (2010). http://optn.transplant.hrsa.gov/.accessed July 27, 2012).

[35] Vitale, A, Boccagni, P, Brolese, A, Neri, D, Srsen, N, Zanus, G, et al. Progression of hepatocellular carcinoma before liver transplantation: dropout or liver transplantation? Transplant Proc. (2009). , 41, 1264-1267.

[36] Pelletier, S. J, Fu, S, Thyagarajan, V, Romero-marrero, C, Batheja, M. J, Punch, J. D, et al. An intention-to-treat analysis of liver transplantation for hepatocellular carcinoma using organ procurement transplant network data. Liver Transpl. (2009). , 15, 859-868.

[37] Facciuto, M. E, Rochon, C, Pandey, M, Rodriguez-davalos, M, Samaniego, S, Wolf, D. C, et al. Surgical dilemma: liver resection or liver transplantation for hepatocellular carcinoma and cirrhosis. Intention-to-treat analysis in patients within and outwith Milan criteria. HPB (Oxford). (2009). , 11, 398-404.

[38] Yao, F. Y, & Roberts, J. P. Applying expanded criteria to liver transplantation for hepatocellular carcinoma: too much too soon, or is now the time? Liver Transpl. (2004). , 10, 919-921.

[39] Poon RTPFan ST, Lo CM, Liu CL, Wong J. Difference in tumor invasiveness in cirrhotic patients with hepatocellular carcinoma fulfilling the Milan criteria treated by resection and transplantation: impact on long-term survival. Ann Surg. (2007). , 245, 51-58.

[40] Cha, C. H, Ruo, L, Fong, Y, Jarnagin, W. R, Shia, J, Blumgart, L. H, et al. Resection of hepatocellular carcinoma in patients otherwise eligible for transplantation. Ann Surg. (2003). discussion 321-3., 238, 315-21.

[41] Del Gaudio MErcolani G, Ravaioli M, Cescon M, Lauro A, Vivarelli M, et al. Liver transplantation for recurrent hepatocellular carcinoma on cirrhosis after liver resection: University of Bologna experience. Am J Transplant. (2008). , 8, 1177-1185.

[42] Fan, S. T. Poon RTP, Yeung C, Lam CM, Lo CM, Yuen WK, et al. Outcome after partial hepatectomy for hepatocellular cancer within the Milan criteria. Br J Surg. (2011). , 98, 1292-1300.

[43] Lim, K. C. Chow PKH, Allen JC, Chia GS, Lim M, Cheow PC, et al. Microvascular invasion is a better predictor of tumor recurrence and overall survival following surgical resection for hepatocellular carcinoma compared to the Milan criteria. Ann Surg. (2011). , 254, 108-113.

[44] Kamiyama, T, Nakanishi, K, Yokoo, H, Kamachi, H, Tahara, M, Suzuki, T, et al. Recurrence patterns after hepatectomy of hepatocellular carcinoma: implication of Milan criteria utilization. Ann Surg Oncol. (2009). , 16, 1560-1571.

[45] Taura, K, Ikai, I, Hatano, E, Yasuchika, K, Nakajima, A, Tada, M, et al. Influence of coexisting cirrhosis on outcomes after partial hepatic resection for hepatocellular carcinoma fulfilling the Milan criteria: an analysis of 293 patients. Surgery. (2007). , 142, 685-694.

[46] Merchant, N, David, C. S, & Cunningham, S. C. Early Hepatocellular Carcinoma: Transplantation versus Resection: The Case for Liver Resection. Int J Hepatol. (2011).

[47] Tanaka, S, Noguchi, N, Ochiai, T, Kudo, A, Nakamura, N, Ito, K, et al. Outcomes and recurrence of initially resectable hepatocellular carcinoma meeting milan criteria: Rationale for partial hepatectomy as first strategy. J Am Coll Surg. (2007). , 204, 1-6.

[48] Sumie, S, Kuromatsu, R, Okuda, K, Ando, E, Takata, A, Fukushima, N, et al. Microvascular invasion in patients with hepatocellular carcinoma and its predictable clinicopathological factors. Ann Surg Oncol. (2008). , 15, 1375-1382.

[49] Belghiti, J, Cortes, A, Abdalla, E. K, Régimbeau, J. M, Prakash, K, Durand, F, et al. Resection prior to liver transplantation for hepatocellular carcinoma. Ann Surg. (2003). discussion 892-3., 238, 885-92.

[50] Makuuchi, M, Imamura, H, Sugawara, Y, & Takayama, T. Progress in surgical treatment of hepatocellular carcinoma. Oncology. (2002). Suppl , 1, 74-81.

[51] Chouillard, E, Cherqui, D, Tayar, C, Brunetti, F, & Fagniez, P. L. Anatomical bi- and trisegmentectomies as alternatives to extensive liver resections. Ann Surg. (2003). , 238, 29-34.

[52] Zhou, X. D, Tang, Z. Y, Yang, B. H, Lin, Z. Y, Ma, Z. C, Ye, S. L, et al. Experience of 1000 patients who underwent hepatectomy for small hepatocellular carcinoma. Cancer. (2001). , 91, 1479-1486.

[53] Bismuth, H. Surgical anatomy and anatomical surgery of the liver. World J Surg. (1982). , 6, 3-9.

[54] Kosuge, T, Makuuchi, M, Takayama, T, Yamamoto, J, Shimada, K, & Yamasaki, S. Long-term results after resection of hepatocellular carcinoma: experience of 480 cases. Hepatogastroenterology. (1993). , 40, 328-332.

[55] Young, A. L, Malik, H. Z, Abu-hilal, M, Guthrie, J. A, Wyatt, J, Prasad, K. R, et al. Large hepatocellular carcinoma: time to stop preoperative biopsy. J Am Coll Surg. (2007). , 205, 453-462.

[56] Wang, B. W, Mok, K. T, Liu, S. I, Chou, N. H, Tsai, C. C, Chen, I. S, et al. Is hepatectomy beneficial in the treatment of multinodular hepatocellular carcinoma? J Formos Med Assoc. (2008). , 107, 616-626.

[57] Ishizawa, T, Hasegawa, K, Aoki, T, Takahashi, M, Inoue, Y, Sano, K, et al. Neither multiple tumors nor portal hypertension are surgical contraindications for hepatocellular carcinoma. Gastroenterology. (2008). , 134, 1908-1916.

[58] Ng, K. K, Vauthey, J. N, Pawlik, T. M, Lauwers, G. Y, Regimbeau, J. M, Belghiti, J, et al. Is hepatic resection for large or multinodular hepatocellular carcinoma justified? Results from a multi-institutional database. Ann Surg Oncol. (2005). , 12, 364-373.

[59] Pawlik, T. M, Poon, R. T, Abdalla, E. K, Ikai, I, Nagorney, D. M, Belghiti, J, et al. Hepatectomy for hepatocellular carcinoma with major portal or hepatic vein invasion: results of a multicenter study. Surgery. (2005). , 137, 403-410.

[60] Choi, D, Lim, H. K, Joh, J. W, Kim, S. J, Kim, M. J, Rhim, H, et al. Combined hepatectomy and radiofrequency ablation for multifocal hepatocellular carcinomas: long-term follow-up results and prognostic factors. Ann Surg Oncol. (2007). , 14, 3510-3518.

[61] Liu, C. L, Fan, S. T, & Lo, C. M. Ng IOL, Poon RTP, Wong J. Hepatic resection for bilobar hepatocellular carcinoma: is it justified? Arch Surg. (2003). , 138, 100-104.

[62] Ikai, I, Yamamoto, Y, Yamamoto, N, Terajima, H, Hatano, E, Shimahara, Y, et al. Results of hepatic resection for hepatocellular carcinoma invading major portal and/or hepatic veins. Surg Oncol Clin N Am. (2003). ix., 12, 65-75.

[63] Rahbari, N. N, Mehrabi, A, Mollberg, N. M, Müller, S. A, Koch, M, Büchler, M. W, et al. Hepatocellular carcinoma: current management and perspectives for the future. Ann Surg. (2011). , 253, 453-469.

[64] Truty, M. J, & Vauthey, J. N. Surgical resection of high-risk hepatocellular carcinoma: patient selection, preoperative considerations, and operative technique. Ann Surg Oncol. (2010). , 17, 1219-1225.

[65] Agrawal, S, & Belghiti, J. Oncologic resection for malignant tumors of the liver. Ann Surg. (2011). , 253, 656-665.

[66] Bruix, J, & Llovet, J. M. Prognostic prediction and treatment strategy in hepatocellular carcinoma. Hepatology. (2002). , 35, 519-524.

[67] Bruix, J, & Llovet, J. M. Locoregional treatments for hepatocellular carcinoma. Baillieres Best Pract Res Clin Gastroenterol. (1999). , 13, 611-622.

[68] Lin, C. T, Hsu, K. F, Chen, T. W, Yu, J. C, Chan, D. C, Yu, C. Y, et al. Comparing hepatic resection and transarterial chemoembolization for Barcelona Clinic Liver Cancer (BCLC) stage B hepatocellular carcinoma: change for treatment of choice? World J Surg. (2010). , 34, 2155-2161.

[69] Delis, S. G, Bakoyiannis, A, Tassopoulos, N, Athanassiou, K, Kechagias, A, Kelekis, D, et al. Hepatic resection for large hepatocellular carcinoma in the era of UCSF criteria. HPB (Oxford). (2009). , 11, 551-558.

[70] Wu, C. C, Hsieh, S. R, Chen, J. T, Ho, W. L, Lin, M. C, Yeh, D. C, et al. An appraisal of liver and portal vein resection for hepatocellular carcinoma with tumor thrombi extending to portal bifurcation. Arch Surg. (2000). , 135, 1273-1279.

[71] Minagawa, M, Makuuchi, M, Takayama, T, & Ohtomo, K. Selection criteria for hepatectomy in patients with hepatocellular carcinoma and portal vein tumor thrombus. Ann Surg. (2001). , 233, 379-384.

[72] Hemming, A. W, Reed, A. I, Langham, M. R, Fujita, S, Van Der Werf, W. J, & Howard, R. J. Hepatic vein reconstruction for resection of hepatic tumors. Ann Surg. (2002). , 235, 850-858.

[73] Kokudo, N, & Makuuchi, M. Evidence-based clinical practice guidelines for hepatocellular carcinoma in Japan: the J-HCC guidelines. J Gastroenterol. (2009). Suppl , 19, 119-121.

[74] Jarnagin, W, Chapman, W. C, Curley, S, Angelica, D, Rosen, M, & Dixon, C. E, et al. Surgical treatment of hepatocellular carcinoma: expert consensus statement. HPB (Oxford). (2010). , 12, 302-310.

[75] Poon, D, Anderson, B. O, Chen, L. T, Tanaka, K, Lau, W. Y, Van Cutsem, E, et al. Management of hepatocellular carcinoma in Asia: consensus statement from the Asian Oncology Summit (2009). Lancet Oncol. 2009;, 10, 1111-1118.

[76] Sano, K, Makuuchi, M, Miki, K, Maema, A, Sugawara, Y, Imamura, H, et al. Evaluation of hepatic venous congestion: proposed indication criteria for hepatic vein reconstruction. Ann Surg. (2002). , 236, 241-247.

[77] Lau, W. Y. Lai ECH, Lau SHY. Methods of vascular control technique during liver resection: a comprehensive review. Hepatobiliary Pancreat Dis Int. (2010). , 9, 473-481.

[78] Winbladh, A, Björnsson, B, Trulsson, L, Offenbartl, K, Gullstrand, P, & Sandström, P. Ischemic preconditioning prior to intermittent Pringle maneuver in liver resections. J Hepatobiliary Pancreat Sci. (2012). , 19, 159-170.

[79] Scatton, O, Zalinski, S, Jegou, D, Compagnon, P, Lesurtel, M, Belghiti, J, et al. Randomized clinical trial of ischaemic preconditioning in major liver resection with intermittent Pringle manoeuvre. Br J Surg. (2011). , 98, 1236-1243.

[80] Van Wagensveld, B. A, Van Gulik, T. M, Gelderblom, H. C, Scheepers, J. J, Bosma, A, Endert, E, et al. Prolonged continuous or intermittent vascular inflow occlusion during hemihepatectomy in pigs. Ann Surg. (1999). , 229, 376-384.

[81] Belghiti, J, Noun, R, Malafosse, R, Jagot, P, Sauvanet, A, Pierangeli, F, et al. Continuous versus intermittent portal triad clamping for liver resection: a controlled study. Ann Surg. (1999). , 229, 369-375.

[82] Murry, C. E, Jennings, R. B, & Reimer, K. A. Preconditioning with ischemia: a delay of lethal cell injury in ischemic myocardium. Circulation. (1986). , 74, 1124-1136.

[83] Jones, R. M, Moulton, C. E, & Hardy, K. J. Central venous pressure and its effect on blood loss during liver resection. Br J Surg. (1998). , 85, 1058-1060.

[84] Smyrniotis, V, Kostopanagiotou, G, Theodoraki, K, Tsantoulas, D, & Contis, J. C. The role of central venous pressure and type of vascular control in blood loss during major liver resections. Am J Surg. (2004). , 187, 398-402.

[85] Johnson, M, Mannar, R, & Wu, A. V. Correlation between blood loss and inferior vena caval pressure during liver resection. Br J Surg. (1998). , 85, 188-190.

[86] Cunningham, J. D, Fong, Y, Shriver, C, Melendez, J, Marx, W. L, & Blumgart, L. H. One hundred consecutive hepatic resections. Blood loss, transfusion, and operative technique. Arch Surg. (1994). , 129, 1050-1056.

[87] Doklestic, K, Karamarkovic, A, Stefanovic, B, Stefanovic, B, Milic, N, Gregoric, P, et al. The efficacy of three transection techniques of the liver resection: a randomized clinical trial. Hepatogastroenterology. (2012). , 59, 1501-1506.

[88] Schindl, M. J, & Redhead, D. N. Fearon KCH, Garden OJ, Wigmore SJ, ELS, et al. The value of residual liver volume as a predictor of hepatic dysfunction and infection after major liver resection. Gut. (2005). , 54, 289-296.

[89] Yigitler, C, Farges, O, Kianmanesh, R, Regimbeau, J. M, Abdalla, E. K, & Belghiti, J. The small remnant liver after major liver resection: how common and how relevant? Liver Transpl. (2003). SS25., 18.

[90] Madoff, D. C, Hicks, M. E, Vauthey, J. N, & Charnsangavej, C. Morello FA Jr, Ahrar K, et al. Transhepatic portal vein embolization: anatomy, indications, and technical considerations. Radiographics. (2002). , 22, 1063-1076.

[91] Farges, O, Belghiti, J, Kianmanesh, R, Regimbeau, J. M, Santoro, R, Vilgrain, V, et al. Portal vein embolization before right hepatectomy: prospective clinical trial. Ann Surg. (2003). , 237, 208-217.

[92] Adam, R, Karam, V, Delvart, V, Grady, O, Mirza, J, & Klempnauer, D. J, et al. Evolution of indications and results of liver transplantation in Europe. A report from the European Liver Transplant Registry (ELTR). J Hepatol. (2012). , 57, 675-688.

[93] Samuel, D, Colombo, M, Serag, H, Sobesky, R, & Heaton, N. Toward optimizing the indications for orthotopic liver transplantation in hepatocellular carcinoma. Liver Transpl. (2011). Suppl 2:S, 6-13.

[94] Pomfret, E. A. Lodge JPA, Villamil FG, Siegler M. Should we use living donor grafts for patients with hepatocellular carcinoma? Ethical considerations. Liver Transpl. (2011). Suppl 2:SS132., 128.

[95] Grant, D, Fisher, R. A, Abecassis, M, Mccaughan, G, Wright, L, & Fan, S. T. Should the liver transplant criteria for hepatocellular carcinoma be different for deceased donation and living donation? Liver Transpl. (2011). Suppl 2:SS138., 133.

[96] Greig, P. D, Geier, A, Alessandro, D, Campbell, A. M, & Wright, M. L. Should we perform deceased donor liver transplantation after living donor liver transplantation has failed? Liver Transpl. (2011). Suppl 2:SS146., 139.

[97] Vakili, K, Pomposelli, J. J, Cheah, Y. L, Akoad, M, Lewis, W. D, Khettry, U, et al. Living donor liver transplantation for hepatocellular carcinoma: Increased recurrence but improved survival. Liver Transpl. (2009). , 15, 1861-1866.

[98] Cronin, D. C. nd, Millis JM. Living donor liver transplantation: The ethics and the practice. Hepatology. (2008). , 47, 11-13.

[99] Mazzaferro, V, Bhoori, S, Sposito, C, Bongini, M, Langer, M, Miceli, R, et al. Milan criteria in liver transplantation for hepatocellular carcinoma: an evidence-based analysis of 15 years of experience. Liver Transpl. (2011). Suppl 2:SS57., 44.

[100] Wiesner, R. H, Mcdiarmid, S. V, Kamath, P. S, Edwards, E. B, Malinchoc, M, Kremers, W. K, et al. MELD and PELD: application of survival models to liver allocation. Liver Transpl. (2001). , 7, 567-580.

[101] Vibert, E, Azoulay, D, Hoti, E, Iacopinelli, S, Samuel, D, Salloum, C, et al. Progression of alphafetoprotein before liver transplantation for hepatocellular carcinoma in cirrhotic patients: a critical factor. Am J Transplant. (2010). , 10, 129-137.

[102] Li, H. Y, Wei, Y. G, Yan, L. N, & Li, B. Salvage liver transplantation in the treatment of hepatocellular carcinoma: a meta-analysis. World J Gastroenterol. (2012). , 18, 2415-2422.

[103] Zimmerman, M. A, Ghobrial, R. M, Tong, M. J, Hiatt, J. R, Cameron, A. M, Hong, J, et al. Recurrence of hepatocellular carcinoma following liver transplantation: a review of preoperative and postoperative prognostic indicators. Arch Surg. (2008). discussion 188., 143, 182-8.

[104] Hsieh, C. B, Chou, S. J, Shih, M. L, Chu, H. C, Chu, C. H, Yu, J. C, et al. Preliminary experience with gemcitabine and cisplatin adjuvant chemotherapy after liver transplantation for hepatocellular carcinoma. Eur J Surg Oncol. (2008). , 34, 906-910.

[105] Taketomi, A, Fukuhara, T, Morita, K, Kayashima, H, Ninomiya, M, Yamashita, Y, et al. Improved results of a surgical resection for the recurrence of hepatocellular carcinoma after living donor liver transplantation. Ann Surg Oncol. (2010). , 17, 2283-2289.

[106] Davis, E, Wiesner, R, Valdecasas, J, Kita, Y, Rossi, M, & Schwartz, M. Treatment of recurrent hepatocellular carcinoma after liver transplantation. Liver Transpl. (2011). Suppl 2:SS166., 162.

Chapter 9

Conditions that Predispose to the Development of HCC: The Role of Tumor Associated Fibroblasts and of microRNA

C. Avellini, D. Cesselli, A.P. Beltrami, M. Orsaria,
S. Marzinotto, F. Morassi and S. Uzzau

Additional information is available at the end of the chapter

http://dx.doi.org/10.5772/56951

1. Introduction

The high frequency of cases of hepatocellular carcinoma (HCC) led to vigorous efforts to identify the biological behavior and the pathogenetic mechanisms of this disease. The estimated 564.000 new cases worldwide and almost the same number of deaths in 2000 make it necessary to understand how to treat and control HCC [1]. This is possible acquiring a deep knowledge of the natural history of the disease, particularly of its initial steps which bring the parenchyma to the first changes and expose the cells to chronic insults, leading to a long standing disease endowed with a high risk of cancer development.

The pathogenesis of HCC is a complex phenomenon-, given the high number of variables and factors involved in liver function and of the possible pathway activation or deregulation during liver disease.

The first valuable step is based upon the death of hepatocytes: different pathological conditions able to induce hepatocyte damage and death will determine recruitment of inflammatory cells and deposition of connective tissue.

On the one hand this fact shows the relatively limited range of liver parenchyma response to various kind of damage. The structure and function of the organ are associated with necroinflammatory, fibrotic and cholestatic changes as the main phenomena which the parenchyma response to damage is able to produce.

On the other hand, this kind of elementary lesions is mostly self-maintaining: in fact, some of the main consequences of hepatocyte destruction and fibrotic parenchymal substitution are the changes in blood flow and in the composition and function of both extracellular matrix and microenvironment of the liver [1], which heavily influence hepatocyte life and function.

There is a strict connection between different phenomena concerning the liver in normal and pathological conditions. Chronic inflammation and fibrosis are well known as the main changes leading to neoplasia harboring in the majority of chronic liver diseases; but some insights into the mechanisms and the cellular types which can act either in organ development, or in regenerative and neoplastic processes represent one of the objective of this text. At this regard, a particular role in the relationship between microenvironment and liver cells proliferation concerns tumor associated fibroblasts (TAFs), considered critical for tumor growth and progression.

Experimental studies in solid tumors other than HCC suggest a possible origin of these cells from mesenchymal stem cells derived from the bone marrow, but in vitro human models lack. These cells exert important functions in cirrhotic and neoplastic liver parenchyma: recently it has been demonstrated the presence in human neoplastic livers of a population of multipotent adult stem cells with properties of tumor associated fibroblasts, while a population of MASCs derived TAFs is already present in cirrhotic, not yet neoplastic parenchyma. Furthermore, mesenchymal stem cells isolated from non-neoplastic and non-cirrhotic livers can acquire a TAF phenotype when grown in a medium conditioned by tumor cell lines [2]

After a brief evaluation of the main factors playing important roles in the pathogenesis and progression of hepatocellular carcinoma (pathways deregulation with respect to morphological changes, molecular factors and pathways cross-talk influencing interplay between different cellular elements, role of extracellular matrix and angiogenesis), the relationship between liver embryogenesis, regeneration and neoplastic growths is considered, inparticular as far as the interplay between parenchymal cells and stromal component in non-neoplastic and neoplastic liver is concerned. Further deeper look is addressed to more recent progresses, which can really offer new important insights in the pathogenesis and treatment of hepatocellular carcinoma: microRNA deregulation and tumor associated fibroblasts. The former show a great potential in targeting a lot of genes involved in the neoplastic process: different tumors in different organs show strict relationships with the effects of groups of miRNA similarly associated for some organs, giving rise to signatures characteristic of neoplastic development, able to predict prognosis and to represent targets for new therapeutic chances. Similar results come from the action of miRNA in hepatocellular carcinoma, where distinct tumor subtypes are associated with different miRNA signature.

Tumor associated fibroblasts represent a population of stromal cells able to influence in crucial ways the parenchymal microenvironment changes which accompany all steps of HCC development, from the origin to progression and diffusion.

1.1. Growth factors and molecular pathways

With the ongoing of the pathological process the proliferation of liver cells accelerates and monoclonal populations occur: this is the hallmark of all preneoplastic lesions and takes places also in HCC. From this point of view the foci of phenotypically altered hepatocytes represent the first discrete step, morphologically identifiable, in the way leading to cancer.

The foci of altered hepatocytes contain differentiated hepatocytes that have acquired molecular aberrations and changed their metabolic properties [3]: this may allow the progress to malignant phenotype. These cells and their morphological and biochemical phenotype are unstable and, given the absence of uniformity in foci, the clonal origin is partly suggested: at least 8 cytomorphological and cytochemical atypical foci types exist [3]. These premalignant changes represent perhaps one of the first effects of viral or environmental damage.

The main etiological agents of HCC are well known: HBV,HCV and Aflatoxin B1 are considered causative agents of about 80% of cases [1]. During last years a lot of genomic aberrations have been identified and the mechanisms of interaction at molecular level between liver cells and etiologic agents in producing gene changes responsible of the development of neoplasia have been studied and often understood [1].

After the production of foci of altered hepatocytes, the subsequent step, morphologically defined, is represented by the formation of dysplastic foci and dysplastic nodules: in these lesions, probably, molecular changes can take further development with a selection of genetic and epigenetic changes leading to a proliferative advantage for altered hepatocytes and to the involvement of several regulatory pathways in simultaneous disorders favoring the passage from dysplastic to neoplastic lesion.

The simple increase in cell proliferation and DNA synthesis associated with increasing enzymatic and metabolic changes is not enough to give rise to carcinogenesis.

The production of growth factors and hormones (e.g. Insulin, IGF2, TGF alfa, TGF beta, HGF, Transferrin, VEGF), of cytokines and chemokines and the activation or deregulation of different pathways give an essential contribution to the development of neoplasia, but the whole mechanism of the transformation from dysplastic to fully neoplastic lesion is not yet completely understood.

A crucial element to consider in this context comes from the interaction between the different cell types present in liver parenchyma.

For example, hepatocyte proliferation is regulated by cytokines (especially IL-6) produced by Kupffer cells as well as by endothelial cells and hepatic stellate cells. On the other hand, hepatocytes modulate sinusoidal endothelium phenotype and its production of prostaglandins, endothelin, IL-1 e IL-6 and Hepatocyte Growth Factor [4]. Moreover, the complexity of cross talk between cellular types is relevant in the relationship between hepatocytes and hepatic stellate cells: the production of peptides stimulating hepatic stellate cells proliferation leads to the increased production of cytokines by hepatic stellate cells. These latter are able either to inhibit or to stimulate hepatocyte proliferation [5]. For example, TGF-beta produced by hepatic stellate cells can act as an inhibitor of liver cells replication; moreover, IL-6 response is downregulated by SOCS-3 (suppressor of cytokine signaling 3) with blocking of JAK mediated STAT-3 activation [4, 5].

Regarding the interaction between hepatocytes and Kupffer cells, growth factors and cytokines activate critical transcription factors, such as AP-1, NFkB, STAT-3, inducing Kupffer cells activation and production of IL-6 thus increasing liver cell DNA synthesis [5].

1.2. Extracellular matrix

The site where the described interactions take place is not a silent structure away from any biochemical activity: the relationship between hepatocytes and extracellular matrix is particularly active and crucial [3].

A lot of adhesion molecules and receptor mediating cell-matrix binding are present.

Extracellular matrix acts as a reservoir and presenter of cell growth factors and cytokines; it undergoes a rapid turnover and significant modifications, often induced by liver parenchymal and non-parenchymal cells, through the production of matrix-degrading enzymes, such as metalloproteinases, and their inhibitors which control the extracellular matrix degradation. Soluble mediators able to influence hepatic stellate cells and Kupffer cells induce the production of proteinases which may initiate the process of matrix degradation. Kupffer cells adhesion on endothelial cells via CD4 and ICAM-1 produce hepatic stellate cells stimulating factors: again, hepatic stellate cells, modulated by hepatocytes, endothelial cells, Kupffer cells, platelets and inflammatory cells play a role in fibrogenesis and liver morphogenesis.

When extracellular matrix at sinusoidal subendothelial level undergoes some kind of disruption, hepatocytes can lose their differentiated function and morphofunctional changes take place: altered porosity in sinusoidal barrier and impaired movement of solutes and macromolecules into and out of Disse spaces favor fibrogenetic progression, with further functional impairment. In particular, extracellular matrix turnover and degradation are under the control of different factors, either at extracellular (metalloproteinases) or intracellular level (lysosomalcathepsins) [3].

Collagenases acting on fibrillar collagen, stromelysins (degrading collagen IV, gelatin, laminin, fibronectin), gelatinase, neutrophilic collagenase (acting on collagen I and III) and so on parallel the activity of molecules expressed by hepatocytes and hepatic stellate cells, functioning as inhibitors of metalloproteinases (tissue inhibitors of metalloproteinases 1 and 2 and alfa 2 macroglobulin), with a regulation of relative gene expression by same cytokines and growth factors as metalloproteinases [3].

Interstitial collagenase activity is increased in liver fibrosis, mainly during the early development of extensive lesions, but diminishes with advanced cirrhosis.

1.3. Angiogenesis

Fibrogenetic progression with Disse spaces fibrosis and sinusoidal capillarization induces great impairment particularly in hepatocellular secretion of proteins (albumin, clotting factors, lipoproteins), associated with dramatic changes in fluid dynamics [3].

Genetic changes and local hypoxia may lead to secretion of soluble angiogenic factors, with a complex interplay between cells, basal membranes and pro-or antiangiogenic factors.

The proangiogenetic factors exert their influence in particular by activating endothelial cells, which, when activated, loose interendothelial cells contacts and breakdown the surrounding basement membrane and extracellular matrix: the associated phenomena of proliferation and migration of endothelial cells are widened by further secretion of angiogenic factors,formerlysequestered in perivascular extracellular matrix. The secretion of protease induces the release of free vascular endothelial growth factor which stimulates endothelial cells [6, 7].

Endothelial cells proliferation and migration is followed by the tendency to assemble in tubular structures, with subsequent basement membrane material production and pericytes (supportive vascular smooth muscle cells) recruitment through the action of PDGF beta: these newly formed vascular channels nevertheless show irregular and variable diameter, with abnormal branching pattern, incomplete structure of basement membrane and only partialpericytes cover, which represent the main characteristics of new vascular channels associated with the development of neoplastic growth at the beginning. The process go on when phenomena ofhypoxia in the central area of the tumoror some viral component if present (for example HBX protein) stimulate the production of Hipoxia Inducible Factor-1alfa, followed by the action of VEGF glycoproteins (A,B,C,D and placental growth factor) on corresponding receptors (flt1 and flk1) on endothelial cells. It has been demonstrated that Trans arterial chemoembolization (TACE) for hepatocellular carcinoma treatment is followed by parallel increase of VEGF expression related to microvascular density and hypoxia [6, 7], which confirms the relationship between ischemia and reactive neoangiogenesis.

Angiogenic stimuli produce different effects in normal, cirrhotic and neoplastic liver parenchyma:within normal and regenerating tissue new functional sinusoids appear, while in chronic liver disease capillarized vascular structures take place [7].

The high number of complex interplays, here rapidly summarized, underlines the crucial connection between parenchymal cells, non-parenchymal cells and extracellular matrix, including vascular component. Again this phenomenon-show significantsimilarities between different physiological and pathological events involving the liver.

2. Liver development, regeneration, neoplasia: The role of stem cells

It has been recognized the existence, in the liver, of a strict connection between development, regeneration, and carcinogenesis [8, 9]. As a consequence, researchers are trying to dissect the molecular mechanisms regulating liver homeostasis, the comprehension of which could open the way to new targeted therapies for liver regeneration, liver cirrhosis and primary liver cancers [8, 9].

Liver development involves complex mechanisms. Multipotent tissue specific progenitor cells, derived from blastocyst inner cell mass stem cells, give rise to the different organs [8]. Specifically, fibroblast growth factor (FGF) from the cardiac mesoderm, through a coordination of signaling with bone morphogenic proteins from the septum transversum mesenchyme, influences the hepatic induction [10-14]. In fact, committed foregut endoderm elements, through WNT signaling, promote liver bud emergence [15-17]: hepatoblasts invade the septum transversum mesenchyme to give rise to liver bud and proliferate under the influence of mesenchymal cells derived cytokines and growth factors, such as FGF, HGF and TGF beta [18-21] and of neighboring endothelial cells signaling.

The hepatoblasts show bipotential characteristic and specific pathways induce their differentiation into hepatocytes or biliary epithelium, respectively. Some studies suggest the ductal plate as the site of fetal liver progenitor cells, with 4 hypothetical anatomic compartments [22]: hepatocytes which meet the canal of Hering, pankeratin positive cells in the canal of Hering, intraductalcholagiocytes, peribiliary" null" cells.

After injury, liver regeneration processes are strictly related to the extent of the loss of liver parenchyma [8] Specifically, after experimental partial hepatectomy, mass restoration is mainly due to mitotic division of mature liver cells [23], while when this regenerative capacity is overwhelmed by massive parenchymal loss, for example in chronic liver disease, mass regeneration implies the activation of a liver progenitor cell compartment [22]. The molecular pathways activated in this latter case suggest a recapitulation of the fetal development [8]. In fact progenitor cells phenotypes and antigenic profiling are similar to fetal liver: these cells are located at the canal of Hering; the presence of label retaining cells within the iuxta portal, proximal biliary tree (slow cycling cells which retain Bromodeoxyuridin (BRDU) label for 8 weeks after experimental injury related cell division) confirm this site as a possible stem cell niche [22]. Similar observations concern peribiliary hepatocytes, mostly identified as BRDU positive very early in post-injury period, at variance with mid-acinar and central acinar hepatocytes, involved in rapid turnover for regenerative response to the loss of parenchyma. On the other hand, intraductalcholangiocytes and peribiliary "null" cells are less likely to take a role in the niche population, due also to the difficult evaluation of their relationship with neighbor liver parenchyma [22].

Liver regeneration takes places within some days or few weeks from the insult. After experimental partial hepatectomy, inflammatory cells produce TNF-alfa which damages surviving cells, but induces DNA synthesis and adult liver cells proliferation; this mechanism needs the presence of a specific receptor on hepatocytes (Tumor necrosis factor Receptor 1). TNFR1-null mice can nevertheless grow to adulthood, demonstrating the possible development also in the absence of this interaction TNF alfa-TNFR1. This is simply one out of several mechanisms (such as the action of drugs or hormones) which increase hepatocyte proliferation, while interaction with TNF is not a unique way for liver development [24]: although TNF production and Glutation (GSH) synthesis represent rapid reaction to experimental hepatectomy, TNF simply activates different factors (such as NFKB and SEK-1, a stress related kinase) that permit hepatocytes to survive to TNF exposure. "Surviving hepatocytes are then surveyed for damage and repaired or deleted" [24]: this is a defensive, initial mechanism that, together with antiapoptotic and antioxidant factors, makepossible subsequent parenchymal regeneration. All these observations show a complex picture of stress regulated intracellular signals that allow adult hepatocytes to proliferate, to survive without proliferation or to dye.

Chronic inflammatory response, growth factors and DNA damaging agents (including ROS) also play a role [25, 26], favoring the involvement of progenitor cells in regenerative / proliferative activity and therefore probably also favoring tumor development.

Type and duration of exposure to ROS, increasing after cellular stress, play a pivotal role in choosing the direction of cells destiny. An acute and transient increase in ROS is necessary for proto-oncogenes and growth factors to induce cellular proliferation [24]. Interestingly, similarly toregenerative response, with H-RAS mediated proliferative activity, malignant transformation also requires K-RAS proto-oncogene activation, inducing ERK 1-2 activation [24]. Surviving hepatocytes surveillance could therefore be overwhelmed by stress induced proliferative stimuli associated to malignant transformation.

On the one hand, normal livers, which undergone experimental hepatectomy, show a regenerative, mitotic response starting from adult hepatocytes. On the other hand, in the presence of a chronic parenchymal damage, the response isbased upon progenitor cells, with molecular signaling patterns that suggest a recapitulation of fetal development [8].

A part from experimental parenchymal damage, chronic ethanol consumption generally increases the death rate of mature hepatocytes. This stimulates a compensatory regenerative response to preserve normal liver mass and function. Nevertheless, most of the mature hepatocytes that survive in alcohol damaged livers are replicatively senescent and hence incapable of proliferating to replace their dead neighbors, given the chronic alcohol exposure which inhibits the induction of DNA synthesis. Hence, regeneration of alcohol damaged livers involves the expansion and differentiation of facultative liver progenitor cells [24]. This regenerative mechanism requires lengthening the time needed for liver mass reconstitution, due to the time necessary for differentiation of progenitor cells.

On the whole, the reparative processes take advantage of two principal strategies of defense, depending on the extent of the damage [8]. While mild injury is mainly repaired through compensatory hyperplasia of hepatocytes, severe damage implies the activation of a liver progenitor cell compartment [27]. In both cases, other non-parenchymal cells (stellate cells, vascular and biliary cells) proliferate as soon as hepatocytes starts to [27]and cooperate to restore morphofunctional competent liver tissue. In rodent experimental models with chronic liver injury.

HGF and EGF promote the upregulation of proliferation rate and expansion of oval cells, while TGF-beta exerts the opposite effect on oval cells [28-31], with an upregulation of the WNT-Beta Catenin pathway in acute and chronic liver injury experimental models [8]. These data again suggest symmetry between fetal development and regenerative mechanisms. Molecular mechanisms involved in fetal development, when identified, can allow to target pathways connected with parenchymal damage: tyrosine kinase inhibitors, for instance, are able to inhibit progenitor cell response, liver fibrosis and liver cancer development in a mouse model of chronic liver injury [32]; C-kit inhibition by imatinibmesylate attenuates progenitor cell expansion and inhibits liver tumor formation in mice [32].

Therefore, the presence of pathways playing a role either in fetal development or in regenerative but also in neoplastic phenomena opens important perspectives: three distinct cell lineages can be found in the liver,susceptible of neoplastic transformation: mature hepatocytes, small proliferating hepatocytes and stem cells [33, 34].

Specifically, hepatocellular carcinoma might result from dedifferentiation of mature hepatocytes, from activation of oval cells, from arrested differentiation of tissue based stem cells, the latter being an expression of blocked ontogeny, linked to hepatocarcinogenesis. Evidence of the fact that hepatocarcinogenesis partly recapitulates fetal development comes from some observations: both progenitor and fetal cells are self-renewing, with heterogeneous progeny and limitless division; bipotent cells, with hepatocytic and cholangiocytic potential are present in fetal livers and have been isolated in a number of HCC cell lines; finally, the strict relationship between tumor cells and fetal program is testified by the fact that HCC cell lines (e.g. Huh1, Huh 7, Hep 3b cell lines) share with fetal liver progenitors several oncofetal markers and that HCC characterized by a gene expression profile similar to fetal hepatoblasts have a poorer prognosis than HCC with an adult-type genomic profile [35-39].

According to the possible origin from progenitor cells or from dedifferentiated adult cells, HCC could assume different phenotypes and be linked to the activation of different pathways, associated to variable parenchymal morphological changes. For instance, significantly fewer HCCs expressing CK7 or CK19 show nuclear beta Catenin expression. The beta catenin pathway could preferentially involve "mature" hepatocytes versus less "mature" (progenitor) phenotype cells, with CK7 and CK19 expression,associated withless advanced fibrosis in non-tumoral parenchyma [40].

CK19 expression in HCC can change with different expression of beta catenin: decreased fibrosis degree in the non-tumoral parenchyma parallels reduced nuclear beta catenin expression [25].

Regarding oval cells, many of the compounds that induce their proliferation are DNA-damaging agents or carcinogens, therefore oval cells can be considered as potential precancerous cells [41]. Oval cells activation with "ductular reaction" represent the expansion of a transit amplifyingcell compartment of small biliary bipotent cells [25].

In cirrhosis, hepatocytes are characterized by senescence determined by telomere shortening, while mesenchymal cells (e.g. endothelial cells and stellate cells) seem not to be affected by replicative senescence [25]. In the hepatocytes this latter can be the result of an enhanced proliferation rate that can persist for 20-30 years of chronic liver disease. It is possible to hypothesize that the parallel proliferative activity of progenitor cells and mesenchymal cells allows an influence of the latter elements on the progenitor cells carcinogenic evolution: it is known that sinusoidal lining cells like hepatic stellate cells proliferate in close anatomical relationship with progenitor cells and are able to produce growth factors for which progenitor cells have the receptors, suggesting an interaction between these cell compartments [26].

"A characteristic of stem cells is to survive to toxic and hypoxic stimuli due to their low cell cycling ".

"One possibility is that HLSC may represent a mesenchymal population modified by the influence of the local environment, reflecting the importance of the niche in establishing the phenotype of MSC" [42].

The "tumor stroma" can be considered as "normal wound healing gone awry [43], able to interact through paracrine and juxtacrine pathways with the tumor stem cells that are influenced by the microenvironment in which they are endowed, with a direct role of micro-environment cells in determining the malignant phenotype [44-52]. In summary, fetal development, regeneration and carcinogenetic processes show some point of similarity in molecular pathways and mechanisms, partly recapitulatedin chronic parenchymal liver damage evolving to advanced stages.

Starting from the concept of chronic liver disease development, with progressive liver cell destruction, reactive fibrosis and general parenchymal organization disarray, it is possible a better comprehension of the whole changes.

These phenomena are all present since the beginning of liver damage, when liver cells are involved by viral or toxic damage and fibrous tissue deposition replace the destroyed cells. This is the beginning of fibrosis development, firstly at sub-sinusoidal level, then within the damaged areas, often associated, in more advanced stages, with a ductular reaction.

Importantly, evolution of liver fibrosis and activation of hepatic stellate cells share some pathways [4]. In fact, the adhesion molecules and receptors mediating cell-extracellular matrix binding and growth factors and cytokines present in ECM influence matrix turnover and modifications and, together with liver cells, endothelium, Kupffer cells and inflammatory cells, modulate hepatic stellate cells. These latter express Integrins, mediating cell adhesion to fibronectin and collagens and modulating metalloproteinases: integrins activate intracellular signaling pathways in response to ECM protein they recognize, influencing hepatocytes differentiation.

As a consequence, any kind of liver parenchymal damage, though mild, induces a regenerative liver cell response, starting from periportal liver cells [25].

Liver cells, ductular cells, stromal cells and perisinusoidal cells all undergo regenerative phenomena: it is a complex sequence associated with progressive collagen deposition with a healing role, involving subsinusoidalDisse spaces, periportal and perilaminarinterstitium, with ECM and parenchymal cells activation and proliferation and with ECM synthesis by stellate cells, fibroblasts and, in some cases, parenchymal cells. In fact, in this context, epithelial-mesenchymal transition and mesenchymal-epithelial transition play a role, with different tissue component phenotypic changes, significantly involving parenchymal structure and function [53].

If chronic inflammation with long standing tissue damage represents a risk condition for neoplastic disease, cirrhosis is the typical predisposing setting for hepatocellular carcinoma. In fact, cirrhosis is characterized by a microenvironment possibly favoring HCC onset: most cases of hepatocellular carcinoma are linked to the presence of cirrhosis [54, 55].

3. Molecular changes in the development of HCC: The novel role of miRNA

During the last years it has been shown a significant correspondence between clinical and humoral parameters (tumor size, differentiation grading, HBV or HCV infection, serum alfafeto protein (AFP)) and different molecular pathways activated in HCC cases: beta-catenin and Axin-1 mutated cases, with early relapse, behave in a different way comparedto cases with c-Myc and AKT activation associated with Interferon target genes inhibition, but also compared to hepatocellular carcinoma with overexpression of p53 and p21, the latter showing better differentiation and lower size [56]. Subclasses S1,S2,S3 defined on the basis of above mentioned clinical, humoraland morphological parametersare oftenassociated with different molecular profiles: S1 show Beta catenin and Axin mutation; S2 activation of c-Myc, AFP overexpression, AKT activation, IFN target genes inhibition; S3 cases are associated with better histological differentiation, overexpression of p53, p21, gene related with glycolipidic and alcohol metabolism, oxygen radical scavenging and coagulation [56]. The effort is the identification of a classification system on the basis or with the contribution of the molecular changes of the tumors.

At this regard, miRNAs can play a crucial role. In fact, each of these small endogenous non-coding RNAs is characterized by the ability to transcriptionally or post-transcriptionally regulate many different target genes, thus being responsible of complex molecular changes [57].

In fact, these sequences favor mRNA degradation through sequence-specific interaction with the 3′ untranslated region (3′-UTR) of targeted mRNAs; when the sequence is totally complementary, miRNA pairing will induce mRNA degradation and are involved in development, apoptosis, proliferation and differentiation processes [58]. Alternatively, sequences partially complementary will more probably induce a stop in translation, without mRNA degradation. Therefore, a single miRNA is able to regulate the genic expression of hundreds of target genes.Its altered expression could cause a "post transcriptional collapse", i.e. the contemporary deregulation of multiple tumor suppressor or oncogenes whose sequences are complementary to the considered miRNA [59], thus deregulating many molecular pathways which could favor a malignant cellular phenotype [57]. In fact, the global effect of inactivation of a miRNA molecule will be the over-expression of its target genes, while its activation will induce the down-regulation of a lot of target genes. If deregulated miRNA target genes are involved in the regulation of important biological processes, such as apoptosis, cell cycle, tumoral cells invasiveness or angiogenesis, then the risk of uncontrolled growth and tumor development will increase [58].

Accordingly, in HCC has been described a deregulation of miRNA expression [57]. The fact that HCC-related changes in miRNA expression are absent in non-neoplastic parenchyma and the association of these changes with other neoplasms confirm the hypothesis of miRNA involvement in HCC pathogenesis.

Interestingly, more than 50% of miRNA genes are located in fragile chromosomal site or in cancer-associated genomic regions [60].

Many experimental evidences support the relationship between fragile sites and DNA instability in cancerous cells. In fact, fragile sites are preferential sites for chromatids exchanges, translocations, deletions, gene amplification or integrations of associated viral sequences, such as HPV [60].

Besides the association with fragile sites, microRNA genes may be involved in tumorigenesis process through other mechanisms, such as point mutation, deletion, amplification, translocation or epigenetic modifications [61]. Most known microRNA have been identified within genomic cancer-associated regions: minimal regions of loss of heterozigosity, where often oncosuppressor genes are present or minimal region of amplification, where often oncogenes have been identified [62]. This strongly suggest that miRNAgenes may behave either as oncogenes or as tumor suppressor genes and, in particular, the same miRNA may behave in different way on the basis of the kind of alteration, cellular type or transcriptional/post-transcriptional regulation of target genes.

miRNA deregulation can also be the consequence of epigenetic changes, In fact, an extensive genomic analysis of miRNA-coding gene sequences showed that about 50% of these loci are CpG island associated [62] makingpossible that an alteration in DNA methylation/acethylation could be responsible for miRNA deregulation in tumors [63].

Regarding the changes in miRNA expression in different tumors, the Volinia study [64], performed a microarray analysis of 20 different miRNAs in 540 specimen obtained from different tumor types (lung, breast, stomach, prostate, colon, pancreas) identifying a miRNA signature common to some different solid tumors). The value of this study, find a confirmation in the similar grouping, between different tumors, of the miRNA expression signature: this suggest a common mechanism of involvement of miRNA in human carcinogenesis. Prostate, colon, stomach, pancreas show mostly similar signature among them, whereas lung and breast are represented by a fairly different signature. Furthermore, within the signature, some miRNA have been found whose association with other human tumors was already known: among them there are miR-17-5p, miR-20a, miR-21, miR-92, miR-106a, e miR-155, and molecular targets of these miRNA are significantly rich in tumor suppressor genes and oncogenes. These data suggest the crucial involvement of miRNA in the pathogenesis of solid tumors and confirm the function of miRNA as dominant and recessive tumoral genes. Furthermore, it has been shown the role of miRNA not only in the early phases of primitive tumors development, but also during the progression and the metastatic diffusion of the neoplastic disease. In fact, many experimental evidences show miRNA involvement in the regulation of biological process leading to the acquisition of metastatic potential, such as adhesion, invasion, migration, epithelial-to-mesenchymal transition and angiogenesis [65, 66].

Among miRNAs with an aberrant expression in both HCC and other solid tumors, we must list: miR221/222 (up-regulated in HCC, colon, pancreas and gastric cancer); miR-21 (up-regulated in HCC, ovarian, lung, breast cancer and glioblastoma); miR-199a, 200b and 214 (down-regulated in HCC and ovarian cancer) and miR-199b (down-regulated in HCC, ovarian and lung cancer). Importantly, genes frequently de-regulated in HCC, such as p27/CDKN1B and p57/CDKN1C or PTEN, have been identified as targets of miR-221/222 and miR-21 targets (see below).

Considering HCC-specific miRNAs, miR-122 is one of the best characterized molecules. miR-122 is, in fact, a liver specific miRNA, representing 70% of all liver expressed miRNAs, and it is down-regulated in most human and murine HCC. Its deregulation induces important changes in the phenotype of adult hepatocytes and in several liver functions, such as lipid metabolism [67] and cholesterol synthesis [68]. These data allow hypothesizing a correlation between the lowered miR-122 expression in HCC and the loss of hepatic differentiation in neoplastic cells. Furthermore, Jopling*et al*have demonstrated that miR-122 is able to bind to 5'-UTR RNA region of HCV [69]: this region is preserved in all six viral genotypes, so suggesting that miR-122 is an essential element for virus replication in hepatocytes. It has been shown that functional inactivation of miR-122 induces the 80% reduction of viral replication, suggesting that miR-122 inactivation in hepatocellular carcinoma could increase neoplastic cells resistance to HCV replication.

Concerning the miRNA involvement in different steps of hepatocellular carcinoma progression, it has been demonstrated a correlation between miR-222, miR-106, miR-92, miR-17-5p, miR-20, miR-18 and hepatocellular carcinoma differentiation grading, suggesting the involvement of a restricted number of miRNA in neoplastic progression [70]. According to this data a 20 miRNAs signature has been reported [71], capable to distinguish primitive hepatocellular carcinoma metastasizing through venous channels from solitary, non-metastatic tumors. Furthermore, a predictive analysis revealed that most of 20 miRNA of HCC signature are associated with patients' survival. These signatures could then represent a simple method for a diagnostic/prognostic profiling, capable of identifying HCC patients at high risk of developing a metastatic disease or a liver relapse.

Other authors evaluate the predictive accuracy in distinguishing neoplastic and non-neoplastic parenchyma equal to97,8% on the basis of 8 miRNAs, while others again identify 18 overexpressed miRNA in hepatocellular carcinoma and only 6 overexpressedin non-neoplastic tissue [72] (and with aberrant miR-21 expression associated with metastasis risk and connected with PTEN targeting; miR-224 could act on genes apoptosis regulating (API-5) [73, 74].

Another miRNA involved in tumor progression and diffusion is miR-34a, a transcriptional target of p53, deleted in many human neoplastic lesions. Besides molecular targets involved in cell cycle progression, miR-34a regulates the expression of the oncoprotein c-Met, a tyrosin kinase receptor activated by the hepatocyte growth factor binding, able to induce the phosphorilation of molecules responsible for signal transduction, such as ERK1/2, thus exerting the function of key factors in tumor invasion and migration regulation.

A recent study [66] reported a significant reduction of miR-34a expression in most carcinomatous liver tissue with respect to non-neoplastic adjacent liver tissue, with an inverse correlation between miR-34a-and c-Met-expression levels. Furthermore, low levels of miR-34a positively relate with the development of metastatic disease and neoplastic vascular invasion. Accordingly, in vitro studies showed a lower migration and metastatic potential of neoplastic cells after miR-34a c-Met dependent suppression.

It is worth noting that another mi-RNA under-expressed in most HCC [75], miR-199a-3p, is capable of regulating c-Met oncogene expression [76]:these data suggest that various deregulated miRNA in a specific neoplasia may modulate the same target gene, leading to strong alteration of the molecular pathways downstream the target gene, thus influencing the tumor progression.

RAS oncogene overexpression is associated to miRNA deregulation without oncogene point mutation. Pathway alteration can be induced by downregulation of let-7 miRNA family component.

Regarding the biological processes controlled by miRNAs, they play a direct role on cellular growth control. As previously mentioned, miR-221 is up-regulated in many neoplasms and influence the expression of the cyclin-dependent kinase inhibitor CDKN1B/p27, which controls the cell cycle progression [57]. The activation of pathways involving PI3K/AKT leads to phosphorylation of proteins that favor cell survival, under the control of tumor suppressor lipid phosphatase PTEN, which is a direct miR-21 target; in vitro studies showed the association between mir-21 inhibition and PTEN overexpression, with subsequent decreased neoplastic cell proliferation and invasion [57]. Moreover, MiR-21 inhibition induces changes in metalloproteinases 2 and 9 expression: both these molecules are downstream PTEN mediators with a known role in cellular migration and invasion [57]. These data suggest that the aberrant miR-21 expression may favor HCC growth and diffusion through the modulation of the expression of PTEN and of PTEN-dependent pathways involved in neoplastic cells phenotype and behavior modulation. Again, cyclin G1 upregulation following miR-122 down-regulation may induce p53 down-regulation, so favoring tumorigenesis [57].

Regarding the role of miRNA as biomarkers, there is evidence that, in HCC, miRNAs could have a prognostic as well as a diagnostic role.

As already underlined, some known molecular factors characterizing HCC may play a role as prognostic factors (for example c-MET or p27); similarly, there is evidence that some deregulated miR [58] may allow, in association with clinical parameters and histological patterns, classifying HCC, thus identifying new criteria for prognostic stratification [57]. This is also possible due to distinct miRNA profiles of different hepatocellular carcinoma subtypes (at variance with similar signature between tumors in different organs)Such a differentiation takes place on the basis of supposed mechanism of origin (cancer stem cells or mature hepatocyte-like): the different groups show distinctbiological behavior. Furthermore,HBV or HCV etiology of basic disease and primary or metastatic nature of the neoplastic lesion are associated with different miRNA signatures in HCC [60].

Regarding the potential role of miRNAs as diagnostic biomarkers, at least 20 miRNAs show different changes between lesions with different origin; cancer stem cells origin is associated with self-renewal capability, differentiation and aggressive tumorigenesis in vivo: miR-181 family members, over-expressed in HCC, favor the origin of neoplasia from progenitor cells through an influence on CDX2 and GATA6, differentiation related genes, and on NLK a WNT/ Beta catenin pathway inhibitor.

MiR-21, miR-10b, miR-222 and miR-224 are highly represented in HCC, while non-malignant hepatic lesions show decreased miR-202 and miR-203 expression. Alcohol consumption related hepatocellular carcinoma shows low miR-126 levels, while high levels of miR-96 are present in neoplastic lesions HBV associated: such alterations have not been shown in non-neoplastic parenchyma [58]. Furthermore, hepatocellular carcinoma cases with high risk of metastatic diffusion and cases without metastasis risk present distinct miRNA groups' expression.

Low miR-375 expression have been shown either in hepatocellular adenoma or in carcinoma with Beta catenin mutation: the significant inverse correlation between miR-375 level and Beta catenin targeted gene expression suggests a direct relationship between Beta catenin activation and miR-375 repression [58]. Recently a role of survival predictor and IFN adjuvant therapy response in hepatocellular carcinoma for miR-26 has been identified [77].

Finally, as previously mentioned, genetic mutations and transcriptional, epigenetic changes may induce miRNA alterations. In the case of HCC it has been shown the role of endoribonuclease III DICER for miRNA maturation: its role in cleavage and maturation of miRNA renders impossible for the cell a full expression of miRNA if endoribonuclease is disrupted. DICER deficient hepatocytes loose the expression of all miRNA, with expression of liver specific fetal genes and deregulation of much genes related to neoplastic development [60].

In conclusion, up to date experimental evidences show that hepatocellular carcinoma subtypes are characterized by distinct miRNA expression profiles, related to grade of aggressiveness, risk factors and genetic changes. MiRNAs may therefore represent not only useful diagnostic and prognostic markers, but important target molecules for potential therapeutic treatment.

4. Tumor associated fibroblast in the development of HCC

If molecular changes take place in liver parenchymal cells undergoing to inflammatory and fibrotic parenchymal damage, leading to the phenomena that characterize tumoral initiation and progression, then, it is also an important matter the evaluation of the role of inflammatory conditions and fibrosis in stromal changes, and, particularly, in tumor associated fibroblasts development.

Among the constituents of the tumor microenvironment, tumor associated fibroblasts (TAF) play a key role in tumor progression, angiogenesis, growth and metastasis: they are characterized by the expression of specific markers [45, 78-82] and seems to assume a role in clinical tumor prognosis.

Recently [83, 84] it has been optimized a method to isolate, from several human adult tissues, a population of primitive cells, named multipotent adult stem cells (MASCs) with mesenchymalimmunophenotype, clonogenicity and multiple in vitro differentiation capacity [83, 84]. MASCs isolated both from neoplastic and from cirrhotic human liver tissue allow to test the hypothesis that liver resident MASCs could generate TAFs in pathological conditions: a population of MASCs with TAFs characteristics both in human hepatocellular carcinoma and cirrhotic liver has been demonstrated, so suggesting a possible role in the development of neoplasia in the adequate environment [2]. On the other hand, TAFs from non-neoplastic and non-cirrhotic livers do not show aberrant growth properties: so, TAFs can originate from resident primitive cells [2].

The in vivo counterpart of MASCs is still undefined, but the interesting data concern their sharing of some feature with activated hepatic stellate cells [85-87]. This aspect is of particular interest, given the hypothesis that stellate cells could be progenitor cells: in fact, the expression of OCT-4 and of markers of all the three germ layers and their ability to give rise in vitro to endothelial cells and hepatocytes offer essential elements [2].

A fate-mapping study showed that stellate cells could become oval cells when activated in liver injury, and that these cells participate in ductular proliferation [88]. This offers a substantial contribution to the discussed sharing of pathways and cells between developmental, regenerative and neoplastic processes in the liver.

All these evidences point to the presence of mesenchymal, widely multipotent cells in adult tissues, which can take part to regenerative as well as inflammatory and neoplastic processes [89].

In the paper by Cesselli et al 2011 [2] it is well documented that MASCs isolated from hepatocellular carcinoma have the main characteristic of TAFs, at variance with cells from non-neoplastic and non-cirrhotic livers. TAFs act on the tumor growth in different ways, which are able to modify the microenvironment in the sense of a more suitable situation for the increase of tumor growth [48, 78, 90]. TAFs are contractile cells, with a strict spatial relation with blood vessels; they produce growth factors (HGF, TGF beta, EGF, bFGF, IGF), cytokines, chemokines, enzymes; they can degrade the extracellular matrix and can behave as immunomodulating cells [48, 78, 90]. Finally, increased metastatic potential and poor prognosis are associated with the presence of TAFs [48].

Tumor cell lines medium can induce in L-MASCs aberrant growth properties and the ability to produce specific TAF markers [47, 48, 78]. The origin of TAFs seems to be connected with four possible sources: epithelial-mesenchymal transition of the neoplastic cells (associated with genetic changes within the TAFs); recruitment and activation of resident fibroblasts; recruitment of circulating/bone marrow derived mesenchymal stem cells; recruitment of mesenchymal stem cells [48, 78, 82]. In the paper from Cesselli, Beltrami et al. it has been shown the origin of TAFs from a population of resident primitive cells with mesenchymal features [2].The Authors also underline that blocking the activation of TAFs and their continuous communication with the cancer cells could, in conjunction with chemotherapy regimens, limit tumor progression and metastasis [45, 82, 91]: the much lower instability of TAFs versus malignant cells seems to make them less likely to undergo the onset of resistance to chemotherapy drugs [81, 92].

5. Conclusions

Liver parenchyma, exposed to long standing viral or toxic damage, undergoes a diffuse, fibrosing rearrangement, developing cirrhosis. In this context, genetic changes in the cellular component, the activation of different pathways, the production of cytokines and growth factors, phenotypic changes of epithelial or mesenchymal cells produce complex phenomena, involving regenerative, preneoplastic and neoplastic changes.The role of liver cells and/or progenitor cells in neoplastic growth is heavily influenced by mesenchymal component, in particular by TAFs. Cirrhotic livers, when not yet neoplastic, already possess a population of multipotent adult stem cells with TAFs properties.

The possible origin of TAFs from a population of primitive mesenchymal stem cells gives to the tumor supporting stroma a more complex and important role. In fact, from " rare resident stem cells, such as multipotent adult stem cells (MASCs) " the entire formation and instruction of the elements of supportive microenvironment could take place [2]. MASCs differentiation potential " into many stromal cell types and their molecular signature consisting of overexpression " of a gene panel involved in extracellular matrix remodeling, immunomodulation, and cytokines and growth factors production [83] offer a key to understand the relationship between liver parenchyma, neoplastic growth and stromal component.

" Multipotent adult stem cells isolated from healthy livers can acquire a TAF phenotype when grown in conditional medium from tumor cell lines, suggesting that multipotent cells residing in the liver may represent a population " able to stroma formation and contributing to tumor progression, in adequate conditions [2]. The effort to identify novel therapies aimed at interfering with the interaction between stroma and cancer cells represent a crucial perspective.

The discovery, in 1993, by Ambros and Ruvkun of this new mechanism of gene regulation, with large mRNA under the control of a small RNA opened a new way to develop the understanding of the regulation of critical cellular process (cell division, metabolism, development and death) by micro RNA. MiRNA can target more than 500 mRNA and a single mRNA can be targeted by multiple miRNA. The specificity of targets depend on the degree of base complementarities to the target mRNA: when the miRNA have perfect base complementarities, than messenger RNA undergo degradation; if there is not perfect complementarity, than posttranslational inhibition occur. Through this mechanism, miRNA can exert an essential control on a lot of processes, in particular in neoplasia harboring and diffusion, opening a crucial field in prognostic prediction and in possible intervention to break the carcinogenetic process and to obtain the disease control through target therapy.

The concepts of multidirectional differentiation of mesenchymal stem cells, of tumor associated fibroblasts, of cancerization fields, epithelial-mesenchymal transition and mesenchymal-epithelial transition, miRNA deregulation,the progress in the identification of reproducible classification criteria on the basis of hepatocellular carcinomamolecular changes offer new insights concerning liver neoplastic growths, with key points concerning the association between developmental, regenerative and neoplastic growth mechanisms and the relationship between parenchymal hepatocytes and stromal component in preneoplastic and neoplastic liver diseases as the main ways for a better understanding of neoplastic liver biology.

http://dx.doi.org/10.5772/56951

Author details

C. Avellini[1*], D. Cesselli[2], A.P. Beltrami[2], M. Orsaria[1], S. Marzinotto[1], F. Morassi[1] and S. Uzzau[3]

*Address all correspondence to: avellini.claudio@aoud.sanita.fvg.it

1 Department of Pathology, University Hospital "S. Maria dellaMisericordia" of Udine, Udine, Italy

2 Department of Medical and Biological Sciences, University of Udine, Udine, Italy

3 Department of Surgery, University Hospital "S. Maria dellaMisericordia" of Udine, Udine, Italy

References

[1] Thorgeirsson SS, Grisham JW. Molecular pathogenesis of human hepatocellular carcinoma. Nat Genet. 2002 Aug;31(4):339-46.

[2] Cesselli D, Beltrami AP, Poz A, Marzinotto S, Comisso E, Bergamin N, et al. Role of tumor associated fibroblasts in human liver regeneration, cirrhosis, and cancer. Int J Hepatol. 2011;2011:120925.

[3] Mcsween. Pathology of the liver. Livingstone C, editor2002.

[4] Patsenker E, Stickel F. Role of integrins in fibrosing liver diseases. Am J PhysiolGastrointest Liver Physiol. 2011 Sep;301(3):G425-34.

[5] Alison MR, Islam S, Lim S. Stem cells in liver regeneration, fibrosis and cancer: the good, the bad and the ugly. J Pathol. 2009 Jan;217(2):282-98.

[6] Semela D, Dufour JF. Angiogenesis and hepatocellular carcinoma. J Hepatol. 2004 Nov;41(5):864-80.

[7] Sanz-Cameno P, Trapero-Marugan M, Chaparro M, Jones EA, Moreno-Otero R. Angiogenesis: from chronic liver inflammation to hepatocellular carcinoma. J Oncol. 2010;2010:272170.

[8] Kung JW, Currie IS, Forbes SJ, Ross JA. Liver development, regeneration, and carcinogenesis. J Biomed Biotechnol. 2010;2010:984248.

[9] Riehle KJ, Dan YY, Campbell JS, Fausto N. New concepts in liver regeneration. J GastroenterolHepatol. 2011 Jan;26Suppl 1:203-12.

[10] Jung J, Zheng M, Goldfarb M, Zaret KS. Initiation of mammalian liver development from endoderm by fibroblast growth factors. Science. 1999 Jun 18;284(5422): 1998-2003.

[11] Rossi JM, Dunn NR, Hogan BL, Zaret KS. Distinct mesodermal signals, including BMPs from the septum transversum mesenchyme, are required in combination for hepatogenesis from the endoderm. Genes Dev. 2001 Aug 1;15(15):1998-2009.

[12] Deutsch G, Jung J, Zheng M, Lora J, Zaret KS. A bipotential precursor population for pancreas and liver within the embryonic endoderm. Development. 2001 Mar;128(6): 871-81.

[13] Shin D, Shin CH, Tucker J, Ober EA, Rentzsch F, Poss KD, et al. Bmp and Fgf signaling are essential for liver specification in zebrafish. Development. 2007 Jun;134(11): 2041-50.

[14] Zhang W, Yatskievych TA, Baker RK, Antin PB. Regulation of Hex gene expression and initial stages of avian hepatogenesis by Bmp and Fgf signaling. Dev Biol. 2004 Apr 15;268(2):312-26.

[15] McLin VA, Rankin SA, Zorn AM. Repression of Wnt/beta-catenin signaling in the anterior endoderm is essential for liver and pancreas development. Development. 2007 Jun;134(12):2207-17.

[16] Monga SP, Monga HK, Tan X, Mule K, Pediaditakis P, Michalopoulos GK. Beta-catenin antisense studies in embryonic liver cultures: role in proliferation, apoptosis, and lineage specification. Gastroenterology. 2003 Jan;124(1):202-16.

[17] Ober EA, Verkade H, Field HA, Stainier DY. Mesodermal Wnt2b signalling positively regulates liver specification. Nature. 2006 Aug 10;442(7103):688-91.

[18] Schmidt C, Bladt F, Goedecke S, Brinkmann V, Zschiesche W, Sharpe M, et al. Scatter factor/hepatocyte growth factor is essential for liver development. Nature. 1995 Feb 23;373(6516):699-702.

[19] Tanimizu N, Miyajima A. Molecular mechanism of liver development and regeneration. Int Rev Cytol. 2007;259:1-48.

[20] Weinstein M, Monga SP, Liu Y, Brodie SG, Tang Y, Li C, et al. Smad proteins and hepatocyte growth factor control parallel regulatory pathways that converge on beta1-integrin to promote normal liver development. Mol Cell Biol. 2001 Aug;21(15): 5122-31.

[21] Zhao R, Duncan SA. Embryonic development of the liver. Hepatology. 2005 May; 41(5):956-67.

[22] Kuwahara R, Kofman AV, Landis CS, Swenson ES, Barendswaard E, Theise ND. The hepatic stem cell niche: identification by label-retaining cell assay. Hepatology. 2008 Jun;47(6):1994-2002.

[23] Fausto N, Campbell JS, Riehle KJ. Liver regeneration. Hepatology. 2006 Feb;43(2 Suppl 1):S45-53.

[24] Diehl AM. Recent events in alcoholic liver disease V. effects of ethanol on liver regeneration. Am J PhysiolGastrointest Liver Physiol. 2005 Jan;288(1):G1-6.

[25] Roskams T. Liver stem cells and their implication in hepatocellular and cholangiocarcinoma. Oncogene. 2006 Jun 26;25(27):3818-22.

[26] Roskams T. Different types of liver progenitor cells and their niches. J Hepatol. 2006 Jul;45(1):1-4.

[27] Riehle KJ, Dan YY, Campbell JS, Fausto N. New concepts in liver regeneration. J GastroenterolHepatol.Jan;26Suppl 1:203-12.

[28] Nagy P, Bisgaard HC, Santoni-Rugiu E, Thorgeirsson SS. In vivo infusion of growth factors enhances the mitogenic response of rat hepatic ductal (oval) cells after administration of 2-acetylaminofluorene. Hepatology. 1996 Jan;23(1):71-9.

[29] Hasuike S, Ido A, Uto H, Moriuchi A, Tahara Y, Numata M, et al. Hepatocyte growth factor accelerates the proliferation of hepatic oval cells and possibly promotes the differentiation in a 2-acetylaminofluorene/partial hepatectomy model in rats. J GastroenterolHepatol. 2005 Nov;20(11):1753-61.

[30] Isfort RJ, Cody DB, Stuard SB, Randall CJ, Miller C, Ridder GM, et al. The combination of epidermal growth factor and transforming growth factor-beta induces novel phenotypic changes in mouse liver stem cell lines. J Cell Sci. 1997 Dec;110 (Pt 24): 3117-29.

[31] Nguyen LN, Furuya MH, Wolfraim LA, Nguyen AP, Holdren MS, Campbell JS, et al. Transforming growth factor-beta differentially regulates oval cell and hepatocyte proliferation. Hepatology. 2007 Jan;45(1):31-41.

[32] Knight B, Tirnitz-Parker JE, Olynyk JK. C-kit inhibition by imatinibmesylate attenuates progenitor cell expansion and inhibits liver tumor formation in mice. Gastroenterology. 2008 Sep;135(3):969-79, 79 e1.

[33] Sell S, Leffert HL. An evaluation of cellular lineages in the pathogenesis of experimental hepatocellular carcinoma. Hepatology. 1982 Jan-Feb;2(1):77-86.

[34] Sell S, Leffert HL. Liver cancer stem cells. J ClinOncol. 2008 Jun 10;26(17):2800-5.

[35] Lee JS, Heo J, Libbrecht L, Chu IS, Kaposi-Novak P, Calvisi DF, et al. A novel prognostic subtype of human hepatocellular carcinoma derived from hepatic progenitor cells. Nat Med. 2006 Apr;12(4):410-6.

[36] Suzuki A, Sekiya S, Onishi M, Oshima N, Kiyonari H, Nakauchi H, et al. Flow cytometric isolation and clonal identification of self-renewing bipotent hepatic progenitor cells in adult mouse liver. Hepatology. 2008 Dec;48(6):1964-78.

[37] Chiba T, Kita K, Zheng YW, Yokosuka O, Saisho H, Iwama A, et al. Side population purified from hepatocellular carcinoma cells harbors cancer stem cell-like properties. Hepatology. 2006 Jul;44(1):240-51.

[38] Yamashita T, Ji J, Budhu A, Forgues M, Yang W, Wang HY, et al. EpCAM-positive hepatocellular carcinoma cells are tumor-initiating cells with stem/progenitor cell features. Gastroenterology. 2009 Mar;136(3):1012-24.

[39] Yamashita T, Forgues M, Wang W, Kim JW, Ye Q, Jia H, et al. EpCAM and alpha-fetoprotein expression defines novel prognostic subtypes of hepatocellular carcinoma. Cancer Res. 2008 Mar 1;68(5):1451-61.

[40] Durnez A, Verslype C, Nevens F, Fevery J, Aerts R, Pirenne J, et al. The clinicopathological and prognostic relevance of cytokeratin 7 and 19 expression in hepatocellular carcinoma. A possible progenitor cell origin. Histopathology. 2006 Aug;49(2):138-51.

[41] Duncan AW, Dorrell C, Grompe M. Stem cells and liver regeneration. Gastroenterology. 2009 Aug;137(2):466-81.

[42] Herrera MB, Bruno S, Buttiglieri S, Tetta C, Gatti S, Deregibus MC, et al. Isolation and characterization of a stem cell population from adult human liver. Stem Cells. 2006 Dec;24(12):2840-50.

[43] Dvorak HF. Tumors: wounds that do not heal. Similarities between tumor stroma generation and wound healing. N Engl J Med. 1986 Dec 25;315(26):1650-9.

[44] Hanahan D, Weinberg RA. The hallmarks of cancer. Cell. 2000 Jan 7;100(1):57-70.

[45] Kalluri R, Zeisberg M. Fibroblasts in cancer. Nat Rev Cancer. 2006 May;6(5):392-401.

[46] Pietras K, Ostman A. Hallmarks of cancer: interactions with the tumor stroma. Exp Cell Res. 2010 May 1;316(8):1324-31.

[47] Rasanen K, Vaheri A. Activation of fibroblasts in cancer stroma. Exp Cell Res. 2010 Oct 15;316(17):2713-22.

[48] Shimoda M, Mellody KT, Orimo A. Carcinoma-associated fibroblasts are a rate-limiting determinant for tumour progression. Semin Cell Dev Biol. 2010 Feb;21(1):19-25.

[49] Anderson AR, Weaver AM, Cummings PT, Quaranta V. Tumor morphology and phenotypic evolution driven by selective pressure from the microenvironment. Cell. 2006 Dec 1;127(5):905-15.

[50] Mishra P, Banerjee D, Ben-Baruch A. Chemokines at the crossroads of tumor-fibroblast interactions that promote malignancy. J Leukoc Biol. 2010 Jan;89(1):31-9.

[51] Polyak K, Haviv I, Campbell IG. Co-evolution of tumor cells and their microenvironment. Trends Genet. 2009 Jan;25(1):30-8.

[52] Chang HY, Sneddon JB, Alizadeh AA, Sood R, West RB, Montgomery K, et al. Gene expression signature of fibroblast serum response predicts human cancer progression: similarities between tumors and wounds. PLoS Biol. 2004 Feb;2(2):E7.

[53] Thiery JP, Sleeman JP. Complex networks orchestrate epithelial-mesenchymal transitions. Nat Rev Mol Cell Biol. 2006 Feb;7(2):131-42.

[54] Farazi PA, DePinho RA. Hepatocellular carcinoma pathogenesis: from genes to environment. Nat Rev Cancer. 2006 Sep;6(9):674-87.

[55] Bruix J, Boix L, Sala M, Llovet JM. Focus on hepatocellular carcinoma. Cancer Cell. 2004 Mar;5(3):215-9.

[56] Hoshida Y, Toffanin S, Lachenmayer A, Villanueva A, Minguez B, Llovet JM. Molecular classification and novel targets in hepatocellular carcinoma: recent advancements. Semin Liver Dis. 2010 Feb;30(1):35-51.

[57] Gramantieri L, Fornari F, Callegari E, Sabbioni S, Lanza G, Croce CM, et al. MicroRNA involvement in hepatocellular carcinoma. J Cell Mol Med. 2008 Dec;12(6A): 2189-204.

[58] Ladeiro Y, Couchy G, Balabaud C, Bioulac-Sage P, Pelletier L, Rebouissou S, et al. MicroRNA profiling in hepatocellular tumors is associated with clinical features and oncogene/tumor suppressor gene mutations. Hepatology. 2008 Jun;47(6):1955-63.

[59] McManus MT. MicroRNAs and cancer. Semin Cancer Biol. 2003 Aug;13(4):253-8.

[60] Ji J, Wang XW. New kids on the block: diagnostic and prognostic microRNAs in hepatocellular carcinoma. Cancer BiolTher. 2009 Sep;8(18):1686-93.

[61] Calin GA, Croce CM. MicroRNA signatures in human cancers. Nat Rev Cancer. 2006;6:857-66.

[62] Weber B, Stresemann C, Brueckner B, Lyko F. Methylation of human microRNA genes in normal and neoplastic cells. Cell Cycle. 2007 May 2;6(9):1001-5.

[63] Fazi F, Racanicchi S, Zardo G, Starnes LM, Mancini M, Travaglini L, et al. Epigenetic silencing of the myelopoiesis regulator microRNA-223 by the AML1/ETO oncoprotein. Cancer Cell. 2007 Nov;12(5):457-66.

[64] Volinia S, Calin GA, Liu CG, Ambs S, Cimmino A, Petrocca F, et al. A microRNA expression signature of human solid tumors defines cancer gene targets. ProcNatlAcadSci U S A. 2006 Feb 14;103(7):2257-61.

[65] Ma L, Teruya-Feldstein J, Weinberg RA. Tumour invasion and metastasis initiated by microRNA-10b in breast cancer. Nature. 2007 Oct 11;449(7163):682-8.

[66] Li N, Fu H, Tie Y, Hu Z, Kong W, Wu Y, et al. miR-34a inhibits migration and invasion by down-regulation of c-Met expression in human hepatocellular carcinoma cells. Cancer Lett. 2009 Mar 8;275(1):44-53.

[67] Esau C, Davis S, Murray SF, Yu XX, Pandey SK, Pear M, et al. miR-122 regulation of lipid metabolism revealed by in vivo antisense targeting. Cell Metab. 2006 Feb;3(2): 87-98.

[68] Krutzfeldt J, Rajewsky N, Braich R, Rajeev KG, Tuschl T, Manoharan M, et al. Silencing of microRNAs in vivo with 'antagomirs'. Nature. 2005 Dec 1;438(7068):685-9.

[69] Jopling CL, Yi M, Lancaster AM, Lemon SM, Sarnow P. Modulation of hepatitis C virus RNA abundance by a liver-specific MicroRNA. Science. 2005 Sep 2;309(5740): 1577-81.

[70] Murakami Y, Yasuda T, Saigo K, Urashima T, Toyoda H, Okanoue T, et al. Comprehensive analysis of microRNA expression patterns in hepatocellular carcinoma and non-tumorous tissues. Oncogene. 2006 Apr 20;25(17):2537-45.

[71] Budhu A, Jia HL, Forgues M, Liu CG, Goldstein D, Lam A, et al. Identification of metastasis-related microRNAs in hepatocellular carcinoma. Hepatology. 2008 Mar; 47(3):897-907.

[72] Pei Y, Zhang T, Renault V, Zhang X. An overview of hepatocellular carcinoma study by omics-based methods. ActaBiochimBiophys Sin (Shanghai). 2009 Jan;41(1):1-15.

[73] Meng F, Henson R, Wehbe-Janek H, Ghoshal K, Jacob ST, Patel T. MicroRNA-21 regulates expression of the PTEN tumor suppressor gene in human hepatocellular cancer. Gastroenterology. 2007 Aug;133(2):647-58.

[74] Wang Y, Lee AT, Ma JZ, Wang J, Ren J, Yang Y, et al. Profiling microRNA expression in hepatocellular carcinoma reveals microRNA-224 up-regulation and apoptosis inhibitor-5 as a microRNA-224-specific target. J Biol Chem. 2008 May 9;283(19): 13205-15.

[75] Ura S, Honda M, Yamashita T, Ueda T, Takatori H, Nishino R, et al. Differential microRNA expression between hepatitis B and hepatitis C leading disease progression to hepatocellular carcinoma. Hepatology. 2009 Apr;49(4):1098-112.

[76] Kim S, Lee UJ, Kim MN, Lee EJ, Kim JY, Lee MY, et al. MicroRNA miR-199a* regulates the MET proto-oncogene and the downstream extracellular signal-regulated kinase 2 (ERK2). J Biol Chem. 2008 Jun 27;283(26):18158-66.

[77] Roessler S, Jia HL, Budhu A, Forgues M, Ye QH, Lee JS, et al. A unique metastasis gene signature enables prediction of tumor relapse in early-stage hepatocellular carcinoma patients. Cancer Res. 2010 Dec 15;70(24):10202-12.

[78] Spaeth EL, Dembinski JL, Sasser AK, Watson K, Klopp A, Hall B, et al. Mesenchymal stem cell transition to tumor-associated fibroblasts contributes to fibrovascular network expansion and tumor progression. PLoS One. 2009;4(4):e4992.

[79] Mishra PJ, Glod JW, Banerjee D. Mesenchymal stem cells: flip side of the coin. Cancer Res. 2009 Feb 15;69(4):1255-8.

[80] Mishra PJ, Humeniuk R, Medina DJ, Alexe G, Mesirov JP, Ganesan S, et al. Carcinoma-associated fibroblast-like differentiation of human mesenchymal stem cells. Cancer Res. 2008 Jun 1;68(11):4331-9.

[81] Mueller MM, Fusenig NE. Friends or foes -bipolar effects of the tumourstroma in cancer. Nat Rev Cancer. 2004 Nov;4(11):839-49.

[82] Wels J, Kaplan RN, Rafii S, Lyden D. Migratory neighbors and distant invaders: tumor-associated niche cells. Genes Dev. 2008 Mar 1;22(5):559-74.

[83] Beltrami AP, Cesselli D, Bergamin N, Marcon P, Rigo S, Puppato E, et al. Multipotent cells can be generated in vitro from several adult human organs (heart, liver, and bone marrow). Blood. 2007 Nov 1;110(9):3438-46.

[84] Cesselli D, Beltrami AP, Rigo S, Bergamin N, D'Aurizio F, Verardo R, et al. Multipotent progenitor cells are present in human peripheral blood. Circ Res. 2009 May 22;104(10):1225-34.

[85] Kordes C, Sawitza I, Haussinger D. Canon-icalWnt signaling maintains the quiescent stage of hepatic stellate cells. BiochemBiophys Res Commun. 2008 Feb 29;367(1): 116-23.

[86] Kordes C, Sawitza I, Muller-Marbach A, Ale-Agha N, Keitel V, Klonowski-Stumpe H, et al. CD133+ hepatic stellate cells are progenitor cells. BiochemBiophys Res Commun. 2007 Jan 12;352(2):410-7.

[87] Kordes C, Sawitza I, Haussinger D. Hepatic and pancreatic stellate cells in focus. Biol Chem. 2009 Oct;390(10):1003-12.

[88] Yang L, Jung Y, Omenetti A, Witek RP, Choi S, Vandongen HM, et al. Fate-mapping evidence that hepatic stellate cells are epithelial progenitors in adult mouse livers. Stem Cells. 2008 Aug;26(8):2104-13.

[89] Slack JM. Origin of stem cells in organogenesis. Science. 2008 Dec 5;322(5907): 1498-501.

[90] Franco OE, Shaw AK, Strand DW, Hayward SW. Cancer associated fibroblasts in cancer pathogenesis. Semin Cell Dev Biol. 2010 Feb;21(1):33-9.

[91] LeBeau AM, Brennen WN, Aggarwal S, Denmeade SR. Targeting the cancer stroma with a fibroblast activation protein-activated promelittinprotoxin. Mol Cancer Ther. 2009 May;8(5):1378-86.

[92] Orimo A, Weinberg RA. Stromal fibroblasts in cancer: a novel tumor-promoting cell type. Cell Cycle. 2006 Aug;5(15):1597-601.

Chapter 10

Signs and Symptoms

Valerio Barghini, Debora Donnini,
Alessandro Uzzau and Giorgio Soardo

Additional information is available at the end of the chapter

http://dx.doi.org/10.5772/56162

1. Introduction

Hepatocellular carcinoma (HCC) is often diagnosed after the tumor manifests clinical signs and symptoms. Early diagnosis is usually performed thanks to HCC screening programs for patients affected by liver cirrhosis or chronic viral hepatopathies using ultrasound and serum alfa-fetoprotien. In most HCC cases, clinical signs and symptoms of this tumor may occur several months after development, when therapy can not be curative, given the advanced tumor stage and underlying liver disease, which preclude curative options, such as ablation, resection, or liver transplantation.

Clinical features of HCC are often similar to those caused by the underlying hepatic disease. It is very hard for physicians to distinguish signs and symptoms of HCC in contests characterized by an advanced liver disease. Advanced liver cancer can be responsible for accelerated liver functions deterioration caused by the intrahepatic tumor growth.

In this chapter, we review the clinical signs and symptoms induced by advanced carcinoma. We also discuss particular clinical scenarios caused by metastases and paraneoplastic syndromes, sometimes described case reports in literature.

2. Non-specific signs and symptoms

Non-specific systemic signs and symptoms as asthenia, anorexia, weight loss, and nausea, are often present in patients with HCC (table 1). HCC should be suspected with the onset of these clinical features in patients at risk for this tumor.

2.1. Clinical aspects of cirrhosis

Clinical signs and symptoms of hepatic cirrhosis that is often present in patients with HCC, usually mask the presence of an underlying early hepatocellular carcinoma [1]. Symptoms and signs of cirrhosis are often the only expression of the disease. Because of this, patients affected by HCC usually present at an advanced stage of the disease with clinical signs as jaundice, ascites, peripheral oedemas, neurologic manifestations of hepatic encephalopathy, bleeding, or infections. Other signs of hepatic cirrhosis include gynecomastia, palmar erythema, spider angiomas, axillary or chest hair loss, hypogonadism (testicular atrophy, loss of libido).

A large HCC can worsen the underlying hepatic disease, therefore in case of clinical worsening of a cirrhotic patient, onset of a HCC should be suspected.

2.2. Hepatomegaly

Hepatomegaly can be an expression of the tumor mass,(table 1) [1,2]. In case of HCC, the palpable edge of the liver is more often irregular, hard, with nodular consistency.

Hepatomegaly is more often present in patients without advanced cirrhosis [2]. In case of large tumors, the mass can cause asymmetry of the abdomen [3]. The costal margin can be deformed and the profile of lower ribs can be asymmetric. The right hemi-diaphragm can be elevated. This alteration of diaphragm profile can be asymptomatic or can cause mild respiratory symptoms. With thorax percussion is possible to detect an area of dullness, while trough auscultation is possible not to hear the vescicular murmur in case of elevation of diaphragm. HCC can also cause a pleural effusion. All these clinical aspects are difficult to be differentiated from signs and symptoms of the underlying chronic liver disease: Right diaphragm elevation is possible in case of hepatopathy not associated to HCC and pleural effusion can be the expression of an ascending ascitic fluid or of the anasarca state caused by cirrhosis and hypoalbuminemia.

2.3. Vascular bruit

Trough auscultation of the abdomen, an arterial bruit can be heard in patients affected by HCC. This bruit is typically heard throughout the liver and it is described to have different characteristic from other vascular abdominal auscultatory findings. In fact, usually, arterial bruit caused by abdominal aortic aneurysm or by renal artery stenosis are soft and short. Arterial bruit caused by HCC is usually a hard bruit and it is more prolonged than those caused by other conditions. This clinical sign is thought to be caused by the presence of an arteriovenous fistula in the context of the tumor [4], suggesting the presence of a highly vascularized HCC [5].

3. Abdominal pain, portal vein thrombosis, rupture of HCC

A frequent manifestation of onset of HCC is abdominal pain. The pain is usually mild, located in right hypochondrium and it can radiate to the right shoulder. Prior reports suggested that

http://dx.doi.org/10.5772/56162

in black South African patients, abdominal pain is frequent in 95% of cases while it is referred by 46%, 51% and 38% of Japanese, Chinese and Italian patients, respectively (table 1).

Abdominal pain is more frequent in non cirrhotic patients, and in case of portal thrombosis [1]. Portal vein thrombosis has been found in (14-44%) of autopsies of patients with HCC [6,7]. Patients with both cirrhosis and hepatic carcinoma have the highest risk to develop portal vein thrombosis [6]. Portal vein thrombosis is reported to be diagnosed during investigation for acute abdominal pain in 18% of cases in cirrhotic patients [8].

Other clinical manifestations of portal vein thrombosis and/or portal hypertension are hematemesis from rupture of esophageal varices, nausea, vomiting, anorexia, weight loss, diarrhea. Splenomegaly has been reported to be present in 75-100% of patients with portal vein thrombosis [9]. Bleeding from esophageal varices or from portal hypertensive gastropathy is the most common presenting symptom of portal vein thrombosis in cirrhotic patients [8,10]. In 43% of cases of Portal vein thrombosis in cirrhotic patients, diagnosis is done during a routine echo-Doppler examination [8].

If a cirrhotic patient present an acute pain, then bleeding from rupture of tumor should be suspected. HCC rupture causes a severe and sudden pain, and the patient can present the clinical features of an acute abdomen, with rebound and tenderness during physician palpation and an abdominal involuntary defense contraction. A hypovolemic state and signs and symptoms of acute anemia can be present. Clinical features of chronic anemia can be present in case of slow blood loss from HCC.

HCC rupture has been reported to be a rare condition in Western countries, occurring only in 3% of Italian patients [11], while spontaneous hemoperitoneum is more frequent in Sub-Saharian Africa and in Southeast Asia, being present in 10% of patients at presentation [12].

Usually,HCC tumors bleedings are spontaneous, but in rare cases, they can be caused by external causes. The protrusion of HCC beyond the liver surface seems to be an important risk factor for HCC rupture [13]: hemorrhages occur more easily and can also be caused by slight external forces. So HCC rupture can be caused by abdominal traumas [14],vigorous muscular exertion, or rarely after forceful physician's palpation [15].

HCC rupture is also a rare complication of therapeutic procedures on HCC. For example after transcatheter arterial chemoembolization (TACE), HCC rupture occurs in less than 1% of patients [16].

The drainage of hematic peritoneal liquid in patient with acute abdominal pain can suggest the presence of a ruptured HCC, not being specific for this condition.

3.1. Gastrointestinal bleeding

A particular manifestation of HCC can be a bleeding from esophageal varices. This presentation is not frequent, occurring as first clinical sign only in 1%-8% of cases of HCC [17,18] (table1). Variceal bleeding is caused by higher pressure in portal district which in turn can be caused by tumor invasion of this venous system and portal hypertension [17]. This portal invasion can be detected radiologically in 44-57% [17,18] of cases of variceal bleeding as presenting clinical manifestation of HCC. If variceal bleeding can be related with portal venous system invasion suggesting an advanced neoplastic disease, it does not seem to exist a relationship between this kind of clinical presentation and the size of the underlying tumor. Bleeding from esophageal varices is obviously a more frequent clinical presentation of HCC in patients with more advanced liver cirrhosis [18] and high degree of portal hypertension. However, HCC can present with variceal bleeding also in patients without a known history of hepatopathy [17].

Variceal bleeding can present with melena or hematemesis. Bleeding can be massive, leading to hypovolemic state and it is one of the known triggers of cirrhotic encephalopathy so that tremors, confusion till to coma, can be present in these patients too. Also infections can be caused by gastrointestinal bleeding in cirrhotic patients (22% of cases) [19], therefore, clinical signs and symptoms of an abdominal infections can be present.

Additionally, 50 % of causes of gastrointestinal hemorrhages are represented by hypertensive gastropathy, peptic ulcer and direct tumoral invasion of digestive tract [20,21].

3.2. Jaundice

Jaundice is a frequent sign of presentation of HCC. Some studies indicated that it is present at the diagnosis of HCC in 28% of African patients, but less frequent in Chinese, Japanese or European countries (table1).

Different pathologic conditions linked to HCC can explain the onset of jaundice. Jaundice can be expression of hepatic failure, due to extensive tumor infiltration of a cirrhotic liver or by worsening of the underlying hepatitis that can occur in presence of HCC. [22].

In other cases, jaundice result from obstruction of bile ducts by HCC. Clinical manifestation are those of typical cholestatic syndrome. In these cases jaundice is usually accompanied by itchiness, caused by elevation of serum level of bile acids, hypocolic stool and dark urine. All these symptoms can be presents also in the underlying liver disease, not being specific for biliary tract invasion.

The neoplastic obstruction can occur due to intraluminal biliary obstruction, extraluminal neoplastic compression or clot formation secondary to hemobilia caused by tumor invasion of biliary tree [23]. The presence of an intraluminal free-floating tumor fragment in the extrahepatic biliary tree may show an intermittent jaundice that can be associated with colicky pain [24]. Also in case of hemobilia a colicky pain can be present [5].

3.3. Fever

Fever of Unknown Origin can be a way of presentation of HCC [25,26]. It can be intermittent, and usually is accompanied by leukocytosis. Imaging studies are often necessary to differentiate an HCC from a liver abscess. Fever occur more frequently in patients with massive HCC and in non cirrhotic individuals [1].

http://dx.doi.org/10.5772/56162

3.4. Caval invasion

If HCC invades the inferior vena cava, signs and symptoms of venous insufficiency can appear. In this case relevant pitting edema can appear, usually bilaterally, affecting both inferior limbs, from the inguinal region. The invasion of the venous district, can worsen ascites and hepatomegaly [24].

Caval tumor thrombus can extend to the right atrium, causing dyspnea and heart failure [27]. When a patient presents signs and symptoms of right heart failure, such as jugular turgor, dyspnea, new onset of inferior limbs edema and worsening of hepatic insufficiency, heart tumoral invasion should always be suspected [28]. Anyway atrial invasion is reported to be also asymptomatic [29]. Pulmonary embolization by venous invasion is a rare, but reported primary manifestation of HCC [30].

4. Age differences in presentation

Patient's age can influence the clinical presentation of HCC. Signs and symptoms at presentation of HCC described in patients affected by hepatitis B are significantly different in patients younger and older than 40 years. Younger patients present more often with pain, hepatomegaly and ruptured HCC. Older patient present more often with ankle oedema and ascites. This is explained by the fact that in patients affected by viral hepatitis, advanced cirrhosis is more frequent in the older ones [2]. In younger patients it is more difficult that cirrhosis masks clinical aspect caused by HCC.

	Clinical signs and symptoms in different geographic regions (%)			
	Black African	Japan	China	Europe (Italy)
Asymtomatic	-	-	29,9	38
Abdominal pain	95	46	51	38
Ascites	51	27	18	12
Palpable mass	92	23	5	-
Hepatomegaly	-	-	54	90
Ankle Edema	-	17	14	-
Jaundice	28	17	9	14
Fever	35	17	2	12
Diarrhea	-	-	1	3
Hemoperitoneum	-	7	3	3
Variceal Bleeding	2	8	-	4

Table 1. [1,2,11,24]

5. Extrahepatic metastases

Metastases from HCC, spread through lymphatic or hematic system, are more frequently placed in abdominal and thoracic lymph nodes, lung, bones, adrenal glands. Less frequent sites of metastases are brain, spleen and breast [31]. Rarely metastases can also be detected in digestive tube, pancreas, seminal vesicle and bladder [32].

When HCC is diagnosed, extrahepatic metastases, are present in more or less 40% of cases, [32,33] and several signs and symptoms can be caused by this condition. Sometimes signs and symptoms caused by metastases are the only clinical manifestation of HCC [34]. Regional lymph nodes are affected in up to 60% of metastatic HCC, while distant lymphatic stations are involved only in 12% of these cases [32]. The frequencies of metastases in different sites are reported in (Table 2).

Pain and pathologic fractures can be caused by osteolytic metastases. Severe pain is present in 90 % of patients with bone metastases [35]. Bone metastases are present in up 66% of patients in some studies, mostly in the transverse skeleton as in thoracic spine, lumbosacral spine, sacrum. Frequently they can also be present in ribs, skull, head of femur and peripheral bones [24,32]. Rarely HCC can have as only presentation pain or other symptoms caused by bone metastases, and this can also occur in non-common bone sites [36,37].

HCC metastases can cause also symptoms linked to nervous system. In fact in case of vertebral fractures, spinal cord compression can occur, causing neurological symptoms, leading to paraplegia in some cases. Clinical features of spinal compression can occur as complication of advanced known HCC, or rarely they can be the clinical presentation of this tumor [38].

Excluding lymph nodes, lung is the most common site of metastases (54% of metastatic HCC) [39].Lung metastases sometimes are causes of dyspnea, cough, hemoptysis, chest pain [40]. Fatal respiratory failure is described in more or less 20% of HCC lung metastatic tumors [39].

Brain metastases are not frequent, but often they cause important neurological symptoms, up to causing paralysis in most of these cases [39].

Peritoneal metastases can cause ascites and abdominal pain and they are present in more or less 10% of metastatic HCC [32]. Rarely, metastases were reported in appendix, and signs and symptoms typical of acute appendicitis, as pain in the right lower quadrant associated with tenderness at the physical examination, can be a clinical presentation of HCC [41].

6. Paraneoplastic syndromes

Paraneoplastic syndromes occur in 19-44% of patients affected by HCC [42,43]. The presence of paraneoplastic syndromes is described to be related with younger patients, with larger size tumor (>10 cm) and with presence of portal vein thrombosis [43].

Among patients that have paraneoplastic syndromes during the clinical course of HCC, most of them have a single paraneoplastic manifestation. Hypercholesterolemia, erythrocytosis,

http://dx.doi.org/10.5772/56162

Frequency of metastases in different sites (%)			
Frequent Sites		**Not Frequent Sites**	
Lungs	55	Brain	2
Lymph Nodes	53	Rectum	1
Regional	41	Spleen	1
Distant	12	Diaphragm	1
Musculoskeletal	28	Duodenum	1
Adrenal	11	Esophagus	1
Peritoneum and/or omenutm	11	Pancreas	1
		Seminal Vescicle	1
		Bladder	1

Table 2. [32]

hypoglycemia and hypercalcemia are some of the most common paraneoplastic manifestations of HCC. Only 7% of patients have 2 of these syndromes, and rarely can be present all of them (<1% of cases) [42].

Below, there are described the most common paraneoplastic syndromes and there are also reported other manifestations described in some case reports. See (Table 3) for some of the reported paraneoplastc syndromes.

6.1. Hypoglycemia

Hypoglycemia is not an infrequent paraneoplastic syndrome caused by HCC, occurring in about 4,6-27% of the patients with advanced HCC [43–45]. Hypoglycemia is caused by the increased demand for glucose by the tumor together with a reduction of gluconeogenesis and glycogenolysis, due to a decreased residual liver tissue coupled with cachectic state and malnutrition that are often present in these patients [46]. Episodes of hypoglycemia caused by an advanced HCC typically occur in the last weeks before the death of the patients.

Another pathologic mechanism involved in causing hypoglycemia is overproduction by the tumor of Insulin-Like Growth Factor II [47]. Hypoglycemia caused by over production of IGF II occurs not only in late stage HCC, but also in the early phases of the neoplastic disease [44].

Hypoglycemia has been also described as the first clinical manifestation of HCC in some reports [44,48].

6.2. Hypercalcemia

Hypercalcemia is described to occur in 7-12% of patients with HCC [43,45,49]. A PTH-like humoral factor is probably responsible of this paraneoplastic syndrome [50]. Hypercalcemia can also be caused by the presence of osteolytic bone metastases [51].

Hypercaclemic coma can occur in patients with HCC and it can be confused with hepatic encephalopathy [52].

6.3. Hypercholesterolemia

Paraneoplastic hypercholesterolemia is present in 11-20% of patients with HCC [43,45,53]. Hypercholesterolemia in patients with HCC has been related with a reduced expression of LDL receptor, as in familiar hypercholesterolemia. Clinical manifestation of hypercholesterolemia in patients with HCC are not reported, but increased cardiovascular risk can be present and manifestations typical of familiar hypercholesterolemia, as xanthelasmas could be possible.

6.4. Erythrocytosis

Erythrocytosis is present in 2-16% of patients with HCC [45,54–58]. Higher levels of erythropoietin, produced by the tumor, have been reported [58]. Local hypoxia has been suggested to be the cause of overproduction of erythropoietin by large HCC tumors [58,59].

Erythrocytosis accompanied by high levels of erythropoietin has been described as a rare primary presentation of HCC [60].

6.5. Thrombocytosis

Thrombocytosis has been reported to be present in 3% of cases of HCC. This paraneoplastic syndrome seems to occur in younger patients (<60 yr), being related with the presence of a larger tumor and main portal vein tumor thrombosis representing an unfavorable prognostic factor [61]. Thrombocytosis has been described to be related with thrombopoietin production by the HCC [62]. A case of HCC associated with both thrombocytosis and acquired Von Willebrand disease has been reported [63].

6.6. Arterial hypertension

Arterial hypertension has been described as a paraneoplastic manifestation of HCC. Some cases of severe arterial blood pressure associated with high plasma level of angiotensin-I, accompanied with hypokalemia have been reported [64]. Elevated concentrations of angiotensinogen have been found, whether or not associated with higher plasma levels of renin. Overproduction of angiotensinogen and renin could both play a role in causing paraneoplastic hypertension in patients affected by HCC [65].

6.7. Diarrhea

Watery diarrhea is another manifestation that can occur in patients with HCC. Overproduction of intestinal peptides as gastrin and vasoactive intestinal peptide (VIP) is one possible explanation of the onset of diarrhea in these patients [66]. Diarrhea was also described to be a possible clinical presentation of HCC [67–69].

6.8. Feminization

Feminization is described to be present in patient with HCC, also in those not affected by liver cirrhosis, showing clinical signs and symptoms as gynecomastia, loss of body hair, loss of libido. Onset of spider naevi can be a sign of an underlying HCC and this finding has been reported more frequently in men than in women [70]. Studies about circulating sex hormones in patients affected by HCC have shown unclear results and a direct role of HCC in causing feminization is still not defined [71–74].

7. Cutaneous manifestaion

Various cutaneous manifestations have been reported as paraneoplastic syndromes caused by HCC. In rare cases, dermatomyositis has been described in patients affected by HCC, either associated or not to viral hepatitis. [75–77]. Also polymyositis can be a paraneoplastic manifestation of HCC. Polymyositis has been described also as a rare presenting manifestation of HCC, sometimes causing severe rhabdomyolysis [78–81].

A relationship between HCC and acquired porphyria cutanea tarda has been reportedin literature, [82–84].

Pityriasis rotunda is a rare cutaneous disease characterized by round/oval, hypo/hyperpigmented rash with scaling. The number of skin lesion is variable and the size is described to be between 1,5 to 25 cm. The localization of the lesions is usually over the trunk, lower back and proximal extremities [85,86].

In South African Black patients with diagnosis of HCC, its prevalence is of 16%, much higher than in patients affected by other diseases associated with pityriasis rotunda. In selected groups of people, the onset of this cutaneous disorder could represent a diagnostic instrument for HCC [87].

The sign of Leser-Trelat defined as the abrupt appearance and rapid increase in size and number of multiple seborrheic keratoses as a result of cancer development has been reported [88]. This sign has been reported also in association to HCC [89].

Also paraneoplastic pemphigus has been related to HCC [90].

8. Neurological manifestations

Neurologic paraneoplasic syndromes are rarely present in patients affected by HCC, such as multifocal necrotizing leukoencephalopathy leading to coma or non-inflammatory cerebral vasculopathy with widespread cortical and subcortical infarcts causing progressive hemiparesis and dysarthria, also in young patients [91,92].

Peripheral polyneuropathy with cranial nerve involvement has been described as a rare presenting manifestation of HCC [93].

9. Other paraneoplastic syndromes

Other paraneoplastic manifestations rarely described in patients with HCC are dysfibrinogennemia [94,95], cryofibrinogenemia [96], carcinoid syndrome [24], myasthenia gravis [97] and membranous glomerulonephritis [98].

Paraneoplastic Syndromes			
Usual Manifestations			
Hypoglycemia	Hypercalcemia	Hypercholesterolemia	Erythrocytosis
Thrombocytosis	Pityriasis Rotunda		
Reported Manifestations			
Arterial Hypertension	Dermatomyositis/ Polymyositis	Porphyria cutanea tarda	Pemphigus
Sign of Leser-Trelat	Diarrhea	Neurological manifestations	Membranous glomerulonephritis
Dysfibrinogenemia	Cryofibrinogenemia	Carcinoid syndrome	Myasthenia grave

Table 3. Add caption

10. Conclusion

Clinical signs and symptoms of HCC are various. In absence of screening programs clinical signs can be helpful for diagnosis. Clinical signs are different depending on tumor size, vascular invasion, presence of cirrhosis and presence of metastases. Several paraneoplastic syndromes are described but our knowledge about some manifestation is limited to few published case reports.

Author details

Valerio Barghini, Debora Donnini, Alessandro Uzzau* and Giorgio Soardo*

*Address all correspondence to: soardo.giorgio@aoud.sanita.fvg.it

Department of Clinical and Experimental Sciences, University of Udine, Italy

References

[1] Trevisani, F, Intino, D, Caraceni, P. E, Pizzo, P, Stefanini, M, & Mazziotti, G. F. A, et al. Etiologic factors and clinical presentation of hepatocellular carcinoma. Differences between cirrhotic and non cirrhotic Italian patients. Cancer. (1995). May 1;, 75(9), 2220-32.

[2] Lam, C-M, Chan, a O. O, Ho, P, Ng, I. O-L, Lo, C. M, Liu, C. L, et al. Different presentation of hepatitis B-related hepatocellular carcinoma in a cohort of 1863 young and old patients- implications for screening. Alimentary pharmacology & therapeutics. (2004). Apr 1;, 19(7), 771-7.

[3] Sanders, C. F. The plain chest radiograph in seventy-five cases of primary carcinoma of the liver. Clinical radiology. (1968). Jul;, 19(3), 341-6.

[4] Sherman, H. I, & Hardison, J. E. The Importance of a Coexistent Hepatic Rub and Bruit: A Clue to the Diagnosis of Cancer in the Liver. JAMA: The Journal of the American Medical Association. (1979). Apr 6;, 241(14), 1495-1495.

[5] Okuda, K O. H. Malignant Tumour. Oxford Textbook of Clinical Hepatology- Bircher, J Benhamou, J-P McIntyre, N Rizzetto, M Rodes, J.E. (1999). , 1505-1507.

[6] Ogren, M, Bergqvist, D, Björck, M, Acosta, S, Eriksson, H, & Sternby, N. H. Portal vein thrombosis: prevalence, patient characteristics and lifetime risk: a population study based on 23,796 consecutive autopsies. World journal of gastroenterology. (2006). Apr 7;, 12(13), 2115-9.

[7] Pirisi, M, Avellini, C, Fabris, C, Scott, C, Bardus, P, Soardo, G, et al. Portal vein thrombosis in hepatocellular carcinoma: age and sex distribution in an autopsy study. Journal of cancer research and clinical oncology. (1998). Jan;, 124(7), 397-400.

[8] Amitrano, L, Guardascione, M. A, Brancaccio, V, Margaglione, M, Manguso, F, Iannaccone, L, et al. Risk factors and clinical presentation of portal vein thrombosis in patients with liver cirrhosis. Journal of hepatology. (2004). May;, 40(5), 736-41.

[9] Sobhonslidsuk, A, & Reddy, K. R. Portal vein thrombosis: a concise review. The American journal of gastroenterology. (2002). Mar;, 97(3), 535-41.

[10] Belli, L, Romani, F, & Sansalone, C. Portal thrombosis in cirrhotics. A retrospective analysis. Annals of surgery. (1986). Mar; , 203(3), 286-91.

[11] Vergara, V, Muratore, A, Bouzari, H, Polastri, R, Ferrero, A, Galatola, G, et al. Spontaneous rupture of hepatocelluar carcinoma: surgical resection and long-term survival. European journal of surgical oncology: the journal of the European Society of Surgical Oncology and the British Association of Surgical Oncology. (2000). Dec;, 26(8), 770-2.

[12] Lai, E, Wu, K, Choi, T, Fan, S, & Wong, J. Spontaneous ruptured hepatocellular carcinoma. An appraisal of surgical treatment. Annals of surgery. (1989). , 24-8.

[13] Hong, S, Kim, J, Wang, H, & Kim, M. Risk Factors and Treatment Strategy of Ruptured Hepatocellular Carcinoma. The Korean Journal of Gastroenterology. (1998). Dec 1;, 32(6), 749-56.

[14] Kew, M. C, & Hodkinson, J. Rupture of hepatocellular carcinoma as a result of blunt abdominal trauma. The American journal of gastroenterology. (1991). Aug;, 86(8), 1083-5.

[15] Okuda, H, & Okuda, K. Carcinome primitif du foie. (1993). , 1010-1053.

[16] Battula, N, Srinivasan, P, Madanur, M, Chava, S. P, Priest, O, Rela, M, et al. Ruptured hepatocellular carcinoma following chemoembolization: a western experience. Hepatobiliary & pancreatic diseases international. (2007). Feb;, 6(1), 49-51.

[17] Chen, C-H, Sjeu, J-C, Huang, G-T, Lee, H-S, Yang, P-M, Wong, J-M, et al. Characteristics of hepatocellular carcinoma presenting with variceal bleeding. Journal of Gastroenterology and Hepatology. (1998). Feb;, 13(2), 170-4.

[18] Lang, B. H, Poon, R. T, Fan, S. T, & Wong, J. Outcomes of patients with hepatocellular carcinoma presenting with variceal bleeding. The American journal of gastroenterology. (2004). Nov;, 99(11), 2158-65.

[19] Bleichner, G, Boulanger, R, Squara, P, Sollet, J. P, & Parent, A. Frequency of infections in cirrhotic patients presenting with acute gastrointestinal haemorrhage. The British journal of surgery. (1986). Sep;, 73(9), 724-6.

[20] Yeo, W, Sung, J. Y, Ward, S. C, Chung, S. C, Lee, W. Y, Li, A. K, et al. A prospective study of upper gastrointestinal hemorrhage in patients with hepatocellular carcinoma. Digestive diseases and sciences. (1995). Dec;, 40(12), 2516-21.

[21] Humbert, P, Sarmiento, J, Boix, J, Planas, R, Quintero, E, Franquet, T, et al. Hepatocellular carcinoma presenting with bleeding due to duodenal perforation by the tumor. Endoscopy. (1987). Jan;, 19(1), 37-8.

[22] Lau, W, Leung, K, Leung, T. W, Liew, C. T, Chan, M. S, Yu, S. C, et al. A logical approach to hepatocellular carcinoma presenting with jaundice. Annals of surgery. (1997). Mar;, 225(3), 281-5.

[23] Lau, W. Y, Leow, C. K, Leung, K. L, Leung, T. W, Chan, M, & Yu, S. C. Cholangiographic features in the diagnosis and management of obstructive icteric type hepatocellular carcinoma. HPB surgery: a world journal of hepatic, pancreatic and biliary surgery. (2000). Jan;, 11(5), 299-306.

[24] Ribero, D, & Morris-stiff, G V. J. Presentation and Diagnosis. Hepatocellular Carcinoma- Lau W. Y. (2007). , 143-158.

[25] Okuda, K, Kondo, Y, Nakano, M, Kage, M, Arakawa, M, Kojiro, M, et al. Hepatocellular carcinoma presenting with pyrexia and leukocytosis: report of five cases. Hepatology (Baltimore, Md.). (1991). Apr;, 13(4), 695-700.

[26] Hayashi, T, Honda, H, Kaneko, K, Fukuya, T, Tateshi, Y, Ro, T, et al. Hepatocellular carcinoma with pyrexia: report of a case. Radiation medicine. (1995). , 13(3), 133-6.

[27] Saïsse, J, Hardwigsen, J, Castellani, P, & Caus, T. Le Treut YP. Budd-Chiari syndrome secondary to intracardiac extension of hepatocellular carcinoma. Two cases treated by radical resection. Hepato-gastroenterology. (2001). , 48(39), 836-9.

[28] Agelopoulou, P, Kapatais, A, Varounis, C, Grassos, C, Kalkandi, E, Kouris, N, et al. Hepatocellular carcinoma with invasion into the right atrium. Report of two cases and review of the literature. Hepato-gastroenterology. (2007). , 54(79), 2106-8.

[29] Ulus, T, Birdane, A, Dündar, E, & Tünerir, B. Asymptomatic course of a metastatic mass completely filling the right atrium in a patient with hepatocellular carcinoma. Türk Kardiyoloji Derneği arşivi: Türk Kardiyoloji Derneğinin yayın organıdır. (2012). Jan;, 40(1), 52-4.

[30] Papp, E, Keszthelyi, Z, Kalmar, N-K, Papp, L, Weninger, C, Tornoczky, T, et al. Pulmonary embolization as primary manifestation of hepatocellular carcinoma with intracardiac penetration: a case report. World journal of gastroenterology. (2005). Apr 21;, 11(15), 2357-9.

[31] Uchino, K, Tateishi, R, Shiina, S, Kanda, M, Masuzaki, R, Kondo, Y, et al. Hepatocellular carcinoma with extrahepatic metastasis: clinical features and prognostic factors. Cancer. (2011). Oct 1;, 117(19), 4475-83.

[32] Katyal, S, Oliver, J, Peterson, M, & Ferris, J. Extrahepatic Metastases of Hepatocellular Carcinoma. Radiology. (2000). , 216(3), 698-703.

[33] Si, M-S, Amersi, F, Golish, S. R, Ortiz, J. A, Zaky, J, Finklestein, D, et al. Prevalence of metastases in hepatocellular carcinoma: risk factors and impact on survival. The American surgeon. (2003). Oct;, 69(10), 879-85.

[34] Liaw, C. C, Ng, K. T, Chen, T. J, & Liaw, Y. F. Hepatocellular carcinoma presenting as bone metastasis. Cancer. (1989). Oct 15;, 64(8), 1753-7.

[35] Natsuizaka, M, Omura, T, Akaike, T, Kuwata, Y, Yamazaki, K, Sato, T, et al. Clinical features of hepatocellular carcinoma with extrahepatic metastases. Journal of gastroenterology and hepatology. (2005). Nov;, 20(11), 1781-7.

[36] Mantonakis, E. I, Margariti, T. S, Petrou, A. S, Stofas, A. C, Lazaris, A. C, Papalampros, A. E, et al. A pathological fracture and a solitary mass in the right clavicle: an unusual first presentation of HCC and the role of immunohistochemistry. World journal of surgical oncology. BioMed Central Ltd; (2012). Jan;10(1):50.

[37] Shim, Y. S, Ahn, J. Y, Cho, J. H, & Lee, K. S. Solitary skull metastasis as initial manifestation of hepatocellular carcinoma. World journal of surgical oncology. (2008). Jan; 6:66.

[38] Doval, D. C, Bhatia, K, Vaid, A. K, Pavithran, K, Sharma, J. B, Hazarika, D, et al. Spinal cord compression secondary to bone metastases from hepatocellular carcinoma. World journal of gastroenterology. (2006). Aug 28;, 12(32), 5247-52.

[39] Natsuizaka, M, Omura, T, Akaike, T, Kuwata, Y, Yamazaki, K, Sato, T, et al. Clinical features of hepatocellular carcinoma with extrahepatic metastases. Journal of gastroenterology and hepatology. (2005). Nov;, 20(11), 1781-7.

[40] Shuangshoti, S. Hepatocellular carcinoma having progressive dyspnea as clinical presentation. Journal of the Medical Association of Thailand = Chotmaihet thangphaet. (1996). Nov;, 79(11), 744-8.

[41] Kim, H. C, Yang, D. M, Jin, W, Kim, G. Y, & Choi, S. I. Metastasis to the appendix from a hepatocellular carcinoma manifesting as acute appendicitis: CT findings. The British journal of radiology. (2008). Jul;81(967):e, 194-6.

[42] Luo, J. C, Hwang, S. J, Wu, J. C, Li, C. P, Hsiao, L. T, Lai, C. R, et al. Paraneoplastic syndromes in patients with hepatocellular carcinoma in Taiwan. Cancer. (1999). Sep 1;, 86(5), 799-804.

[43] Huh, U, Kim, J, Kim, B, & Nam, K. The incidence and clinical significance of paraneoplastic syndromes in patients with hepatocellular carcinoma. Korean Journal of Hepatology. (2005). , 11(3), 275-83.

[44] Sorlini, M, Benini, F, Cravarezza, P, & Romanelli, G. Hypoglycemia, an atypical early sign of hepatocellular carcinoma. Journal of gastrointestinal cancer. (2010). Sep;, 41(3), 209-11.

[45] Teniola, S. O, & Ogunleye, I. O. Paraneoplastic syndromes in primary liver cell carcinoma in Nigeria. Tropical and geographical medicine. (1994). Jan;, 46(1), 20-2.

[46] Mcfadzean, A. J, & Yeung, R. T. Further observations on hypoglycaemia in hepatocellular carcinoma. The American journal of medicine. (1969). Aug;, 47(2), 220-35.

[47] Wu, J. C, Daughaday, W. H, Lee, S. D, Hsiao, T. S, Chou, C. K, Lin, H. D, et al. Radioimmunoassay of serum IGF-I and IGF-II in patients with chronic liver diseases and hepatocellular carcinoma with or without hypoglycemia. The Journal of laboratory and clinical medicine. (1988). Nov;, 112(5), 589-94.

[48] Nikeghbalian, S, Bananzadeh, A, & Yarmohammadi, H. Hypoglycemia, the first presenting sign of hepatocellular carcinoma. Saudi medical journal. (2006). Mar;, 27(3), 387-8.

[49] Panesar, N. S, Au, K. M, Leung, N. W, Shek, C. C, & Swaminathan, R. Nephrogenous cyclic AMP in primary hepatocellular carcinoma patients with or without hypercalcaemia. Clinical endocrinology. (1991). Dec;, 35(6), 527-32.

[50] Yen, T. C, Hwang, S. J, Wang, C. C, Lee, S. D, & Yeh, S. H. Hypercalcemia and parathyroid hormone-related protein in hepatocellular carcinoma. Liver. (1993). Dec;, 13(6), 311-5.

[51] Clines, G. A. Mechanisms and treatment of hypercalcemia of malignancy. Current opinion in endocrinology, diabetes, and obesity. (2011). Dec;, 18(6), 339-46.

[52] Tudela, P, Soldevila, B, Mòdol, J. M, & Domènech, E. Hypercalcemic encephalopathy in a patient with hepatocellular carcinoma. Digestive diseases and sciences. (2007). Nov;, 52(11), 3296-7.

[53] Hwang, S. J, Lee, S. D, Chang, C. F, Wu, J. C, Tsay, S. H, Lui, W. Y, et al. Hypercholesterolaemia in patients with hepatocellular carcinoma. Journal of gastroenterology and hepatology. (2008). , 7(5), 491-6.

[54] Hwang, S. J, Lee, S. D, Wu, J. C, Chang, C. F, Lu, C. L, Tsay, S. H, et al. Clinical evaluation of erythrocytosis in patients with hepatocellular carcinoma. Zhonghua yi xue za zhi = Chinese medical journal; Free China ed. (1994). May;, 53(5), 262-9.

[55] Sawabe, Y, Iida, S, Tabata, Y, & Yonemitsu, H. Serum erythropoietin measurements by a one-step sandwich enzyme linked immunosorbent assay in patients with hepatocellular carcinoma and liver cirrhosis. Japanese journal of clinical oncology. (1993). Oct;, 23(5), 273-7.

[56] Mcfadzean, A. J, Todd, D, & Tsang, K. C. Polycythemia in primary carcinoma of the liver. Blood. (1958). May;, 13(5), 427-35.

[57] Jacobson, R. J, Lowenthal, M. N, & Kew, M. C. Erythrocytosis in hepatocellular cancer. South African medical journal = Suid-Afrikaanse tydskrif vir geneeskunde. (1978). Apr 29;, 53(17), 658-60.

[58] Matsuyama, M, & Yamazaki, O. Erythrocytosis caused by an erythropoietin- producing hepatocellular carcinoma. Journal of surgical oncology. (2000). May):, 197-202.

[59] Tso, S. C, & Hua, A. S. Erythrocytosis in hepatocellular carcinoma: a compensatory phenomenon. British journal of haematology. (1974). Dec;, 28(4), 497-503.

[60] Chang, P-E, & Tan, C-K. Paraneoplastic erythrocytosis as a primary presentation of hepatocellular carcinoma. Indian journal of medical sciences [Internet]. Medknow Publications; (2009). May 1;63(5):202-3. Available from: http://www.indianjmedsci.org/article.asp?issn=0019-5359;year=2009;spage=202;epage=203;aulast=Chang

[61] Hwang, S-J, Luo, J-C, Li, C-P, Chu, C-W, Wu, J-C, Lai, C-R, et al. Thrombocytosis: a paraneoplastic syndrome in patients with hepatocellular carcinoma. World journal of gastroenterology. (2004). Sep 1;, 10(17), 2472-7.

[62] Ryu, T, Nishimura, S, Miura, H, Yamada, H, Morita, H, Miyazaki, H, et al. Thrombopoietin-producing hepatocellular carcinoma. Internal medicine (Tokyo, Japan). (2003). Aug;, 42(8), 730-4.

[63] Chen, C-C, Chang, J-Y, Liu, K-J, Chan, C, Ho, C-H, Lee, S-C, et al. Hepatocellular carcinoma associated with acquired von Willebrand disease and extreme thrombocytosis. Annals of oncology. (2005). Jun;, 16(6), 988-9.

[64] Arai, H, Saitoh, S, Matsumoto, T, Makita, F, Mitsugi, S, Yuasa, K, et al. Hypertension as a paraneoplastic syndrome in hepatocellular carcinoma. Journal of gastroenterology. (1999). Aug;, 34(4), 530-4.

[65] Kew, M. C, Leckie, B. J, & Greeff, M. C. Arterial hypertension as a paraneoplastic phenomenon in hepatocellular carcinoma. Archives of internal medicine. (1989). Sep;, 149(9), 2111-3.

[66] Bialecki, E. S. Di Bisceglie AM. Diagnosis of hepatocellular carcinoma. HPB: the official journal of the International Hepato Pancreato Biliary Association. (2005). Jan;, 7(1), 26-34.

[67] Steiner, E, Velt, P, Gutierrez, O, Schwartz, S, & Chey, W. Hepatocellular carcinoma presenting with intractable diarrhea. A radiologic-pathologic correlation. Archives of surgery (Chicago, Ill.: 1960). (1986). Jul;, 121(7), 849-51.

[68] Bruix, J, Castells, A, Calvet, X, Feu, F, Bru, C, Solé, M, et al. Diarrhea as a presenting symptom of hepatocellular carcinoma. Digestive diseases and sciences. (1990). Jun;, 35(6), 681-5.

[69] Giannelli, G, Pierri, F, Schiraldi, O, & Antonaci, S. Diarrhea as first clinical manifestation of hepatocellular carcinoma. Recenti progressi in medicina. (2002). Sep;, 93(9), 478-81.

[70] Lai, C, Gregory, P, Wu, P, & Lok, A. Hepatocellular carcinoma in Chinese males and females. Possible causes for the male predominance. Cancer. (1987). , 60(5), 1107-10.

[71] Pignata, S, Daniele, B, Galati, M. G, Esposito, G, Vallone, P, Fiore, F, et al. Oestradiol and testosterone blood levels in patients with viral cirrhosis and hepatocellular carcinoma. European journal of gastroenterology & hepatology. (1997). Mar;, 9(3), 283-6.

[72] Olubuyide, I. O, & Ola, O. S. Clinical feminisation and sex hormone concentrations in Nigerian men with cirrhosis with and without hepatocellular carcinoma. The British journal of clinical practice. (1994). , 48(2), 70-2.

[73] Salles, G. Vital Durand D, Mackiewicz R, Pugeat M, Levrat R. Hepatocellular carcinoma and hyperestrogenia in a male. Gastroentérologie clinique et biologique. (1987).

[74] Lampropoulou-karatzas, C, Goritsas, P, & Makri, M. G. Low serum testosterone: a special feature of hepatocellular carcinoma. The European journal of medicine. (1993). Jan;, 2(1), 23-7.

[75] Toshikuni, N, Torigoe, R, Mitsunaga, M, Omoto, A, & Nakashima, K. Dermatomyositis associated with hepatocellular carcinoma in an elderly female patient with hepatitis C virus-related liver cirrhosis. World journal of gastroenterology. (2006). Mar 14;, 12(10), 1641-4.

[76] Kee, S-J, Kim, T-J, Lee, S-J, Cho, Y-N, Park, S-C, Kim, J-S, et al. Dermatomyositis associated with hepatitis B virus-related hepatocellular carcinoma. Rheumatology international. (2009). Mar;, 29(5), 595-9.

[77] Apostolidis, L, Kahlert, C, Siegmund, A, Thom, R, Horstmann, S, Jäger, D, et al. Remission of paraneoplastic dermatomyositis associated with hepatocellular carcinoma under prednisolone and azathiopin, and concommittant sorafenib. Onkologie. (2009). Feb;32(1-2):50-3.

[78] Kim, M-J, Kim, J-A, Sung, M-S, & Min, J-K. Hepatocellular carcinoma,polymyositis,rhabdomyolysis,and acute renal failure. Journal of Korean medical science. (2004). Dec;, 19(6), 891-4.

[79] Tekaya, R, Abdelghni, K, & Abdelmoula, L. Ben Hadj Yahia C, Chaabouni L, Zouari R. Hepatocellular carcinoma with polymyositis as an initial symptom: a case report. Acta clinica Belgica. (2011). , 66(1), 53-4.

[80] Hasegawa, K, Uesugi, H, Kubota, K, Ugawa, Y, Murayama, S, Kobayashi, T, et al. Polymyositis as a paraneoplastic manifestation of hepatocellular carcinoma. Hepato-gastroenterology. (2000). , 47(35), 1425-7.

[81] Kishore, D, Khurana, V, Raj, A, Gambhir, I. S, & Diwaker, A. Hepatocellular carcinoma presenting as polymyositis: a paraneoplastic syndrome. Annals of Saudi medicine [Internet]. (2011). Available from: http://www.pubmedcentral.nih.gov/articlerender.fcgi?artid=3183691&tool=pmcentrez&rendertype=abstract, 31(5), 533-5.

[82] Ishibashi, H, Matsunaga, T, & Dohmen, K. Association of cirrhosis and hepatocellular carcinoma with porphyria cutanea tarda. Nihon rinsho. Japanese journal of clinical medicine. (1995). Jun;, 53(6), 1474-8.

[83] Huang, W. S, Liao, L. Y, Wang, C. S, & Chen, P. H. Hepatocellular carcinoma presenting with acquired porphyria: a case report and review of the literature. Changgeng yi xue za zhi / Changgeng ji nian yi yuan = Chang Gung medical journal / Chang Gung Memorial Hospital. (1999). Mar;, 22(1), 111-6.

[84] Fracanzani, A. L, Taioli, E, Sampietro, M, Fatta, E, Bertelli, C, Fiorelli, G, et al. Liver cancer risk is increased in patients with porphyria cutanea tarda in comparison to matched control patients with chronic liver disease. Journal of hepatology. (2001). Oct 1;, 35(4), 498-503.

[85] Gupta, S. Pityriasis rotunda mimicking tinea cruris/corporis and erythrasma in an Indian patient. The Journal of dermatology. (2001). Jan;, 28(1), 50-3.

[86] DiBisceglie AMHodkinson HJ, Berkowitz I, Kew MC. Pityriasis rotunda. A cutaneous marker of hepatocellular carcinoma in South African blacks. Archives of dermatology. (1986). Jul;, 122(7), 802-4.

[87] Berkowitz, I, Hodkinson, H. J, & Kew, M. C. DiBisceglie AM. Pityriasis rotunda as a cutaneous marker of hepatocellular carcinoma: a comparison with its prevalence in other diseases. The British journal of dermatology. (1989). Apr;, 120(4), 545-9.

[88] Schwartz, R. A. Sign of Leser-Trélat. Journal of the American Academy of Dermatology. (1996). Jul;, 35(1), 88-95.

[89] Tajima, H, Mitsuoka, S, Ohtsuka, E, Nakamura, Y, Nakayama, T, Satoh, Y, et al. A case of hepatocellular carcinoma with the sign of Leser-Trelat: a possible role of a cutaneous marker for internal malignancy. Japanese journal of medicine. (1991). , 30(1), 53-6.

[90] Yokokura, H, Demitsu, T, Kakurai, M, Umemoto, N, Azuma, R, Yamada, T, et al. Paraneoplastic pemphigus mimicking erosive mucosal lichen planus associated with primary hepatocellular carcinoma. The Journal of dermatology. (2006). Dec;, 33(12), 842-5.

[91] Phanthumchinda, K, & Rungruxsirivorn, S. Encephaloradiculopathy: a non-metastatic complication of hepatocellular carcinoma. Journal of the Medical Association of Thailand = Chotmaihet thangphaet. (1991). May;, 74(5), 288-91.

[92] Norris, S, Rajendiran, S, Sheahan, K, Murphy, S, Royston, D, Alyusuf, R, et al. Noncirrhotic hepatoma presenting with paraneoplastic neurologic manifestations: two cases. The American journal of gastroenterology. (1997). Oct;, 92(10), 1923-6.

[93] Hatzis, G. S, Delladetsima, I, & Koufos, C. Hepatocellular carcinoma presenting with paraneoplastic neurologic syndrome in a hepatitis B surface antigen-positive patient. Journal of clinical gastroenterology. (1998). Mar;, 26(2), 144-7.

[94] Von Felten, A, Straub, P. W, & Frick, P. G. Dysfibrinogenemia in a patient with primary hepatoma. First observation of an acquired abnormality of fibrin monomer aggregation. The New England journal of medicine. (1969). Feb 20;, 280(8), 405-9.

[95] Gralnick, H. R, Givelber, H, & Abrams, E. Dysfibrinogenemia associated with hepatoma. Increased carbohydrate content of the fibrinogen molecule. The New England journal of medicine. (1978). Aug 3;, 299(5), 221-6.

[96] CryofibrinogenemiaMultiple Dysproteinemias, and Hypervolemia in a Patient with a Primary Hepatoma. Annals of Internal Medicine. (1966). Mar 1;, 64(3), 658-64.

[97] Vautravers, C, Rat, P, Cercueil, J-P, Moreau, T, Horiot, J-C, & Chauffert, B. Hepatocellular carcinoma presenting as paraneoplastic myasthenia gravis. European journal

of internal medicine. European Federation of Internal Medicine; (2008). Dec;19(8):e, 86-7.

[98] Texier, F, Dharancy, S, Provot, F, Augusto, D, Mortier, P-E, Mathurin, P, et al. Membranous glomerulonephritis complicating hepatocellular carcinoma. Gastroentérologie clinique et biologique. (2004). Pt 1):605-7.

Chapter 11

Sorafenib in the Continuum of Care for Hepatocellular Carcinoma: Challenges in Defining Optimal Practice

Ahmed O. Kaseb and Laura M. Kulik

Additional information is available at the end of the chapter

http://dx.doi.org/10.5772/56952

1. Introduction

Globally, liver cancer represents a major health care burden, accounting for almost 700,000 deaths annually. [1] Hepatocellular carcinoma (HCC) comprises 70% to 85% of primary liver cancers in most regions. [2] Although the incidence of HCC has historically been lower in the US than in many other countries, age-adjusted rates tripled between 1975 and 2005. [3] In fact, liver cancer is the fastest-growing cause of cancer-related death in American men. [4] Most patients with HCC are diagnosed at advanced stages and are ineligible for potentially curative treatments such as surgical resection and liver transplantation. [5] Prior to the introduction of sorafenib in 2007, systemic treatments were unavailable for patients with HCC.

In defining optimal treatment for patients with HCC, several questions remain unanswered. Clinical data are needed to evaluate sorafenib safety in patients with advanced liver disease (i.e., those with Child-Pugh [CP] B disease) and in those with HCC-associated portal hypertension. In addition, how best to utilize sorafenib in combination with sequential locoregional therapies (LRT) or post-surgery remains unclear. These challenges are further compounded by the ongoing uncertainties in determining the value of the modified Response Evaluation Criteria In Solid Tumors (mRECIST) and understanding the optimal timing for response assessment in patients treated with sorafenib and/or LRT. Proactive management of adverse events (AEs) associated with sorafenib also remains an area of active investigation. Finally, although sorafenib has demonstrated a clear benefit to patients with advanced HCC, the majority of patients will ultimately experience disease progression. Efforts are underway to evaluate the best approaches to treating these patients in a manner that minimizes the risk of mortality from deterioration of the underlying liver disease. In this review, we describe the current understanding of sorafenib's efficacy and safety, and ongoing approaches to defining even better treatment options for patients with HCC.

2. Late-phase clinical development of sorafenib for unresectable, advanced HCC: Pivotal trials and subanalyses

Clinical trial design in HCC is challenging owing to the complex nature of the disease. The coexistence of cancer, liver disease, and other comorbidities, and the prior or concomitant use of locoregional therapies make selection and recruitment of an appropriately homogeneous patient cohort difficult. Geographical heterogeneities in disease etiology, patient characteristics, and practice patterns are significant and contribute to the need for, and confound, multi-institutional studies.

Both pivotal trials of sorafenib, the Sorafenib Hepatocellular Carcinoma Assessment Randomized Protocol (SHARP) and Asia-Pacific (AP), were designed to elucidate the effect of the drug in a specific population of patients with preserved liver function (CP A). In these trials, sorafenib produced a significant survival advantage over placebo in patients with advanced HCC; these results led to regulatory approval of sorafenib [6,7] (Table 1).

In subanalyses of these pivotal trials, the safety profile of sorafenib was similar regardless of baseline liver function. In the SHARP trial, sorafenib treatment consistently improved overall survival (OS), time to progression (TTP), and disease control rate (DCR) irrespective of Eastern Cooperative Oncology Group performance status (ECOG PS); tumor burden, as evidenced by macroscopic vascular invasion or extrahepatic spread; tumor stage (Barcelona Clinic Liver Cancer [BCLC] stage B or C); prior curative treatments (including surgery, radiofrequency ablation, or percutaneous ethanol injection); or prior transarterial chemoembolization (TACE) [8] (Figure 1). However, patients with tumors confined to the liver, with no vascular invasion or metastases, had better outcomes. Substantially similar results were obtained in subanalyses of the AP trial, with the exception of patients with ECOG PS 0, who had a slightly reduced OS in the sorafenib treatment group [9] (Figure 2). In both studies, sorafenib also improved OS over placebo irrespective of baseline serum alanine aminotransferase/aspartate aminotransferase, alpha-fetoprotein (AFP), and bilirubin levels. [9, 10] Notably, in the SHARP trial, hepatitis B virus (HBV) surface antigen positivity was associated with a longer median OS but shorter TTP in patients treated with sorafenib; however, DCR was similar in sorafenib- and placebo-treated groups.

It is interesting to note that in the SHARP trial, patients positive for HCV antibody derived more benefit from sorafenib treatment than patients with other etiologies [8] (Figure 1) Consistent with this notion, preclinical data suggest that sorafenib may inhibit Raf-dependent HCV replication and HCV-induced increases in vascular endothelial growth factor (VEGF) expression. [11, 12] However, in a small clinical study in 33 HCV-infected patients, viral load was not reduced during treatment, even among those who showed a tumor response; notably, VEGF levels were not measured. [13]

Study Phase N	Treatment Schema	Patient Population	Efficacy Results	Safety Results
Llovet [7] Phase 3 SHARP N=602	400 mg BID continuous SOR vs PBO	CP: A, 97%; B, 3% BCLC stage: B, 17%, C, 82% ECOG PS: 0, 54%; 1, 38%; 2, 8% Hepatitis virus status: HBV, 18%; HCV, 28%	Median OS: 10.7 mo SOR vs 7.9 mo PBO; HR 0.69 (95% CI 0.55-0.87; *P*<.001) Median time to symptomatic progression: 4.1 mo SOR vs 4.9 mo PBO; *P*=.77) Median time to radiologic progression: 5.5 mo SOR vs 2.8 mo PBO (*P*<.001) Response, by RECIST (SOR vs PBO): CR: 0% vs 0% PR: 2% vs 1% (*P*=.05) SD: 71% vs 67% (*P*=.17) DCR (≥SD for ≥28 days): 43% vs 32% (*P*=.002)	Gr 3/4 drug-related AEs (SOR vs PBO): HFSR: 8% vs <1% (*P*<.001) Diarrhea: 8% vs 2% (*P*<.001) Fatigue: 4% vs 3%-4% (*P*=1.0)
Cheng [6] Phase 3 N=226	Randomized 2:1 to 400 mg BID continuous SOR vs PBO	CP: A, 97%; B, 3% BCLC stage: C, 96% ECOG PS: 0, 26%; 1, 69%; 2, 5% Hepatitis virus status: HBV, 73%; HCV, 8%	Median OS: 6.5 mo SOR vs 4.2 mo PBO (HR 0.68 [95% CI 0.50-0.93]; *P*=.014) Median TTP: 2.8 mo SOR vs 1.4 mo PBO (HR 0.57 [95% CI 0.42-0.79]; *P*=.0005) Response by RECIST (SOR vs PBO): CR: 0% vs 0% PR: 3% vs 1% SD: 54% vs 28% PD: 31% vs 54% Not accessible: 12% vs 17% DCR (≥SD for ≥28 days): 35% vs 16% (*P*=.002)	Gr 3/4 drug-related AEs (SOR vs PBO): HFSR: 11% vs 0% Diarrhea: 6% vs 0% Fatigue: 3% vs 1%
Lencioni [15] Phase 4 GIDEON N=1571 for 2nd interim analysis	Prospective, non-interventional study of pts with unresectable HCC treated with SOR	CP: A, 61%; B, 23%; C, 2% BCLC stage: A, 7%; B, 19%; C, 54%; D, 6% ECOG PS: 0, 40%; 1, 43%; 2, 9%; 3-4, 3% HCC etiology: HBV, 37%; HCV, 32%; alcohol, 29%	Median OS by initial dose: 400 mg/d: 7.1 mo (95% CI 5.8-8.1) 800 mg/d: 9.3 mo (95% CI 8.6-10.2) Median TTP by initial dose: 400 mg/d: 3.6 mo (95% CI 2.8-4.1) 800 mg/d: 4.5 mo (95% CI 4.1-5.1) Median OS by CP status: A, 10.3 mo; B, 4.8 mo; C, 2.0 mo Median TTP by CP status: A, 4.2 mo; B, 3.6 mo; C, 2.1 mo	Gr 3/4 drug-related AEs: HFSR: 5% Fatigue: 3%-4% Diarrhea: 3% Drug-related serious AEs: 9% AEs leading to SOR discontinuation: 28%

AE, adverse event; BCLC, Barcelona Clinic Liver Cancer; BID, twice daily; CI, confidence interval; CP, Child-Pugh; CR, complete response; DCR, disease control rate; ECOG PS, Eastern Cooperative Oncology Group performance status; GIDEON, Global Investigation of Therapeutic DEcisions in Hepatocellular Carcinoma and Of its Treatment with SorafeNib; gr, grade; HBV, hepatitis B virus; HCC, hepatocellular carcinoma; HCV, hepatitis C virus; HFSR, hand-foot skin reaction; HR, hazard ratio; OS, overall survival; PBO, placebo; PD, progressive disease; PR, partial response; pt, patient; RECIST, Response Evaluation Criteria in Solid Tumors; SD, stable disease; SHARP, Sorafenib Hepatocellular Carcinoma Assessment Randomized Protocol; SOR, sorafenib; TTP, time to progression

Table 1. Key phase 3 and phase 4 trials evaluating the safety and efficacy of sorafenib in advanced HCC

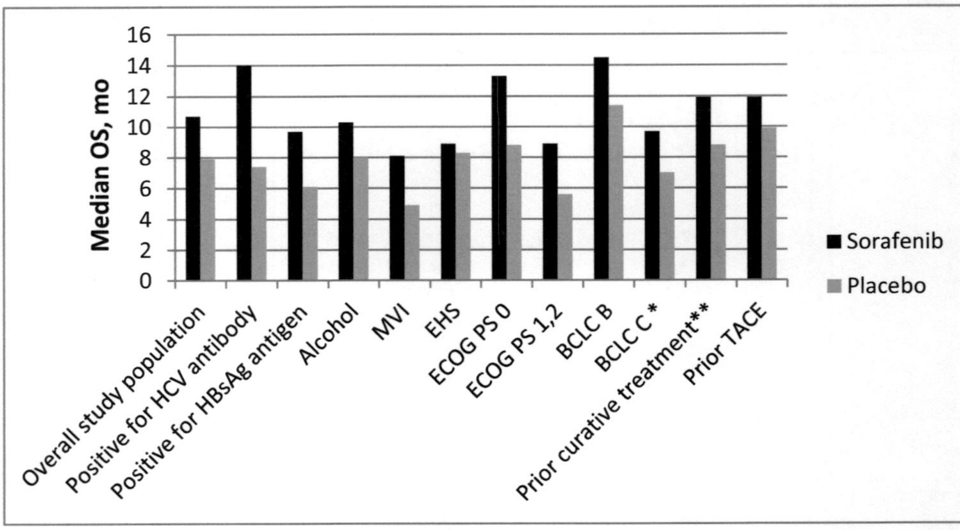

BCLC, Barcelona Clinic Liver Cancer; ECOG PS, Eastern Cooperative Oncology Group performance status; EHS, extrahepatic spread; HBsAG, hepatitis B surface antigen; HCV, hepatitis C virus; MVI, macroscopic vascular invasion; OS, overall survival; TACE, transarterial chemoembolization.

Figure 1. Median survival in the SHARP trial population overall and by subgroups. [8] *Includes 1 sorafenib-treated patient with BCLC D. **Resection/local ablation, percutaneous ethanol injection, or radiofrequency ablation.

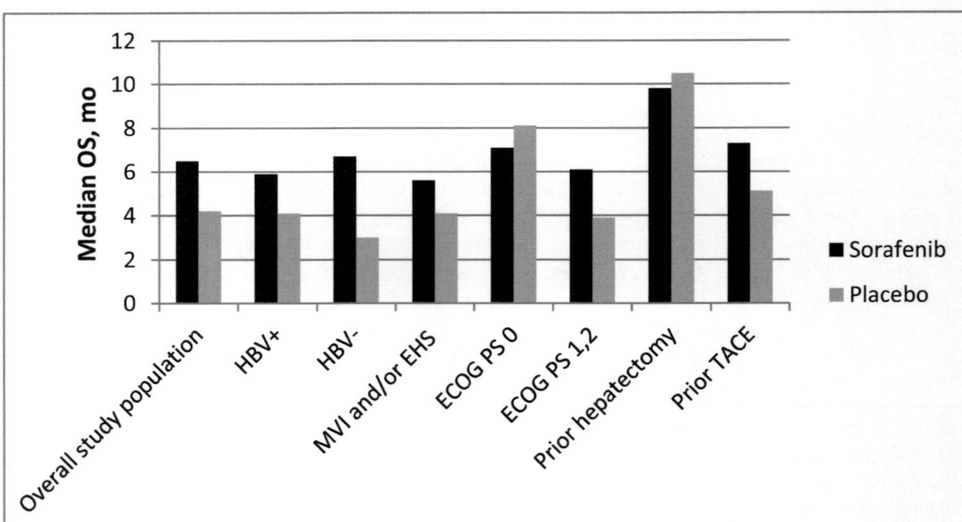

ECOG PS, Eastern Cooperative Oncology Group performance status; EHS, extrahepatic spread; HBV, hepatitis B virus; MVI, macroscopic vascular invasion; OS, overall survival; TACE, transarterial chemoembolization.

Figure 2. Median survival in the AP trial population overall and by various subgroups. [9]

3. Understanding sorafenib efficacy and safety in advanced liver disease

The Global Investigation of Therapeutic DEcisions in Hepatocellular Carcinoma and Of its Treatment with SorafeNib (GIDEON) was initiated in 2009 as a global, prospective, post-marketing non-interventional study to further evaluate the safety of sorafenib in patients with unresectable HCC and CP B liver function. This study of more than 3000 patients was designed to assess a variety of patient subsets under real-life practice conditions. [14] At a second interim analysis in 2011, grade ≥3 AEs and drug-related serious AEs were similar across BCLC stages and were consistent with those reported in the SHARP and AP trials (i.e., hand-foot skin reaction [HFSR], diarrhea, fatigue). [15, 16] The GIDEON data are consistent with those from another study by Abou-Alfa and colleagues, who observed comparable AE rates in CP A and CP B patients with the exception of all-grade elevated bilirubin levels (67% vs 86%, respectively), grade ≥3 hyperbilirubinemia (14% vs 53%, respectively), and grade ≥3 encephalopathy (3% vs 13%, respectively). [17]

In both the GIDEON second interim analysis and the study by Abou-Alfa, patients with CP B status exhibited shorter median OS compared with patients with CP A, supporting the prognostic significance of this classification. [17, 18] Nonetheless, data suggest that CP B patients derive benefit from sorafenib. A retrospective study compared the outcomes of 148 patients with unresectable HCC treated with sorafenib to those of a similar cohort of 78 patients receiving best supportive care (BSC). [19] Sorafenib significantly extended the median OS over BSC in patients with CP A (11.3 vs 6.4 months, respectively; *P*=.01) and patients with CP B (5.5 vs 1.9 months, respectively; *P*=.02). An ongoing randomized phase 3 trial (BOOST, NCT 01405573) comparing sorafenib plus BSC to BSC in patients with CP B will further explore efficacy outcomes in this population; this study is estimated to be completed in March 2014.

4. Trials comparing sorafenib to other potential first-line agents in advanced HCC

The American Association for the Study of Liver Diseases (AASLD) recommends sorafenib for the treatment BCLC stage C disease, [20] and it remains the only approved systemic treatment for unresectable HCC. Although several other targeted therapies have been investigated, to date, none have improved on the outcomes of sorafenib in randomized controlled trials. Cheng and colleagues compared sunitinib and sorafenib in 1073 patients with advanced HCC similar to those in the SHARP and AP trials. [21] Although TTP was comparable, sorafenib-treated patients experienced significantly longer OS (10.0 vs 8.1 months; *P*=.002) than sunitinib-treated patients, possibly due to greater sunitinib-related toxicity, and the trial was terminated early. Employing a non-inferiority statistical design, a recent trial comparing first-line brivanib to sorafenib in advanced HCC (BRISK-FL; N=1155) did not meet its primary OS objective. [22] A phase 3 study evaluating linifanib and sorafenib in CP A patients with advanced HCC (N=1035) failed to show an advantage for linifanib in this setting. [23] OS was 9.8 and 9.1 months in sorafenib- and linifanib-treated patients, respectively. Although secondary end-

points of TTP and overall response rate favored treatment with linifanib, sorafenib was better tolerated in this study population.
αβ

Agent	Molecular Targets
Sorafenib	BRAF, mutant BRAF, CRAF, FLT3, KIT, PDGFRβ, RET, VEGFR1, VEGFR2, VEGFR3 [70]
Sunitinib	CSF1R, FLT3, PDGFRα, PDGFRβ, RET, VEGFR1, VEGFR2, VEGFR3, KIT [71]
Brivanib	FGFR1, VEGFR [72]
Linifanib	CSFR1, FLT3, KIT, PDGFRβ, VEGFR1, VEGFR3 [73]
Dovitinib	CSFR1, FGFR1, FGFR2, FGFR3, FLT3, KIT, PDGFRβ, RET, TrkA, VEGFR1, VEGFR2, VEGFR3 [74]
Nintedanib	FGFR1, FGFR2, FGFR3, FGFR4, PDGFRα, PDGFRβ, VEGFR1, VEGFR2, VEGFR3 [75]

CSF1R, colony-stimulating factor 1 receptor; FGFR, fibroblast growth factor receptor; HCC, hepatocellular carcinoma; PDGFR, platelet-derived growth factor receptor; VEGFR, vascular endothelial growth factor receptor.

Table 2. Specificities of targeted inhibitors investigated in clinical trials of HCC

It is remarkable that despite significant overlap in molecular target specificity— particularly the VEGF receptors (Table 2)— none of these agents have, as yet, demonstrated superior OS benefit compared with sorafenib. One explanation may be that a unique molecular activity of sorafenib accounts for its consistently improved benefit. For example, among these agents, sorafenib is the only reported inhibitor of BRAF; overexpression of Raf1 has been detected in 49-100% of HCC biopsies and is an independent risk factor for death [24, 25] (Table 2). It is also possible that tolerance of sorafenib is a factor in improving OS or that the clinical trial designs (e.g., dosing, patient criteria) were suboptimal for demonstrating comparator activity. Two additional agents, dovitinib and nintedanib (BIBF1120), which have significant activity against fibroblast growth factor receptor, are currently being evaluated as first-line agents in phase 2 trials (NCT01232296, NCT01004003).

5. Addressing HCC management dilemmas: Ongoing studies

The introduction of sorafenib has unveiled a number of new challenges in the real-world setting. Patient management is complicated by the concurrence of underlying hepatic dysfunction. Given the complexity of managing both liver cancer and hepatic impairment, the value of a multidisciplinary approach to HCC care has become increasingly apparent. Patients may have undergone or be candidates for procedures such as TACE, surgery, or radiofrequency ablation. Questions remain as to whether sorafenib use is safe and beneficial in these settings and when it should be used in the continuum of care. Similar questions arise in the context of transplantation. Compounding these scientific quandaries is the fact that these patients may initially be seen by surgeons or interventional radiologists, who typically do not prescribe oncology medications. By the time patients are evaluated by an oncologist or hepatologist, clinical deterioration may prohibit the initiation of sorafenib therapy. Moreover, while institutional standards exist with respect to implementation of these procedures, substantial regional variations occur, making clinical trial design difficult. Significant challenges persist in defining appropriate response guidelines (e.g., RECIST) for specific therapies [26] and in defining the role of sorafenib in the treatment of patients with HCC progression.

5.1. Combination with locoregional therapy

The rationale for combining sorafenib with TACE is to mitigate the VEGF surge in response to hypoxemia associated with embolization of the hepatic artery supplying the tumor. [27, 28] Because increased circulating VEGF post-TACE has been linked to more aggressive disease, [29] blocking angiogenesis following embolization is hypothesized to improve outcomes and provides rationale for further studies.

Two large placebo-controlled studies evaluated the efficacy and safety of sorafenib combined with TACE. The first trial (N=458) evaluated sorafenib in Japanese and Korean patients with unresectable HCC, good performance status (88% ECOG PS 0), preserved liver function (100% CP A), and prior radiologic response to TACE. [30] The median time from TACE to initiating treatment with sorafenib was 9.3 weeks. This interrupted sequencing did not significantly prolong OS or median TTP (5.4 and 3.7 months in the sorafenib and placebo groups, respectively). Hypothetically, the delay between TACE and sorafenib initiation and the relatively low daily dose of sorafenib (median 386 mg, range 112-794.5 mg) may have contributed to the lack of superiority for combined treatment. Notably, significant differences in outcomes were observed among patient groups stratified by geographic region, likely reflecting regional variations in HCC treatment.

Sorafenib may exert its greatest benefit when administered before or concurrent with TACE treatment. The second trial, Sorafenib or Placebo in combination with transarterial chemoembolization with doxorubicin-eluting beads for intermediate-stage HCC (SPACE), examined this strategy. This global phase 2 study randomized 307 patients (CP A, ECOG PS 0) with intermediate-stage HCC to TACE with doxorubicin-eluting beads (DEB-TACE) plus sorafenib or placebo. DEB-TACE was administered 3-7 days after initiating sorafenib or placebo and subsequently on the first day of cycles 3, 7, and 13, and every 6 cycles thereafter. [31] While TTP was similar between the DEB-TACE/sorafenib and DEB-TACE/placebo arms, interpretation of the results is limited by the study design (scheduled DEB-TACE treatments are not routinely employed in clinical practice) and challenges inherent with assessing response to locoregional therapies. A third, single-center, phase 2 randomized controlled study (N=80) examined TACE with or without sorafenib exclusively in HCV-infected patients. [32] In this study, in which sorafenib was administered 30 days after TACE, TTP was significantly delayed in the sorafenib-treated group (9.2 months vs 4.9 months; *P*=.001). This result is interesting in light of the SHARP trial results in which patients with HCV may have derived more benefit from sorafenib treatment than patients with other HCC etiologies.

Several additional trials are currently recruiting patients to evaluate the combined use of LRT and sorafenib. A phase 3 (N=412) TACE-2 trial (NCT01324076) is examining the benefit of initiating sorafenib treatment 2-5 weeks prior to DEB-TACE. Patients may undergo further TACE based on their clinician's evaluation. Another phase 3 (N=400) trial, ECOG 1208 (NCT01004978), will also evaluate initiating sorafenib prior to TACE, with TACE treatment occurring every 4 weeks with up to 4 courses of treatment. In this trial, the TACE protocol may use conventional chemoembolization comprising doxorubicin hydrochloride only or DEB-TACE. Finally, the phase 3 (N=400) STOP-HCC trial (NCT01556490) is evaluating the use of radioembolization followed 30 days later by sorafenib (R. Salem, personal communication). The large number of trials assessing the combination of LRT with sorafenib attests to the perceived potential of this approach. However, the wide variations in trial design underscore the difficulties in evaluating the true benefit of this combination. Variations in the timing of sorafenib dosing and the type of LRT (conventional TACE, DEB-TACE, or radioembolization) and frequency employed, coupled with a lack of reliable standardized methods for evaluating response, make trial design and treatment decision-making very challenging.

5.2. Is there a potential role for adjuvant sorafenib?

Despite intervention with potentially curative resection or ablation, HCC recurrence remains at 15-20% annually, with the 5-year recurrence rate reaching 80–90%. [33] Addressing residual disease and preventing or delaying recurrence remain key unmet needs; proven adjuvant therapies do not yet exist. A phase 3 randomized, double-blind, placebo-controlled study of sorafenib as an adjuvant treatment after surgical resection or local ablation (STORM: NCT00692770) is underway. If sorafenib can substantially delay HCC recurrence, survival may be impacted in a clinically meaningful way.

5.3. Could neoadjuvant sorafenib facilitate surgery or transplantation?

Liver transplantation is the accepted best curative option for HCC patients meeting the Milan criteria. However, organ availability is limited, and in one study, dropout while on the waiting list was found to be the sole prognostic factor in patients selected for orthotopic liver transplantation (OLT). [34] Sorafenib may represent a potential "bridge" option for patients awaiting OLT. Evaluating the benefit of sorafenib treatment in the transplant setting faces many of the same hurdles as for TACE, especially with respect to when it should be used in the continuum of care. Using a sensitivity analysis, one study showed that neoadjuvant sorafenib improved survival over no therapy, providing a cost benefit in T2-HCC patients waiting for liver transplant for ≤6 months; however, further safety assessments in the pre-transplant population are needed. [35]

In a pilot cohort study (N=33) of patients undergoing liver transplantation for HCC, overall death rates were similar between sorafenib-treated patients and controls (20% vs 9%, respectively; *P*=NS). [36] Despite the small sample size, the incidence of post-transplant biliary complications (67% vs 17%, respectively; *P*=.01) and acute cellular rejection (67% vs 22%, respectively; *P*=.04) were significantly higher in the sorafenib group than in controls. Notably, in this study, sorafenib was continued until the day of transplant. Some practitioners recommend that sorafenib be discontinued before a surgical procedure due to potential risks for bleeding, impaired wound healing, and liver dysfunction in the perioperative period. [37] However, limited notice of organ availability challenges the ability to implement defined and controlled pre-transplant regimens. Consequently, patients may be required to remain off therapy for a protracted period of time, with the impact on HCC recurrence unknown.

In another study, investigators reviewed 59 consecutive HCC patients (10 treated with sorafenib and 49 controls) who underwent liver transplantation at a single center and concluded that pre-transplant sorafenib did not increase the rate of surgical complications. [38] The frequency of post-transplant AEs, including biliary complications, strictures, wound infection, and bleeding, was similar in both groups.

Two case reports describe successful outcomes associated with sorafenib followed by curative treatment for HCC. In one report of two patients with locally advanced HCC with portal vein thrombosis (PVT), neoadjuvant sorafenib administered for 10 and 12 months, respectively, produced sufficient tumor shrinkage to reverse PVT, normalize alpha-fetoprotein (AFP), and enable curative surgical resection. In both patients, sorafenib was stopped one week prior to surgery without post-operative complications. [39] However, in the SHARP and AP trials, response rates were <5%; therefore, chances of consistently downsizing HCC are very slim, and multimodality therapies need to be studied in this setting. In another report, a patient with relapsed HCC following hepatic resection was treated for 5 months prior to salvage transplant without complications. Three months after transplant (at the time of the report), the patient had normal liver function and no evidence of recurrence. [40]

5.4. Sorafenib in the post-transplant setting

Only a few small studies have addressed treatment options for post-transplant HCC recurrence. Preliminary data from a phase 1 trial show that sorafenib treatment in high-risk HCC patients post-transplant is feasible, with no dose-limiting toxicities to date; 12 patients have received sorafenib (200 mg once daily [QD] escalating thus far to 400/200 mg QD) for a median 167 days (range 21-170 days) and 3 patients experienced HCC recurrence. [41]

In a retrospective case-controlled study of 17 patients outside Milan criteria who underwent OLT, adjuvant or palliative sorafenib was administered to 5 and 6 patients, respectively. Patients treated adjuvantly demonstrated significantly improved disease-free survival at 6 months (100% vs 37.5%, *P*=.034), 12 months (66.7% vs 9.4%, *P*=.026), and 18 months (68% vs 0%, *P*=.011). All 5 patients treated with adjuvant sorafenib were alive at 24 months, while OS for patients treated with palliative sorafenib was 66.7% at 12 months (vs 40% for controls, *P*=.248) and 50% at 18 months (vs 20%, *P*=.17). [42]

In a single-center retrospective analysis of 24 patients with HCC recurrence post-transplant, treatment with sorafenib (N=8) for disseminated disease outside the liver produced a mean OS of 6.7 months (95% confidence interval [CI], 4.8-8.6). [43] These data require confirmation through further study with larger cohorts and a more rigorous trial design. A randomized phase 2 trial (N=356) of sorafenib versus placebo in high-risk patients after liver transplant

(NCT01624285) is ongoing; 2-year recurrence-free survival (RFS) is the primary endpoint, with secondary endpoints of OS, safety, and RFS at 1 year.

5.5. Potential for combination with other targeted systemic therapies

Although sorafenib significantly improves OS in patients with advanced HCC, patients ultimately experience disease progression. Disease progression may result from the lack of inhibition of, or compensatory activation of, alternate signaling pathways that promote tumor regrowth. Adjunct treatment with other systemic agents may provide additive or synergistic effects. Table 3 summarizes several phase 2 and 3 trials examining combinations of sorafenib with inhibitors of HMG-CoA reductase, mTOR, and angiopoietins-1 and -2 in the first-line setting. SEARCH (Sorafenib and Erlotinib, a rAndomized tRial protocol for the treatment of patients with Hepatocellular carcinoma) (N=720) compared the efficacy of sorafenib plus the epidermal growth factor receptor inhibitor erlotinib with sorafenib alone. This trial did not achieve its primary endpoint of a 33% improvement in OS (9.5 vs 8.5 months, *P*=0.204). [44]

5.6. Sorafenib benefit in portal hypertension remains controversial

Preliminary data suggest a beneficial effect of sorafenib on portal hypertension (PHT) in patients with cirrhosis and HCC. [45, 46] Increased splanchnic circulation combined with increased hepatic vascular resistance and hyperperfusion are the principal mechanisms leading to PHT. Angiogenesis is crucial in mediating increased splanchnic blood flow, and the ability of sorafenib to inhibit angiogenesis may account for the observed effects. This finding may be most relevant in patients with an HCV etiology due to a higher frequency of coexisting cirrhosis and PHT, but additional studies are needed to confirm a benefit in this setting.

5.7. Optimization of sorafenib therapy and patient selection

Prognostic HCC staging may be used for (1) predicting survival; (2) guiding therapy decisions; and (3) stratifying patients in clinical trials. Unlike other cancers, risk factors and underlying chronic liver disease (CLD) in HCC patients may have a greater impact on OS than tumor biology. This syndrome of "two diseases" directly affects patient survival, which in turn influences prognostic stratification in clinical trials and clinical decision-making. Therefore, HCC staging systems generally consider multiple prognostic factors related to CLD status and tumor stage.

The CP score is the standard assessment for classifying liver function in HCC patients. BCLC tumor staging, which also serves as a treatment algorithm, is most commonly used in the US and Europe. BCLC staging is endorsed by the AASLD and the European Association for the Study of the Liver and is most commonly used in therapeutic decision-making and in clinical trials. The prognostic power of the BCLC and other staging systems may potentially be improved by incorporating criteria based on plasma concentrations of biologic factors related to liver reserve and tumor biology.

Study phase N	Study identifier	Title	Secondary agent	Secondary agent target	Primary/secondary outcome measures
Phase 3 N=474	NCT01075555	Randomized Phase III Trial Sorafenib-Pravastatin Versus Sorafenib Alone for the Palliative Treatment of CP A Hepatocellular Carcinoma	Pravastatin	HMG-CoA reductase	OS/PFS, TTP, QOL
Phase 2 N=106	NCT01005199	Sorafenib Alone or in Combination With Everolimus in Patients With Unresectable Hepatocellular Carcinoma. A Randomized Multicenter Phase II Trial.	Everolimus	mTOR	PFS/OR, DS, PFS, TTP, OS
Phase 2 N=28	NCT01687673	Phase II Trial of the Combination of Temsirolimus and Sorafenib in Advanced Hepatocellular Carcinoma	Temsirolimus	mTOR	TTP/RR, PFS, OS, TTF
Phase 2 N=216	NCT01418729	Phase-II, Multicenter, Randomized, Double-Blind, Parallel-Group Trial to Compare the Efficacy and Safety of Sorafenib Plus Pravastatin Against Sorafenib Plus Placebo in Patients With Advanced Hepatocarcinoma	Pravastatin	HMG-CoA reductase	OS/TTP, TTSP
Phase 2 N=60	NCT00872014	Phase 2 Open-label Multi-Center Study to Evaluate the Efficacy and Safety of AMG 386 and Sorafenib as First Line Therapy for Subjects With Advanced or InoperableHepatocellular Carcinoma	AMG386	angiopoietins -1 and -2	PFS/OR,DCR,OS,TTP

CP, Child-Pugh; DCR, disease control rate; DS, disease stabilization; OR, objective response; OS, overall survival; PFS, progression-free survival; QoL, quality of life; RR, response rate; TTF, time to treatment failure; TTP, time to progression; TTSP, time to symptomatic progression

Table 3. Prospective ongoing clinical trials evaluating sorafenib in combination with other agents in the first-line setting

In clinical studies, plasma levels of angiopoietin-2, [47] VEGF, [47]- [50] hepatic growth factor (HGF), [47] insulin-like growth factor (IGF)-1, [48, 51] and IGF-2 [47] have shown prognostic value. In the SHARP study population, 10 plasma biomarkers implicated in HCC pathogenesis were measured in 491 patients at baseline and 305 patients after 12 weeks of treatment. VEGF and ang2 were found to be strong, independent predictors of survival. [47] Similar results were demonstrated in other studies in which elevated expression of angiopoietin-2 [52] and upregulation of its mRNA [53, 54] in HCC tissues were associated with advanced pathologic features and poor outcome. Elevated HGF was also found to be indicative of poor prognosis, though its significance was not retained in multivariate modeling. [55] Kaseb et al have found that integrating plasma IGF-1 as an indicator of liver reserve and VEGF as a measure of tumor burden improves the prognostic stratification of BLCL stage C patients. [51] These results represent promising steps in improving patient stratification but will require further validation.

Biomarkers predicting response to sorafenib have yet to be identified. In the SHARP analysis, low baseline HGF or high baseline s-c-KIT levels were independent predictors of survival in sorafenib-treated patients but showed only a non-significant trend as predictors of response. [55] In another study, an AFP response (>20% decline over baseline) at 6 weeks was associated with improvements in clinical benefit and PFS, and marginally improved OS. [56] Ueshima et al reported that a ≥2-fold increase in serum des-γ-carboxyprothrombin (DCP) at 2 weeks was observed in HCC patients with significantly extended TTP (P=.029). [57] However, the use of this marker is confounded by that fact that chronically elevated DCP levels are associated with poorer prognosis. [58] Finally, preliminary data indicate that reductions in carbonic anhydrase-9 at 1 month after initiating sorafenib may be associated with delayed disease progression (P=.031). [59] Identifying and validating predictive biomarkers of response to sorafenib has been challenging, at least in part, because markers explored to date are not directly affected by sorafenib, and their levels often reflect a combined measure of tumor response and liver reserve.

Studies suggest that AEs occurring during sorafenib treatment may provide prognostic and predictive information. In a single-center prospective study of 40 Asian, predominantly HBV-positive patients with unresectable HCC, the presence of any AE was associated with longer OS than the absence of an AE (21.5 vs 7.6 months, respectively; P=.014) and was also predictive of stable disease (hazard ratio [HR] 0.345 [95% CI 0.991-0.120]; P=.048). [60] In a retrospective study of 112 sorafenib-treated patients with advanced HCC, the onset of diarrhea was an independent predictor for prolonged OS (14.1 vs 7.1 months, P=.011, HR 0.41; P=.001), [61] whereas, the occurrence of HFSR was not associated with prolonged OS or TTP. In contrast, in a retrospective study of 65 sorafenib-treated patients, multivariate analysis found that those developing any-grade HFSR or a rash within 1 month of initiating treatment demonstrated a markedly reduced risk of progression (median TTP, 8.1 vs 4.0 months for patients without skin toxicity; P=.006). [62]

6. Perspective in the management of sorafenib-treated patients with HCC

When sorafenib treatment is initiated, several factors may be considered regarding dose selection, including age, ECOG PS, and status of underlying liver disease. Sorafenib should be continued until unacceptable toxicity or lack of clinical benefit is documented; this latter endpoint is challenged by the suboptimal tools available to assess response in HCC [24] and therefore relies heavily on the discretion of the treating physician. If a patient demonstrates radiologic progression only, sorafenib may be continued at least until symptomatic progression. In a recently published nonrandomized study (N=36), Miyahara et al found that metastatic tumor growth rates increased in patients who discontinued sorafenib after radiologic progression, but remained unchanged in patients who continued sorafenib. Survival beyond first radiologic progression was also significantly longer in patients who continued sorafenib. [63] In the SHARP trial, both clinical and radiologic assessments were performed; OS did not correlate with radiologic response, and patients continued sorafenib until both clinical and radiologic progression. It is important to note that symptomatic progression may be related to tumor growth and/or deteriorating liver status.

Management of side effects is critical for promoting uninterrupted treatment. It is well known that sorafenib is associated with skin reactions, diarrhea, and fatigue, but with proactive management and diligent follow-up in the early months of therapy, long-term treatment is feasible. HFSR often contributes to early discontinuation of sorafenib. In one study, the median onset of HFSR-associated symptoms was 18.4 days after initiating therapy (range 3-56 days). [64] A recent meta-analysis of 24 trials in patients with solid tumors reported a 9% incidence of high-grade HFSR in sorafenib-treated patients. [65] Prophylactic measures may minimize the onset and intensity of HFSR. A large, randomized, controlled phase 2 study (N=868) demonstrated that prophylaxis with urea-based cream over a 12-week period significantly reduced the incidence of all grades of HFSR compared to BSC in sorafenib-treated patients (56% vs 74%; *P*<.0001). [66] Other interventions may include removing hyperkeratotic tissue; applying emollients, creams, and exfoliating agents; limiting exposure to hot water; and protecting the feet with soft, well-fitting shoes and cotton socks [65, 67]; as well as sorafenib dose reduction or interruption until resolution to grade 1 or 0. [68, 69]

7. Conclusion

Sorafenib is an orally active multikinase inhibitor approved for the treatment of advanced, unresectable HCC. In randomized, double-blind, placebo-controlled, multicenter trials, sorafenib monotherapy prolonged median OS and delayed median TTP. With its acceptable safety profile and demonstrated survival benefit, sorafenib remains the only standard of care systemic therapy for unresectable HCC. However, additional trials of new molecules or combination therapy including sorafenib are needed to improve the outcomes of patients with unresectable HCC. Critical to HCC management is the establishment of surveillance programs to facilitate identification and referral in earlier-stage HCC, as well as the introduction of novel approaches to reducing the size of HCC tumors to increase the utilization and success of curative options such as resection or transplantation.

Acknowledgements

The authors acknowledge the medical writing and editorial support provided by Percolation Communications, LLC and funded by Onyx Pharmaceuticals, Inc. and Bayer Healthcare. Dr. Kaseb has received support from Bayer Healthcare and Onyx Pharmaceuticals, Inc. Dr. Kulik has received support from Bayer Healthcare and Nordion.

Author details

Ahmed O. Kaseb[1*] and Laura M. Kulik[2]

*Address all correspondence to: akaseb@mdanderson.org

1 Hepatocellular Carcinoma Program, Department of Gastrointestinal Medical Oncology, The University of Texas M. D., Anderson Cancer Center, Houston, USA

2 Division of Hepatology, Northwestern University's Feinberg School of Medicine, USA

References

[1] Ferlay J, Shin HR, Bray F, Forman D, Mathers C, Parkin DM. GLOBOCAN 2008 v1.2, Cancer Incidence and Mortality Worldwide: IARC CancerBase No. 10. Lyon, France: International Agency for Research on Cancer; 2010. Available at: http: //globocan.iarc.fr/. Accessed July 19, 2013.

[2] El-Serag HB. Epidemiology of hepatocellular carcinoma. Clin Liver Dis 2001; 5: 87-107, vi.

[3] Altekruse SF, McGlynn KA, Reichman ME. Hepatocellular carcinoma incidence, mortality, and survival trends in the United States from 1975 to 2005. J Clin Oncol 2009; 27: 1485-1491.

[4] El-Serag HB, Rudolph KL. Hepatocellular carcinoma: epidemiology and molecular carcinogenesis. Gastroenterology 2007; 132: 2557-2576.

[5] Llovet JM, Burroughs A, Bruix J. Hepatocellular carcinoma. Lancet 2003 ; 362: 1907-1917.

[6] Cheng AL, Kang YK, Chen Z, Tsao CJ, Qin S, Kim JS, et al. Efficacy and safety of sorafenib in patients in the Asia-Pacific region with advanced hepatocellular carcinoma: a phase III randomised, double-blind, placebo-controlled trial. Lancet Oncol 2009; 10: 25-34.

[7] Llovet JM, Ricci S, Mazzaferro V, Hilgard P, Gane E, Blanc JF, et al. Sorafenib in advanced hepatocellular carcinoma. N Engl J Med 2008; 359: 378-390.

[8] Bruix J, Raoul JL, Sherman M, Mazzaferro V, Bolondi L, Craxi A, et al. Efficacy and safety of sorafenib in patients with advanced hepatocellular carcinoma: subanalyses of a phase III trial. J Hepatol 2012; 57: 821-829.

[9] Cheng AL, Guan Z, Chen Z, Tsao CJ, Qin S, Kim JS,.et al. Efficacy and safety of sorafenib in patients with advanced hepatocellular carcinoma according to baseline status: subset analyses of the phase III Sorafenib Asia-Pacific trial. Eur J Cancer 2012; 48: 1452-1465.

[10] Raoul JL, Bruix J, Greten TF, Sherman M, Mazzaferro V, Hilgard P, et al. Relationship between baseline hepatic status and outcome, and effect of sorafenib on liver function: SHARP trial subanalyses. J Hepatol 2012; 56: 1080-1088.

[11] Himmelsbach K, Sauter D, Baumert TF, Ludwig L, Blum HE, Hildt E. New aspects of an anti-tumour drug: sorafenib efficiently inhibits HCV replication. Gut 2009; 58: 1644-1653.

[12] Mee CJ, Farquhar MJ, Harris HJ, Hu K, Ramma W, Ahmed A, et al. Hepatitis C virus infection reduces hepatocellular polarity in a vascular endothelial growth factor-dependent manner. Gastroenterology 2010; 138: 1134-1142.

[13] Cabrera R, Limaye AR, Horne P, Soldevila-Pico C, Clark V, Morelli G, et al. The antiviral effect of sorafenib in hepatitis C-related hepatocellular carcinoma. Aliment Pharmacol Ther 2013; 37: 91-97.

[14] Lencioni R, Marrero J, Venook A, Ye SL, Kudo M. Design and rationale for the non-interventional Global Investigation of Therapeutic DEcisions in Hepatocellular Carcinoma and Of its Treatment with Sorafenib (GIDEON) study. Int J Clin Pract 2010; 64: 1034-1041.

[15] Lencioni R, Venook A, Marrero J, Kudo M, Ye SL, Nakajima K, et al. Second interim results of the GIDEON (Global Investigation of therapeutic DEcisions in HCC and Of its Treatment with sorafeNib) study: Barcelona-Clinic Liver Cancer (BCLC) stage subgroup analysis. European Multidisciplinary Cancer Congress (ECCO-ESMO); September 23-27, 2011; Stockholm, Sweden.

[16] Marrero J, Lencioni R, Kudo M, Ye S, Nakajima K, Cihon F, et al. Global Investigation of Therapeutic Decisions in Hepatocellular Carcinoma and of its Treatment with Sorafenib (GIDEON) second interim analysis in more than 1,500 patients: Clinical findings in patients with liver dysfunction. J Clin Oncol 2011; 29(15s May 20 suppl): 4001.

[17] Abou-Alfa GK, Amadori D, Santoro A, Figer A, De Greve J, Lathia C, et al. Safety and efficacy of sorafenib in patients with hepatocellular carcinoma (HCC) and Child-Pugh A versus B cirrhosis. Gastrointest Cancer Res 2011; 4: 40-44.

[18] Marrero J, Venook A, Kudo M, "Ye S, Nakajima K, Cihon F, et al. Second interim analysis of GIDEON (Global Investigation of therapeutic DEcisions in unresectable hepatocellular carcinoma and Of its treatment with sorafeNib): subgroup analysis by initial sorafenib dose. Presented at the 62nd Annual Meeting of the American Association for the Study of Liver Diseases, November 4-8, 2011; San Francisco, CA. Abstract 2192.

[19] Pinter M, Sieghart W, Hucke F, Graziadei I, Vogel W, Maieron A, et al. Prognostic factors in patients with advanced hepatocellular carcinoma treated with sorafenib. Aliment Pharmacol Ther 2011; 34: 949-959.

[20] Bruix J, Sherman M. Management of hepatocellular carcinoma: an update. Hepatology 2011; 53: 1020-1022,

[21] Cheng A, Kang Y, Lin D, Park J, Kudo M, Qin S, et al. Phase III trial of sunitinib (Su) versus sorafenib (So) in advanced hepatocellular carcinoma (HCC). J Clin Oncol 2011; 29(15 May 20 suppl): 4000.

[22] Johnson P, Qin S, Park JW, Poon RT. Brivanib versus sorafenib as first-line therapy in patients with unresectable, advanced heaptocellular carcinoma: results form the phase 3 BRISK-FL study. 63rd Annual Meeting of the American Association for the Study of Liver Diseases; November 9-19, 2012; Boston, MA. Abstract LB-6.

[23] Cainap C, Qin S, Huang WT, Chung IJ, Pan H, Cheng Y, et al. Phase III trial of linifanib versus sorafenib in patients with advanced hepatocellular carcinoma (HCC). J Clin Oncol 2013; 31(suppl 4): 249.

[24] Chen L, Shi Y, Jiang CY, Wei LX, Wang YL, Dai GH. Expression and prognostic role of pan-Ras, Raf-1, pMEK1 and pERK1/2 in patients with hepatocellular carcinoma. Eur J Surg Oncol 37: 2011; 513-520.

[25] Hwang YH, Choi JY, Kim S, Chung ES, Kim T, Koh SS, et al. Over-expression of c-raf-1 proto-oncogene in liver cirrhosis and hepatocellular carcinoma. Hepatol Res 2004; 29: 113-121.

[26] Riaz A, Memon K, Miller FH, Nikolaidis P, Kulik LM, Lewandowski RJ, et al. Role of the EASL, RECIST, and WHO response guidelines alone or in combination for hepatocellular carcinoma: radiologic-pathologic correlation. J Hepatol 2011; 54: 695-704.

[27] Sergio A, Cristofori C, Cardin R, Pivetta G, Ragazzi R, Baldan A, et al. Transcatheter arterial chemoembolization (TACE) in hepatocellular carcinoma (HCC): the role of angiogenesis and invasiveness. Am J Gastroenterol 2008; 103: 914-921.

[28] Wang B, Xu H, Gao ZQ, Ning HF, Sun YQ, Cao GW. Increased expression of vascular endothelial growth factor in hepatocellular carcinoma after transcatheter arterial chemoembolization. Acta Radiol 2008; 49: 523-529.

[29] Shim JH, Park JW, Kim JH, An M, Kong SY, Nam BH, et al. Association between increment of serum VEGF level and prognosis after transcatheter arterial chemoembolization in hepatocellular carcinoma patients. Cancer Sci 2008; 99: 2037-2044.

[30] Kudo M, Imanaka K, Chida N, Nakachi K, Tak WY, Takayama T, et al. Phase III study of sorafenib after transarterial chemoembolisation in Japanese and Korean patients with unresectable hepatocellular carcinoma. Eur J Cancer 2011; 47: 2117-2127.

[31] Lencioni R, Llovet J, Han G, Tak WY, Yang J, Leberre MA, et al. Sorafenib or placebo in combination with transarterial chemoembolization (TACE) with doxorubicin-eluting beads (DEBDOX) for intermediate-stage hepatocellular carcinoma (HCC): Phase II, randomized, double-blind SPACE trial. J Clin Oncol 2012; 30(4 suppl Feb): LBA154.

[32] Sansonno D, Lauletta G, Russi S, Conteduca V, Sansonno L, Dammacco F. Transarterial chemoembolization plus sorafenib: a sequential therapeutic scheme for HCV-related intermediate-stage hepatocellular carcinoma: a randomized clinical trial. Oncologist 2012; 17: 359-366.

[33] Kudo M. Adjuvant therapy after curative treatment for hepatocellular carcinoma. Oncology 2011; 81(suppl 1): 50-55.

[34] Llovet JM, Fuster J, Bruix J. Intention-to-treat analysis of surgical treatment for early hepatocellular carcinoma: resection versus transplantation. Hepatology 1999; 30: 1434-1440.

[35] Vitale A, Volk ML, Pastorelli D, Lonardi S, Farinati F, Burra P, et al. Use of sorafenib in patients with hepatocellular carcinoma before liver transplantation: a cost-benefit analysis while awaiting data on sorafenib safety. Hepatology 2010; 51: 165-173.

[36] Truesdale AE, Caldwell SH, Shah NL, Argo CK, Al-Osaimi AM, Schmitt TM, et al. Sorafenib therapy for hepatocellular carcinoma prior to liver transplant is associated with increased complications after transplant. Transpl Int 2011; 24: 991-998.

[37] Di Benedetto F, Tarantino G, Montalti R, Ballarin R, D'Amico G, Berretta M, et al. Sorafenib before liver transplantation for hepatocellular carcinoma: risk or give up. Transpl Int 2011; 24: e97; author reply e98-99.

[38] Frenette C. Sorafenib prior to liver transplant does not result in increased surgical complications. Presented at the 62nd Annual Meeting of the American Association for the Study of Liver Disease; November 4-8, 2011; San Francisco, CA. Abstract 562.

[39] Irtan S, Chopin-Laly X, Ronot M, Faivre S, Paradis V, Belghiti J. Complete regression of locally advanced hepatocellular carcinoma induced by sorafenib allowing curative resection. Liver Int 2011; 31: 740-743.

[40] Kim R, Menon N, Aucejo F. Safe use of sorafenib in a patient undergoing salvage liver transplantation for recurrent hepatocellular carcinoma after hepatic resection. Med Oncol 2011; 28: 1044-1047.

[41] Siegel AB, El-Khoueiry AB, Finn RS, Blanke CD, Hidalgo R, Brown RS. Phase I trial of sorafenib in high-risk hepatocellular carcinoma (HCC) patients after liver transplantation. J Clin Oncol 2012; 30(suppl 34): 280.

[42] Teng CL, Hwang WL, Chen YJ, Chang KH, Cheng SB. Sorafenib for hepatocellular carcinoma patients beyond Milan criteria after orthotopic liver transplantation: a case control study. World J Surg Oncol 2012; 10: 41.

[43] Pfiffer TE, Seehofer D, Nicolaou A, Neuhaus R, Riess H, Trappe RU. Recurrent hepatocellular carcinoma in liver transplant recipients: parameters affecting time to recurrence, treatment options and survival in the sorafenib era. Tumori 2011; 97: 436-441.

[44] Zhu AX, Rosmorduc O, Evans J, Ross P. Santoro A, Carrilho FJ, et al. Search: A phase III, randomized, double-blind, placebo-controlled trial of sorafenib plus erlotinib in patients with hepatocellular carcinoma (HCC). Ann Oncol 2012; 23(suppl 9): 11.

[45] Hidaka H, Nakazawa T, Kaneko T, Minamino T, Takada J, Tanaka Y, et al. Portal hemodynamic effects of sorafenib in patients with advanced hepatocellular carcinoma: a prospective cohort study. J Gastroenterol 2012; 47: 1030-1035.

[46] Pinter M, Sieghart W, Reiberger T, Rohr-Udilova N, Ferlitsch A, Peck-Radosavljevic M. The effects of sorafenib on the portal hypertensive syndrome in patients with liver cirrhosis and hepatocellular carcinoma--a pilot study. Aliment Pharmacol Ther 2012; 35: 83-91.

[47] Llovet JM, Pena CE, Lathia CD, Shan M, Meinhardt G, Bruix J, et al. Plasma biomarkers as predictors of outcome in patients with advanced hepatocellular carcinoma. Clin Cancer Res 2012; 18: 2290-2300.

[48] Kaseb AO, Abbruzzese JL, Vauthey JN, et al. I-CLIP: improved stratification of advanced hepatocellular carcinoma patients by integrating plasma IGF-1 into CLIP score. Oncology 80: 373-381, 2011

[49] Kaseb AO, Hassan MM, Lin E, Aloia TA, Abdalla EK, Hassan MM, et al. V-CLIP: Integrating plasma vascular endothelial growth factor into a new scoring system to stratify patients with advanced hepatocellular carcinoma for clinical trials. Cancer 2011; 117: 2478-2488.

[50] Schoenleber SJ, Kurtz DM, Talwalkar JA, Roberts LR, Gores GJ. Prognostic role of vascular endothelial growth factor in hepatocellular carcinoma: systematic review and meta-analysis. Br J Cancer 2009; 100: 1385-1392.

[51] Kaseb AO, Morris JS, Hassan MM, Siddiqui AM, Lin E, Xiao L, et al. Clinical and prognostic implications of plasma insulin-like growth factor-1 and vascular endothe-

lial growth factor in patients with hepatocellular carcinoma. J Clin Oncol 2011; 29: 3892-3899.

[52] Yu Q, Stamenkovic I. Angiopoietin-2 is implicated in the regulation of tumor angiogenesis. Am J Pathol 2001; 158: 563-570.

[53] Moon WS, Rhyu KH, Kang MJ, Lee DG, Yu HC, Yeum JH, et al. Overexpression of VEGF and angiopoietin 2: a key to high vascularity of hepatocellular carcinoma? Mod Pathol 2003; 16: 552-557.

[54] Scholz A, Rehm VA, Rieke S, Derkow K, Schulz P, Neumann K, et al. Angiopoietin-2 serum levels are elevated in patients with liver cirrhosis and hepatocellular carcinoma. Am J Gastroenterol 2007; 102: 2471-2481.

[55] Llovet J, Pena C, Shan M, Lathia C, Bruix J. Plasma biomarkers as predictors of outcome in patients with advanced hepatocellular carcinoma: results from the randomized phase III trial. Presented at the EASL Annual Meeting; April 22-26, 2009; Copenhagen, Denmark.

[56] Yau T, Yao TJ, Chan P, Wong H, Pang R, Fan ST, et al. The significance of early alpha-fetoprotein level changes in predicting clinical and survival benefits in advanced hepatocellular carcinoma patients receiving sorafenib. Oncologist 2011; 16: 1270-1279.

[57] Ueshima K, Kudo M, Takita M, Nagai T, Tatsumi C, Ueda T, et al. Des-gamma-carboxyprothrombin may be a promising biomarker to determine the therapeutic efficacy of sorafenib for hepatocellular carcinoma. Dig Dis 2011; 29: 321-325.

[58] Bertino G, Ardiri A, Malaguarnera M, Malaguarnera G, Bertino N, Calvagno GS. Hepatocellualar carcinoma serum markers. Semin Oncol 2012; 39: 410-433.

[59] Reig M, Boix L, Forner A, BCLC Group, Hospital Clinic. Forner 1, and BCLC Group, Hospital Clinic. Serum carbonic anhydrase 9 is a valuable biomarker to predict the outcome in patients with hepatocellular carcinoma treated with sorafenib. Presented at the International Liver Cancer Association Annual Meeting; September 1-3, 2011; Hong Kong, China.

[60] Song T, Zhang W, Wu Q, Kong D, Ma W. A single center experience of sorafenib in advanced hepatocellular carcinoma patients: evaluation of prognostic factors. Eur J Gastroenterol Hepatol 2011; 23: 1233-1238.

[61] Bettinger D, Schultheiss M, Knuppel E, Thimme R, Blum HE, Spangenberg HC. Diarrhea predicts a positive response to sorafenib in patients with advanced hepatocellular carcinoma. Hepatology, 2012; 56: 789-790.

[62] Vincenzi B, Santini D, Russo A, Addeo R, Giuliani F, Montella L, et al. Early skin toxicity as a predictive factor for tumor control in hepatocellular carcinoma patients treated with sorafenib. Oncologist 2010; 15: 85-92.

[63] Miyahara K, Nouso K, Morimoto Y, Takeuchi Y, Hagihara H, Kuwaki K, et al. Efficacy of sorafenib beyond first progression in patients with metastatic hepatocellular carcinoma. Hepatol Res 2013 Apr 2 (Epub ahead of print).

[64] Lee WJ, Lee JL, Chang SE, Lee MW, Kang YK, Choi JH, et al. Cutaneous adverse effects in patients treated with the multitargeted kinase inhibitors sorafenib and sunitinib. Br J Dermatol 2009; 161: 1045-1051.

[65] Zhang T, Ding X, Wei D, Cheng P, Su X, Liu H, et al. Sorafenib improves the survival of patients with advanced hepatocellular carcinoma: a meta-analysis of randomized trials. Anticancer Drugs 2010; 21: 326-332.

[66] Ren Z, Zhu K, Kang H, Lu M, Qu Z, Lu L, et al. A randomized controlled phase II study of the prophylactic effect of urea-based cream on the hand-foot skin reaction associated with sorafenib in advanced hepatocellular carcinoma. J Clin Oncol 2012; 30(May 20 suppl): 4008.

[67] Anderson R, Jatoi A, Robert C, Wood LS, Keating KN, Lacouture ME. Search for evidence-based approaches for the prevention and palliation of hand-foot skin reaction (HFSR) caused by the multikinase inhibitors (MKIs). Oncologist 2009; 14: 291-302.

[68] Autier J, Escudier B, Wechsler J, Spatz A, Robert C. Prospective study of the cutaneous adverse effects of sorafenib, a novel multikinase inhibitor. Arch Dermatol 2008; 144: 886-892.

[69] Lacouture ME, Wu S, Robert C, Atkins MB, Kong HH, Guitart J, et al. Evolving strategies for the management of hand-foot skin reaction associated with the multitargeted kinase inhibitors sorafenib and sunitinib. Oncologist 2008; 13: 1001-1011.

[70] Wilhelm S, Chien DS. BAY 43-9006: preclinical data. Curr Pharm Des 2002; 8: 2255-2257.

[71] SUTENT® (sunitinib malate) [prescribing information]. New York, NY: Pfizer Labs; 2012.

[72] Bhide RS, Cai ZW, Zhang YZ, Qian L, Wei D, Barbosa S, et al. Discovery and preclinical studies of (R)-1-(4-(4-fluoro-2-methyl-1H-indol-5-yloxy)-5- methylpyrrolo [2,1-f][1,2,4]triazin-6-yloxy)propan- 2-ol (BMS-540215), an in vivo active potent VEGFR-2 inhibitor. J Med Chem 2006; 49: 2143-2146.

[73] Albert DH, Tapang P, Magoc TJ, Pease LJ, Reuter DR, Wei RQ, et al. Preclinical activity of ABT-869, a multitargeted receptor tyrosine kinase inhibitor. Mol Cancer Ther 2006; 5: 995-1006.

[74] Lee SH, Lopes de Menezes D, Vora J, Harris A, Ye H, Nordahl L, et al. In vivo target modulation and biological activity of CHIR-258, a multitargeted growth factor receptor kinase inhibitor, in colon cancer models. Clin Cancer Res 2005; 11: 3633-3641.

[75] Hilberg F, Roth GJ, Krssak M, Kautschitsch S, Sommergruber W, Tontsch-Grunt U, et al. BIBF 1120: triple angiokinase inhibitor with sustained receptor blockade and good antitumor efficacy. Cancer Res 2008; 68: 4774-4782.

Chapter 12

Sorafenib-Inhibited Signaling: Emerging Evidence of RAF-Independent Pathways as Potential Therapeutic Targets in Hepatocellular Carcinoma

Yasunobu Matsuda, Toshifumi Wakai,
Masayuki Kubota, Mami Osawa and Shun Fujimaki

Additional information is available at the end of the chapter

http://dx.doi.org/10.5772/55201

1. Introduction

Hepatocellular carcinoma (HCC) is one of the most common malignancies worldwide [Serag et al., 2007, Liovet et al., 2003, Yang et al., 2010]. More than 500,000 people are diagnosed with HCC every year, and it remains the leading cause of death among patients with hepatitis B virus (HBV), hepatitis C virus (HCV) and alcohol-induced liver cirrhosis. One of the main obstacles for treating HCC is late diagnosis of patients. Many unresectable HCC patients are treated with loco-regional therapies such as radiofrequency ablation and transarterial chemo-embolization (TACE), but the prognosis remains poor [Bruix et al., 2005]. A recent study in multiple clinical facilities in Japan reported that 5-year survival of patients treated with TACE was less than 30% [Takayasu et al., 2006]. Moreover, HCC is poorly responsive to chemotherapeutic drugs and radiotherapy [Arii et al., 2000, Kuwahara et al., 2009]; thus, effective therapeutic tools for HCC are long-awaited.

Sorafenib (Nexavar, BAY 43-9006, Bayer HealthCare Pharmaceuticals) is a new type of drug designed to target RAF signaling, and represents a new era of HCC treatment. However, accumulating evidence has revealed the limited effect of sorafenib, and many clinical trials of sorafenib-based combination therapy are now underway. It should be noted that, while sorafenib was originally designed to target RAF-mediated signaling, recent studies have strongly indicated that its effect is closely involved in various types of non-RAF signaling [Matsuda et al., 2011]. To explore safe and effective therapies combined with sorafenib, full understanding of the functional mechanism of sorafenib is necessary. Herein, we review recent findings from studies of sorafenib-mediated inhibition of RAF and non-

RAF signaling pathways. We also discuss the possibility of administering sorafenib with other drugs in combination therapy, which might become a promising approach in the treatment of advanced HCC.

2. Clinical perspectives of sorafenib

2.1. The effects and limitations of sorafenib

Sorafenib is an orally bioavailable inhibitor of multiple kinases including RAF, vascular endothelial growth factor receptor (VEGFR), platelet-derived growth factor (PDGF) receptor, and the v-kit Hardy-Zuckerman 4 feline sarcoma viral oncogene (*KIT*) and fms-like tyrosine kinase 3 (*FLT-3*) oncogene [Wilhelm et al., 2004, Hochhaus et al., 2011]. At present, sorafenib is the only oral drug shown to improve the survival of unresectable HCC. The SHARP trial (the Sorafenib HCC Assessment Randomized Protocol), a multicenter double-blind phase III trial in Europe, North America, South America, and Australasia conducted in 2008, reported overall survival in the sorafenib-treated group was significantly longer than in the placebo group (10.7 *vs.* 7.9 months) [Llovet et al., 2008]. An Asia-Pacific study, which was conducted in China, South Korea, and Taiwan in 2009, also reported that the median overall survival in the sorafenib-treated group was improved (6.5 *vs.* 4.2 months) [Cheng et al., 2009], suggesting that the effect of sorafenib is universal among different ethnic backgrounds. Unfortunately however, subsequent clinical studies have highlighted several issues. First, sorafenib treatment rarely results in tumor shrinkage [Jubb et al., 2010]. A partial tumor response was seen in only 2% and 3.3% of the SHARP and the Asia-Pacific studies, respectively, and there have been few reported cases that achieved complete remission after sorafenib treatment [SO et al., 2008, Yeganeh et al., 2009, Wang et al., 2010, Sacco et al., 2011]. Second, sorafenib is less effective when the patients are affected with medium to severe liver dysfunction (Child-Pugh class B and C) [Pinter et al., 2009, Schütte et al., 2011]. The reason for the influence of liver function on the efficacy of sorafenib should be determined in the near future. Because liver cirrhosis is a unique condition in which excessive inflammatory cytokines is produced, it is plausible that cancer microenvironment in liver disease might affect the sorafenib efficacy (Fig. 1). Third, sorafenib causes many side-effects, including diarrhea, skin eruption, and bone marrow dysfunction. All these lines of evidence strongly suggest that safer and more effective sorafenib therapy should be established for HCC patients.

2.2. Clinical trial of sorafenib-based combination therapy

To improve the limited efficacy of sorafenib, many clinical trials of sorafenib-based combination treatment have been undertaken. For example, a phase II multicenter study in Italy reported that the combination of sorafenib and long-acting octreotide (an analogue of somatostatin) resulted in a better survival rate as compared with sorafenib monotherapy [Prete et al., 2010]. This report suggests a possible synergic tumor killing effect by sorafenib, because octreotide monotherapy has been regarded as less effective in advanced HCC [Becker et al.,

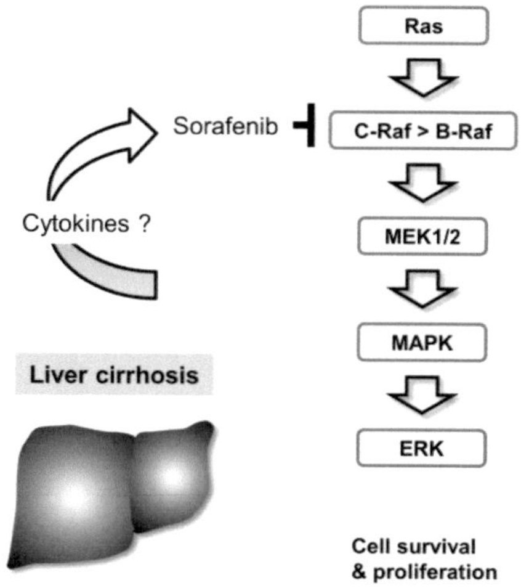

Figure 1. Sorafenib and Raf signaling. Sorafenib inhibits C-Raf rather than B-Raf, and attenuates the activation of MAPK/ERK signaling. However, the effect of sorafenib might be influenced by the cancer microenvironment in liver cirrhosis. MEK, mitogen-activated protein kinase kinase; MAPK, mitogen-activated protein kinase; ERK, extracellular signal-regulated kinase.

2007]. Furthermore, combination of sorafenib and the chemotherapeutic drug doxorubicin was found to be effective in HCC [Abou-Alfa et al., 2010].

Basic studies have now evaluated the preclinical protocols of the combination of sorafenib with other therapeutic agents. The most prospective method for treating HCC is a combination of sorafenib with rapamycin, an inhibitor of the mammalian target of rapamycin (mTOR) pathway. mTOR is known to be activated in many types of cancer cells, and around half of human HCC cases showed aberrant mTOR signaling [Villanueva et al., 2008]. Several studies using a human HCC xenograft mouse model have reported that the combination of rapamycin and sorafenib synergistically enhanced the anti-tumor effect, and resulted in tumor shrinkage [Wang et al., 2008, Huynh et al., 2009, Newell et al., 2009]. Thus far, a phase I trial of the combination therapy of sorafenib and temsirolimus (a rapamycin analog) is in progress for treating advanced HCC [Kelley et al., 2010].

3. Sorafenib affects both RAF and non-RAF signaling pathways

3.1. RAF signaling

3.1.1. RAF signaling and HCC

The *RAS* oncogene encodes a small guanosine triphosphate-binding protein (GTPase) that plays a central role in promoting the cell proliferation, survival and transformation [Karnoub et al., 2008]. Four proteins, including H-RAS, N-RAS, K-RASA and K-RASB are encoded by the *RAS* gene, and all of these mutant forms have been known to lead to increased GTP-bound RAS (RAS-GTP). Of these, K-RAS is frequently activated by gene mutation in many types of cancer cells [Karnoub et al., 2008], indicating that *RAS* is a common oncogene in various cell types. Several growth factors such as epidermal growth factor (EGF), insulin-like growth factor-I (IGF-1) and PDGF induce cell proliferation through enhanced exchange of guanine nucleotides on RAS. RAS has a guanosine diphosphate (GDP) binding domain, and GDP-bound RAS (RAS-GDP) is activated when converted into RAS-GTP. Downstream mediators of RAS (RAF, PI3K-bound RAL-GEF) bind RAS-GTP with higher affinity than RAS-GDP [Herrmann et al., 1995]. RAS recruits members of the RAF serine/threonine kinase family to the plasma membrane, whereupon they are activated by phosphorylation. The RAF kinase family is composed of three members: A-RAF, B-RAF, and RAF-1 (also termed C-RAF). Of these, many studies have suggested that RAF-1 plays a critical role in the early step of carcinogenesis. It has now been widely accepted that RAF signaling exerts a critical role on the progression in many of the incurable diseases. Good example might be an autosomal dominant polycystic kidney disease (ADPKD). Recent studies have unveiled that Ras/Raf signaling is hyper-activated in cyst epithelial cells in this disease, and both sorafenib and a novel Raf kinase inhibitor PLX5568 can attenuate the proliferation of ADPKD cyst epithelial cells [Yamaguchi T et al., 2010, Buchholz et al., 2011].

In the case of HCC, point mutations of *RAS* have been reported to be infrequent in HCC [Challen et al., 1992]. However, it has been revealed that its downstream signaling is frequently activated during hepatocarcinogenesis. Hepatitis B virus X protein (HBx) and HCV core protein, both of which have been considered as strong promoters of hepatocarcinogenesis, increase the kinase activity of RAF-1 [Aoki et al., 2000, Chen et al., 2007]. It has been also reported that the C-terminal of HCV-encoded nonstructural protein 5A (NS5A) binds to and activates RAF-1 [Bürckstümmer et al., 2006]. More importantly, activated RAF-1 has been found in around 90% of liver cirrhosis cases and in 100% of HCC cases [Hwang et al., 2004].

3.1.2. RAF signaling and sorafenib

RAF-1 is a mitogen-activated protein kinase (MAPK) kinase, which phosphorylates and activates the serine/threonine-specific extracellular signal-regulated protein kinases ERK1 and ERK2 [Avruch et al., 1994]. In the nucleus, phosphorylated ERK activates transcription factors such as ELK-1 and c-JUN, leading to cell proliferation and survival. RAF-1 has been also reported to form a complex with Cdc25 and activates the cyclin E-Cdk2 complex, leading to progression through the G1-S phase transition [Kerkhoff et al., 1998, Hindley et al., 2002]. When activated, RAF members form homologous and heterologous complexes, leading to activation of the MEK/ERK pathway. It should be noted that the kinase activity of RAF complexes is defined by the type of RAF constituents. It has been reported that the kinase activity of B-RAF and c-RAF heterodimers is higher than that of B-RAF or C-RAF homodimers [Rushworth et al., 2006]. Moreover, when B-RAF is mutated at V600E (B-RAFV 600E), as observed in some types of cancer cells, it acquires strong kinase activity and can directly stimulate the MEK/ERK pathway [Wan et al., 2004, Garnett et al., 2005]. In turn, the kinase activity of a heterologous complex consisting of C-RAF and B-RAFV600E becomes decreased as compared with C-RAF and non-mutated B-RAF heterodimers [Garnett et al., 2005].

Intriguingly, the difference in the kinase activities of each RAF complex affects the therapeutic effect of sorafenib. Sorafenib inhibits C-RAF at low doses, while it inhibits wild-type and mutated B-RAF at high doses [Wilhelm et al., 2004]. Therefore, high doses of sorafenib can inhibit the activities of both C-RAF and B-RAF (either wild-type or V600E), while at lower doses, sorafenib only inhibits C-RAF, resulting in disinhibition of B-RAF [Garnett et al., 2005]. More importantly, low doses of sorafenib has the unique ability in that it induces the formation of heterologous complexes between B-RAFV600E and wild-type B-RAF, leading to the enhancement of the kinase ability of B-RAFV600E [Garnett et al., 2005]. It has been recently reported that cells expressing oncogenic *RAS* are selectively inhibited, B-RAF, B-RAF-C-RAF heterodimers are induced, and RAF/MEK/ERK signaling is activated [Heidorn et al., 2010]. It has been also shown that B-RAF-ERK signaling and C-RAF signaling play dominant roles in the regulation of proliferation of lung cancer cells with wild-type or mutant *KRAS*, respectively. Intriguingly however, sorafenib can inhibit both cell types by targeting B-RAF-mediated ERK phosphorylation in cells with wild-type *KRAS*, and by targeting C-RAF in the cells with mutant *KRAS* [Takezawa et al., 2009]. These lines of evidence strongly suggest that clinicians should decide the dosage of sorafenib in reference to the level of each RAF kinase in the tumors.

3.1.3. Apoptotic pathways and sorafenib

Recently, several studies have reported that sorafenib has a significant effect on non-RAF-signaling pathways, as well as RAF-mediated signaling, particularly caspase-mediated apoptotic signaling. Apoptosis is mainly regulated by two major pathways; (1) tumor necrosis factor- alpha receptors (TNFRs) or the Fas-mediated caspase-8 signaling pathway, and (2) BCL-2 family members-regulated caspase-9 pathway [Ashkenazi, 2008, Leber et al., 2010]. It has been recently reported that sorafenib kills tumor cells by regulating MCL-1, which is a member of the BCL2 protein family [Akgul, 2009, Thomas et al., 2010]. MCL-1 is a repressor of apoptotic cell death via its interactions with the cell death inducer BAX, and overproduction of MCL-1 inhibits cell apoptosis induced by growth factor withdrawal, MYC overexpression, or cytotoxic agents. MCL-1 has been known to be overexpressed in many types of malignancies, and many studies have suggested that the levels of MCL-1 expression may determine the therapeutic efficacy of anti-tumor agents.

Recent studies have led to the suggestion that MCL-1 might be one of the main targets for MEK/ERK-independent mechanisms of action of sorafenib. Sorafenib reduces MCL-1 in various types of cancer cells by proteasome-mediated degradation [Yo et al., 2005], and sorafenib-mediated MCL-1 downregulation is associated with MCL-1-translation and cytochrome-c release into the cytosol. [Rahmani et al., 2005] Intriguingly, MCL-1 might be a promising biomarker of therapeutic efficacy, because it was found to be upregulated in sorafenib-resistant cells [Ulivi et al., 2009]. It has also been reported that HCV can increase therapeutic response to sorafenib by miR-193b-dependent modulation of MCL-1 [Braconi et al., 2010], suggesting that MCL-1 might be involved in the virus-associated drug response in cancer cells.

3.1.4. Endoplasmic reticulum stress and sorafenib

Another RAF-independent mechanism involved in sorafenib-inhibited signaling is endoplasmic reticulum (ER) stress [Rahmani et al., 2007]. The endoplasmic reticulum (ER) is a central organelle in each eukaryotic cell that serves many general functions, including lipid synthesis, protein folding and protein maturation, transportation of synthesized proteins, and activation of chaperone proteins. When cells are exposed to various types of stress such as hypoxia, oxidative stress, hypoglycemia and viral infection, unfolded protein aggregates (unfolded protein response, UPR) accumulate to interfere the function of ER, which is generally called ER stress [Tsukada et al., 1993, Kim et al., 2008]. ER stress causes decreased protein translation to prevent further accumulation of unfolded proteins. It should be noted, however, that the function of ER stress is complex because it can induce either cell survival or autophagy-related cell death [Schleicher et al., 2010]. Several UPR-involving signaling molecules have been identified; the PKR-like kinase (PERK) is an important inhibitor of protein translation through phosphorylation of eukaryotic initiation factor 2 (eIF2α). The kinase activity of PERK is induced by ER stress, and phosphorylation of PERK at Thr980 is regarded as a marker for ER stress. Endoplasmic oxidoreductin-1 (Ero1) is an ER membrane-associated N-glycoprotein that provides oxidizing potential and protein folding. Inositol requiring-1 (IRE1) and activating transcription factor-6 (ATF6) induce calcium-dependent protein chaperones such as GRP78/BiP to maintain correct protein folding [Kim et al., 2008, McConkey et al., 2008]. Calnexin is a calcium-binding protein that retains the synthesized glycoproteins inside the ER. CAAT/enhancer binding protein (C/EBP) homologous protein (CHOP) is a dominant-negative inhibitor of C/EBP and LAP, which plays a role in cell cycle arrest during G1 to S phase. During ER stress, the level of CHOP is increased to induce the activation of GADD34, a downstream protein of P53 tumor suppressor that causes DNA excision repair and cell arrest, and ERO-1 expression. ERO-1 promotes oxidative stress inside the ER, leading to programmed cell death.

Several studies have reported that sorafenib strongly induces ER stress. Sorafenib results in the phosphorylation of PERK and eIF2α, leading to decreases in protein synthesis [Tsukada, 1993]. ERK cannot rescue this cellular reaction, indicating that sorafenib-induced ER stress is RAF-independent [Rahmani et al., 2007]. It has been also reported that sorafenib-induced apoptosis is associated with the increase in the level of CHOP expression [Niessner et al., 2011]; therefore ER stress might be another important mechanism of sorafenib efficacy.

3.1.5. Oxidative stress and sorafenib

It is well known that reactive oxygen species (ROS) is an important player in the process of various types of cellular process. ROS is unique in its dual role; and it plays a critical role in maintaining cancer phenotype, cell proliferation and genetic instability [Radisky et al., 2005, Chen et al., 2005]. In turn, when produced at high concentrations, it activates the caspases to induce apoptosis. Although the functional mechanisms of these opposing effects of ROS is unknown, recent studies have revealed that the effect of cytotoxic anti-tumor agents is exclusively caused by elevated ROS production. Recently it was revealed that sorafenib induces mitochondria-dependent ROS production to induce hepatoma cell death. Chiou et al. reported that ROS could be generated just 30 minutes after cells were treated with sorafenib, suggesting that sorafenib-induced oxidative stress might not be the secondary phenomenon during cell death [Chiou et al., 2009]. Chiou et al. also reported that glutathione (GSH), an intracellular non-protein-thiol antioxidant, was decreased after treatment with sorafenib. Currently it is not known that why sorafenib results in the dysregulated balance of oxidants and anti-oxidants. Park et al. reported that low doses of sorafenib and vorinostat, a histone deacetylase inhibitor (HDACI) that has shown preclinical evidence of anti-tumor activity against hepatoma, rapidly increase ROS, Ca (2+), and ceramide levels in gastrointestinal tumor cells [Park et al., 2010]. In turn, Banerjee et al. reported that the anti-oxidant enzyme heme oxygenase-1 (HO-1) protected apoptosis of cells treated with sorafenib [Banerjee et al., 2012]. HO-1 was found to induce the expression of anti-apoptotic BCL-$_X$L and decreased the expression of autophagic proteins Beclin-1 and LC3B-II, indicating that ROS might determine the therapeutic efficacy of sorafenib. To improve the efficacy of sorafenib, further investigation of the relationship between ROS and sorafenib should be performed.

4. Future perspectives of combination treatment with sorafenib

Because accumulating evidence strongly indicated that the anti-tumor effect of sorafenib is mediated by both RAF and non-RAF signaling, recent studies have investigated the usefulness of sorafenib-based combination therapy via targeting of non-RAF signaling pathways [Peck-Radosavljevic et al., 2010, Shen et al., 2010, Kudo et al., 2010]. Some studies have reported that targeting non-RAF signaling such as TNF-related apoptosis-inducing ligand (TRAIL) [Meng et al., 2007, Rosato et al., 2007, Ricci et al., 2007, Kudo et al., 2010], histone deacetylase [Dasmahapatra et al., 2007] and BCL-2 [Lin et al., 2007] might be effective when combined with sorafenib. Moreover, several clinically available agents such as sulforaphane (SF) [Rausch et al., 2010], zoledronic acid [Zhang et al., 2010], and vitamin K1, K2, and K5 [Wei et al., 2010a, 2010b] have been also reported to be useful for combination treatment. Recently we found that caffeine, which is a well-known inhibitor of DNA damage-response kinase ataxia telangiectasia mutated (ATM), can effectively enhance the effect of sorafenib [Fujimaki et al., 2012]. ATM is a widely known DNA damage-stimulated serine/threonine kinase that phosphorylates several of the DNA damage checkpoint molecules [Lavin, 2008]. We found that ATM is activated by sorafenib-mediated non-genotoxic ROS production, resulting in the sorafenib-induced reciprocal activation of AKT signaling to help the cells to acquire drug resistance [Fujimaki et al., 2012]. Interestingly, it has been recently reported that intra-arterial local administration of caffeine could potentiate cisplatin-based chemotherapy, without severe side-effects [Takeuchi et al., 2007]. Together with our finding, it would be intriguing to investigate if caffeine could enhance the effect of sorafenib in HCC patients.

5. Conclusions

At present, sorafenib is the only molecular targeting agent proven to have a significant effect on the survival of patients with advanced HCC. Although its tumor-killing effect has been found to be limited, recent basic studies have revealed that this new agent acts upon multiple non-RAF signaling pathways as well as RAF-mediated signaling. More interestingly, recent studies have unveiled that sorafenib might also act as preventive agents against liver fibrosis. Wang et al. reported that sorafenib treatment attenuated liver fibrosis in rat liver fibrosis model, possibly due to its inhibitory role on the cell proliferation of hepatic satellite cells [Wang at al., 2010]. Thus, to further identify an efficient protocol for sorafenib treatment, clinicians should pay more attention to non-RAF signaling in cancer cells.

Author details

Yasunobu Matsuda[1*], Toshifumi Wakai[2], Masayuki Kubota[3], Mami Osawa[3] and Shun Fujimaki[1]

*Address all correspondence to: yasunobu@med.niigata-u.ac.jp

1 Department of Medical Technology, Niigata University Graduate School of Health Sciences, Japan

2 Division of Digestive and General Surgery, Niigata University Graduate School of Medical and Dental Sciences, Japan

3 Division of Pediatric Surgery, Niigata University Graduate School of Medical and Dental Sciences, Japan

References

[1] Abou-alfa, G. K, Johnson, P, Knox, J. J, Capanu, M, Davidenko, I, Lacava, J, Leung, T, Gansukh, B, & Saltz, L. B. (2010). Doxorubicin plus sorafenib vs doxorubicin alone in patients with advanced hepatocellular carcinoma: a randomized trial. *JAMA*, , 304, 2154-2160.

[2] Akgul, C. (2009). Mcl-1 is a potential therapeutic target in multiple types of cancer. *Cell Mol Life Sci, 66* , 1326-1336.

[3] Aoki, H, Hayashi, J, Moriyama, M, Arakawa, Y, & Hino, O. (2000). Hepatitis C virus core protein interacts with 14-3-3 protein and activates the kinase Raf-1. *J Virol*, , 74, 1736-1741.

[4] Arii, S, Yamaoka, Y, Futagawa, S, Inoue, K, Kobayashi, K, Kojiro, M, Makuuchi, M, Nakamura, Y, Okita, K, & Yamada, R. (2000). Results of surgical and nonsurgical treatment for small-sized hepatocellular carcinomas: a retrospective and nationwide survey in Japan. The Liver Cancer Study Group of Japan. *Hepatology*, , 32, 1224-1229.

[5] Ashkenazi, A. (2008). Directing cancer cells to self-destruct with pro-apoptotic receptor agonists. *Nat Rev Drug Discov*, , 7, 1001-1012.

[6] Banerjee, P, Basu, A, Wegiel, B, Otterbein, L. E, Mizumura, K, Gasser, M, Waaga-gasser, A. M, Choi, A. M, & Pal, S. (2012). Heme oxygenase-1 promotes survival of renal cancer cells through modulation of apoptosis- & autophagy-regulating molecules. *J Biol Chem*, , 287, 32113-32123.

[7] Becker, G, Allgaier, H. P, Olschewski, M, Zähringer, A, & Blum, H. E. HECTOR Study Group. ((2007). Long-acting octreotide versus placebo for treatment of advanced HCC: a randomized controlled double-blind study. *Hepatology*, , 45, 9-15.

[8] Braconi, C, Valeri, N, Gasparini, P, Huang, N, Taccioli, C, Nuovo, G, Suzuki, T, Croce, C. M, & Patel, T. (2010). Hepatitis C virus proteins modulate microRNA expression and chemosensitivity in malignant hepatocytes. *Clin Cancer Res*, , 16, 957-966.

[9] Bruix, J, & Sherman, M. (2005). Management of hepatocellular carcinoma. Hepatology , 42, 1208-1236.

[10] Buchholz, B, Klanke, B, Schley, G, Bollag, G, Tsai, J, Kroening, S, Yoshihara, D, Wallace, D. P, Kraenzlin, B, Gretz, N, Hirth, P, Eckardt, K. U, & Bernhardt, W. M. (2011). The Raf kinase inhibitor PLX5568 slows cyst proliferation in rat polycystic kidney disease but promotes renal and hepatic fibrosis. *Nephrol Dial Transplant, 26* , 3458-3465.

[11] Bürckstümmer, T, Kriegs, M, Lupberger, J, Pauli, E. K, Schmittel, S, & Hildt, E. (2006). Raf-1 kinase associates with Hepatitis C virus NS5A and regulates viral replication. *FEBS Lett*, , 580, 575-580.

[12] Challen, C, Guo, K, Collier, J. D, Cavanagh, D, & Bassendine, M. F. (1992). Infrequent point mutations in codons 12 and 61 of ras oncogenes in human hepatocellular carcinomas. *J Hepatol*, , 14, 342-346.

[13] Chen, J, & Siddiqui, A. (2007). Hepatitis B virus X protein stimulates the mitochondrial translocation of Raf-1 via oxidative stress. *J Virol*, , 81, 6757-6760.

[14] Chen, Z, Trotman, L. C, Shaffer, D, Lin, H. K, Dotan, Z. A, Niki, M, Koutcher, J. A, Scher, H. I, Ludwig, T, Gerald, W, Cordon-cardo, C, & Pandolfi, P. P. (2005). Crucial role of cellular senescence in suppression of Pten-deficient tumorigenesis. *Nature*, 436: 725-730, 53.

[15] Cheng, A. L, Kang, Y. K, Chen, Z, Tsao, C. J, Qin, S, Kim, J. S, Luo, R, Feng, J, Ye, S, Yang, T. S, Xu, J, Sun, Y, Liang, H, Liu, J, Wang, J, Tak, W. Y, Pan, H, Burock, K, Zou, J, Voliotis, D, & Guan, Z. (2009). Efficacy and safety of sorafenib in patients in the Asia-Pacific region with advanced hepatocellular carcinoma: a phase III randomised, double-blind, placebo-controlled trial. *Lancet Oncol*, , 10, 25-34.

[16] Chiou, J. F, Tai, C. J, Wang, Y. H, Liu, T. Z, Jen, Y. M, & Shiau, C. Y. (2009). Sorafenib induces preferential apoptotic killing of a drug- and radio-resistant Hep G2 cells

through a mitochondria-dependent oxidative stress mechanism. *Cancer Biol Ther*, , 8, 1904-1913.

[17] Dasmahapatra, G, Yerram, N, Dai, Y, Dent, P, & Grant, S. (2007). Synergistic interactions between vorinostat and sorafenib in chronic myelogenous leukemia cells involve Mcl-1 and down-regulation. *Clin Cancer Res*, 13: 4280-4290, 21CIP1.

[18] El Serag, H. B, & Rudolph, K. L. (2007). Hepatocellular carcinoma: epidemiology and molecular carcinogenesis. *Gastroenterology*, , 132, 2557-2576.

[19] Fujimaki, S, Matsuda, Y, Wakai, T, Sanpei, A, Kubota, M, Takamura, M, Yamagiwa, S, Yano, M, Ohkoshi, S, & Aoyagi, Y. (2012). Blockade of ataxia telangiectasia mutated sensitizes hepatoma cell lines to sorafenib by interfering with Akt signaling. *Cancer Lett*, , 319, 98-108.

[20] Garnett, M. J, Rana, S, Paterson, H, Barford, D, & Marais, R. (2005). Wild-type and mutant B-RAF activate C-RAF through distinct mechanisms involving heterodimerization. *Mol Cell*, , 20, 963-969.

[21] Heidorn, S. J, Milagre, C, Whittaker, S, Nourry, A, Niculescu-duvas, I, Dhomen, N, Hussain, J, Reis-filho, J. S, Springer, C. J, Pritchard, C, & Marais, R. (2010). Kinase-dead BRAF and oncogenic RAS cooperate to drive tumor progression through CRAF. *Cell*, , 140, 209-221.

[22] Herrmann, C, Martin, G. A, & Wittinghofer, A. (1995). Quantitative analysis of the complex between and the Ras-binding domain of the human Raf-1 protein kinase. *J Biol Chem*, 270: :2901-2905, 21ras.

[23] Hindley, A, & Kolch, W. (2002). Extracellular signal regulated kinase (ERK)/mitogen activated protein kinase (MAPK)-independent functions of Raf kinases. *J Cell Sci*, , 115, 1575-1581.

[24] Hochhaus, A, Rosée, P. L, Müller, M. C, Ernst, T, & Cross, N. C. (2011). Impact of BCR-ABL mutations on patients with chronic myeloid leukemia. *Cell Cycle, 10* , 250-260.

[25] Huynh, H, Ngo, V. C, Koong, H. N, Poon, D, Choo, S. P, Thng, C. H, Chow, P, Ong, H. S, Chung, A, & Soo, K. C. (2009). Sorafenib and rapamycin induce growth suppression in mouse models of hepatocellular carcinoma. *J Cell Mol Med*, , 13, 2673-2683.

[26] Hwang, Y. H, Choi, J. Y, Kim, S, Chung, E. S, Kim, T, Koh, S. S, Lee, B, Bae, S. H, Kim, J, & Park, Y. M. (2004). Over-expression of c-raf-1 proto-oncogene in liver cirrhosis and hepatocellular carcinoma. *Hepatol Res*, , 29, 113-121.

[27] Jubb, A. M, & Harris, A. L. (2010). Biomarkers to predict the clinical efficacy of bevacizumab in cancer. *Lancet Oncol, 11* , 1172-1183.

[28] Karnoub, A. E, & Weinberg, R. A. (2008). Ras oncogenes: split personalities. *Nat Rev Mol Cell Biol*, , 9, 517-531.

[29] Kelley, R. K, Nimeiri, H. S, Vergo, M. T, Bergsland, E. K, Ko, A. H, Munster, P. N, Reinert, A, Mulcahy, M. F, Benson, A. B, & Venook, A. P. A Phase I trial of the combination of temsirolimus (TEM) and sorafenib (SOR) in advanced hepatocellular carcinoma (HCC). *J Clin Oncol*, 28 (suppl.):TPS213

[30] Kerkhoff, E, & Rapp, U. R. (1998). Cell cycle targets of Ras/Raf signaling. *Oncogene*, , 17, 1457-1462.

[31] Kim, I, Xu, W, & Reed, J. C. (2008). Cell death and endoplasmic reticulum stress: disease relevance and therapeutic opportunities. *Nat Rev Drug Discov*, , 7, 1013-1030.

[32] Kudo, M, & Ueshima, K. (2010). Positioning of a molecular-targeted agent, sorafenib, in the treatment algorithm for hepatocellular carcinoma and implication of many complete remission cases in Japan. *Oncology*, 78 Suppl , 1, 154-166.

[33] Kuwahara, Y, Li, L, Baba, T, Nakagawa, H, Shimura, T, Yamamoto, Y, Ohkubo, Y, & Fukumoto, M. (2009). Clinically relevant radioresistant cells efficiently repair DNA double-strand breaks induced by X-rays. *Cancer Sci*, , 100, 747-752.

[34] Lavin, M. F. (2008). Ataxia-telangiectasia: from a rare disorder to a paradigm for cell signalling and cancer. *Nat Rev Mol Cell Biol*, , 9, 759-669.

[35] Leber, B, Geng, F, Kale, J, & Andrews, D. W. (2010). Drugs targeting Bcl-2 family members as an emerging strategy in cancer. *Expert Rev Mol Med*, 12: e28

[36] Lin, X, Morgan-lappe, S, Huang, X, Li, L, Zakula, D. M, Vernetti, L. A, Fesik, S. W, & Shen, Y. (2007). Seed' analysis of off-target siRNAs reveals an essential role of Mcl-1 in resistance to the small-molecule Bcl-2/Bcl-XL inhibitor ABT-737. *Oncogene*, , 26, 3972-3979.

[37] Llovet, J. M, Burroughs, A, & Bruix, J. (2003). Hepatocellular carcinoma. Lancet, , 362, 1907-191.

[38] Llovet, J. M, Ricci, S, Mazzaferro, V, Hilgard, P, Gane, E, Blanc, J. F, De Oliveira, A. C, Santoro, A, Raoul, J. L, Forner, A, Schwartz, M, Porta, C, Zeuzem, S, Bolondi, L, Greten, T. F, Galle, P. R, Seitz, J. F, Borbath, I, Häussinger, D, Giannaris, T, Shan, M, Moscovici, M, Voliotis, D, & Bruix, J. SHARP Investigators Study Group ((2008). Sorafenib in advanced hepatocellular carcinoma. *N Engl J Med*, , 359, 378-390.

[39] Matsuda, Y, & Fukumoto, M. (2011). Sorafenib: complexities of Raf-dependent and Raf-independent signaling are now unveiled. *Med Mol Morphol*, , 44, 183-189.

[40] Mcconkey, D. J, & Zhu, K. (2008). Mechanisms of proteasome inhibitor action and resistance in cancer. *Drug Resist Updat*, , 11, 164-179.

[41] Meng, X. W, Lee, S. H, Dai, H, Loegering, D, Yu, C, Flatten, K, Schneider, P, Dai, N. T, Kumar, S. K, Smith, B. D, Karp, J. E, Adjei, A. A, & Kaufmann, S. H. (2007). Mcl-1

as a buffer for proapoptotic Bcl-2 family members during TRAIL-induced apoptosis: a mechanistic basis for sorafenib (Bay 43-9006)-induced TRAIL sensitization. *J Biol Chem*, , 282, 29831-29846.

[42] Newell, P, Toffanin, S, Villanueva, A, Chiang, D. Y, Minguez, B, Cabellos, L, Savic, R, Hoshida, Y, Lim, K. H, Melgar-lesmes, P, Yea, S, Peix, J, Deniz, K, Fiel, M. I, Thung, S, Alsinet, C, Tovar, V, Mazzaferro, V, Bruix, J, Roayaie, S, Schwartz, M, Friedman, S. L, & Llovet, J. M. (2009). Ras pathway activation in hepatocellular carcinoma and anti-tumoral effect of combined sorafenib and rapamycin in vivo. *J Hepatol*, , 51, 725-733.

[43] Niessner, H, Beck, D, Sinnberg, T, Lasithiotakis, K, Maczey, E, Gogel, J, Venturelli, S, Berger, A, Mauthe, M, Toulany, M, Flaherty, K, Schaller, M, Schadendorf, D, Proikas-cezanne, T, Schittek, B, Garbe, C, Kulms, D, & Meier, F. (2011). The farnesyl transferase inhibitor lonafarnib inhibits mTOR signaling and enforces sorafenib-induced apoptosis in melanoma cells. *J Invest Dermatol*, , 131, 468-479.

[44] Park, M. A, Mitchell, C, Zhang, G, Yacoub, A, Allegood, J, Häussinger, D, Reinehr, R, Larner, A, Spiegel, S, Fisher, P. B, Voelkel-johnson, C, Ogretmen, B, Grant, S, & Dent, P. (2010). Vorinostat and sorafenib increase CD95 activation in gastrointestinal tumor cells through a Ca(2+)-de novo ceramide-oxygen species-dependent signaling pathway. *Cancer Res*, 70: 6313-6324, 2A.

[45] Peck-radosavljevic, M, Greten, T. F, Lammer, J, Rosmorduc, O, Sangro, B, Santoro, A, & Bolondi, L. (2010). Consensus on the current use of sorafenib for the treatment of hepatocellular carcinoma. *Eur J Gastroenterol Hepatol*, , 22, 391-398.

[46] Pinter, M, Sieghart, W, Graziadei, I, Vogel, W, Maieron, A, Königsberg, R, Weissmann, A, Kornek, G, Plank, C, & Peck-radosavljevic, M. (2009). Sorafenib in unresectable hepatocellular carcinoma from mild to advanced stage liver cirrhosis. *Oncologist*, , 14, 70-76.

[47] Prete, S. D, Montella, L, Caraglia, M, Maiorino, L, Cennamo, G, Montesarchio, V, Piai, G, Febbraro, A, Tarantino, L, Capasso, E, Palmieri, G, Guarrasi, R, Bianco, M, Mamone, R, Savastano, C, Pisano, A, Vincenzi, B, Sabia, A, Agostino, D, Faiola, A, & Addeo, V. R. ((2010). Sorafenib plus octreotide is an effective and safe treatment in advanced hepatocellular carcinoma: multicenter phase II So.LAR. study. *Cancer Chemother Pharmacol*, , 66, 837-844.

[48] Radisky, D. C, Levy, D. D, Littlepage, L. E, Liu, H, Nelson, C. M, Fata, J. E, Leake, D, Godden, E. L, Albertson, D. G, Nieto, M. A, Werb, Z, & Bissell, M. J. Rac1b and reactive oxygen species mediate MMP-3-induced EMT and genomic instability. *Nature*, , 436, 123-127.

[49] Rahmani, M, Davis, E. M, Bauer, C, Dent, P, & Grant, S. (2005). Apoptosis induced by the kinase inhibitor BAY 43-9006 in human leukemia cells involves down-regulation of Mcl-1 through inhibition of translation. *J Biol Chem*, , 280, 35217-35227.

[50] Rahmani, M, Davis, E. M, Crabtree, T. R, Habibi, J. R, Nguyen, T. K, Dent, P, & Grant, S. (2007). The kinase inhibitor sorafenib induces cell death through a process involving induction of endoplasmic reticulum stress. *Mol Cell Biol*, , 27, 5499-5513.

[51] Rausch, V, Liu, L, Kallifatidis, G, Baumann, B, Mattern, J, Gladkich, J, Wirth, T, Schemmer, P, Büchler, M. W, Zöller, M, Salnikov, A. V, & Herr, I. (2010). Synergistic activity of sorafenib and sulforaphane abolishes pancreatic cancer stem cell characteristics. *Cancer Res*, , 70, 5004-5013.

[52] Ricci, M. S, Kim, S. H, Ogi, K, Plastaras, J. P, Ling, J, Wang, W, Jin, Z, Liu, Y. Y, Dicker, D. T, Chiao, P. J, Flaherty, K. T, Smith, C. D, & Deiry, W. S. (2007). Reduction of TRAIL-induced Mcl-1 and cIAP2 by c-Myc or sorafenib sensitizes resistant human cancer cells to TRAIL-induced death. *Cancer Cell*, , 12, 66-80.

[53] Rosato, R. R, Almenara, J. A, Coe, S, & Grant, S. (2007). The multikinase inhibitor sorafenib potentiates TRAIL lethality in human leukemia cells in association with Mcl-1 and cFLIPL down-regulation. *Cancer Res*, , 67, 9490-9500.

[54] Rushworth, L. K, Hindley, A. D, Neill, O, Kolch, E, & , W. (2006). Regulation and role of Raf-1/B-Raf heterodimerization. *Mol Cell Biol*, , 26, 2262-2272.

[55] Sacco, R, Bargellini, I, Giannelli, G, Bertini, M, Bozzi, E, Altomare, E, Battaglia, V, Romano, A, Bertoni, M, Capria, A, Bresci, G, & Bartolozzi, C. (2011). Complete response for advanced liver cancer during sorafenib therapy: Case Report. *BMC Gastroenterol*, 11: 4

[56] Schleicher, S. M, Moretti, L, Varki, V, & Lu, B. (2010). Progress in the unraveling of the endoplasmic reticulum stress/autophagy pathway and cancer: implications for future therapeutic approaches. *Drug Resist Updat*, , 13, 79-86.

[57] Schütte, K, Zimmermann, L, Bornschein, J, Csepregi, A, Rühl, R, Ricke, J, & Malfertheiner, P. (2011). Sorafenib Therapy in Patients with Advanced Hepatocellular Carcinoma in Advanced Liver Cirrhosis. *Digestion*, , 83, 275-282.

[58] Shen, Y. C, Hsu, C, & Cheng, A. L. (2010). Molecular targeted therapy for advanced hepatocellular carcinoma: current status and future perspectives. *J Gastroenterol*, , 45, 794-807.

[59] So, B. J, Bekaii-saab, T, Bloomston, M. A, & Patel, T. (2008). Complete clinical response of metastatic hepatocellular carcinoma to sorafenib in a patient with hemochromatosis: a case report. *J Hematol Oncol*, 1:18

[60] Takayasu, K, Arii, S, Ikai, I, Omata, M, Okita, K, Ichida, T, Matsuyama, Y, Nakanuma, Y, Kojiro, M, Makuuchi, M, & Yamaoka, Y. (2006). Liver Cancer Study Group of Japan. Prospective cohort study of transarterial chemoembolization for unresectable hepatocellular carcinoma in 8510 patients. *Gastroenterology*, , 131, 461-469.

[61] Takeuchi, A, Tsuchiya, H, Yamamoto, N, Hayashi, K, Yamauchi, K, Kawahara, M, Miyamoto, K, & Tomita, K. (2007). Caffeine-potentiated chemotherapy for patients

with high-grade soft tissue sarcoma: long-term clinical outcome. *Anticancer Res*, , 27, 3489-3495.

[62] Takezawa, K, Okamoto, I, Yonesaka, K, Hatashita, E, Yamada, Y, Fukuoka, M, & Nakagawa, K. (2009). Sorafenib inhibits non-small cell lung cancer cell growth by targeting B-RAF in KRAS wild-type cells and C-RAF in KRAS mutant cells. *Cancer Res*, , 69, 6515-6521.

[63] Tang, Z. Y. (2008). Effect of rapamycin alone and in combination with sorafenib in an orthotopic model of human hepatocellular carcinoma. *Clin Cancer Res, 14* , 5124-5130.

[64] Thomas, L. W, Lam, C, & Edwards, S. W. (2010). Mcl-1; the molecular regulation of protein function. *FEBS Lett*, , 584, 2981-2989.

[65] Tsukada, M, & Oshumi, Y. (1993). Isolation and characterization of autophagy-defective mutants of Saccharomyces cerevisiae. *FEBS Lett*, , 333, 169-174.

[66] Ulivi, P, Arienti, C, Amadori, D, Fabbri, F, Carloni, S, Tesei, A, Vannini, I, Silvestrini, R, & Zoli, W. (2009). Role of RAF/MEK/ERK pathway, p-STAT-3 and Mcl-1 in sorafenib activity in human pancreatic cancer cell lines. *J Cell Physiol,220* , 214-221.

[67] Villanueva, A, Chiang, D. Y, Newell, P, Peix, J, Thung, S, Alsinet, C, Tovar, V, Roayaie, S, Minguez, B, Sole, M, Battiston, C, Van Laarhoven, S, & Fiel, M. I. Di Feo, A., Hoshida, Y., Yea, S., Toffanin, S., Ramos, A., Martignetti, JA., Mazzaferro, V., Bruix, J., Waxman, S., Schwartz, M., Meyerson, M., Friedman, SL., Llovet, JM. ((2008). Pivotal role of mTOR signaling in hepatocellular carcinoma. *Gastroenterology*, , 135, 1972-1983.

[68] Wan, P. T, Garnett, M. J, Roe, S. M, Lee, S, Niculescu-duvaz, D, Good, V. M, Jones, C. M, Marshall, C. J, Springer, C. J, Barford, D, & Marais, R. (2004). Mechanism of activation of the RAF-ERK signaling pathway by oncogenic mutations of B-RAF. *Cell*, , 116, 855-867.

[69] Wang, S. X, Byrnes, A, Verma, S, Pancoast, J. R, & Rixe, O. (2010). Complete remission of unresectable hepatocellular carcinoma treated with reduced dose of sorafenib: a case report. *Target Oncol*, , 5, 59-63.

[70] Wang, Y, Gao, J, Zhang, D, Zhang, J, Ma, J, & Jiang, H. (2010). New insights into the antifibrotic effects of sorafenib on hepatic stellate cells and liver fibrosis. *J Hepatol*, , 53, 132-144.

[71] Wei, G, Wang, M, & Carr, B. I. (2010a). Sorafenib combined vitamin K induces apoptosis in human pancreatic cancer cell lines through RAF/MEK/ERK and c-Jun NH2-terminal kinase pathways. *J Cell Physiol*, , 224, 112-119.

[72] Wei, G, Wang, M, Hyslop, T, Wang, Z, & Carr, B. I. (2010b). Vitamin K enhancement of sorafenib-mediated HCC cell growth inhibition in vitro and in vivo. Int J Cancer, , 127, 2949-295.

[73] Wilhelm, S. M, Carter, C, Tang, L, Wilkie, D, Mcnabola, A, Rong, H, Chen, C, Zhang, X, Vincent, P, Mchugh, M, Cao, Y, Shujath, J, Gawlak, S, Eveleigh, D, Rowley, B, Liu, L, Adnane, L, Lynch, M, Auclair, D, Taylor, I, Gedrich, R, Voznesensky, A, Riedl, B, Post, L. E, Bollag, G, & Trail, P. A. (2004). BAY 43-9006 exhibits broad spectrum oral antitumor activity and targets the RAF/MEK/ERK pathway and receptor tyrosine kinases involved in tumor progression and angiogenesis. *Cancer Res, 64* , 7099-7109.

[74] Yamaguchi, T, Reif, G. A, Calvet, J. P, & Wallace, D. P. (2010). Sorafenib inhibits cAMP-dependent ERK activation, cell proliferation, and in vitro cyst growth of human ADPKD cyst epithelial cells. *Am J Physiol Renal Physiol,* 299: FF951, 944.

[75] Yang, J. D, & Roberts, L. R. (2010). Hepatocellular carcinoma: A global view. *Nat Rev Gastroenterol Hepatol,* , 7, 448-458.

[76] Yeganeh, M, Finn, R. S, & Saab, S. (2009). Apparent remission of a solitary metastatic pulmonary lesion in a liver transplant recipient treated with sorafenib. *Am J Transplant,* , 9, 2851-2854.

[77] Yu, C, Bruzek, L. M, Meng, X. W, Gores, G. J, Carter, C. A, Kaufmann, S. H, & Adjei, A. A. (2005). The role of Mcl-1 downregulation in the proapoptotic activity of the multikinase inhibitor BAY 43-9006. *Oncogene,* , 24, 6861-6869.

[78] Zhang, W, Zhu, X. D, Sun, H. C, Xiong, Y. Q, Zhuang, P. Y, Xu, H. X, Kong, L. Q, Wang, L, Wu, W. Z, & Tang, Z. Y. (2010). Depletion of tumor-associated macrophages enhances the effect of sorafenib in metastatic liver cancer models by antimetastatic and antiangiogenic effects. *Clin Cancer Res,* , 16, 3420-3430.

Chapter 13

Insulin-Like Growth Factor-II: Molecular-Targeted Therapy for Hepatocellular Carcinoma

Min Yao, Li Wang, Meijuan Yan, Xiaodi Yan and Dengfu Yao

Additional information is available at the end of the chapter

http://dx.doi.org/10.5772/55418

1. Introduction

Hepatocellular carcinoma (HCC) is the third deadliest and 5th most common cancer worldwide. It ranks the second in China among all malignancies, and its mortality is almost equal to its morbidity [1-3]. Carcinogenesis of HCC is a multi-factor, multi-step and complex process, which is associated with a background of chronic and persistent infection of hepatitis B virus (HBV) or hepatitis C virus (HCV) [4-6]. Their infections along with alcohol and aflatoxin B1 intake are widely recognized etiological agents in HCC [7, 8]. Multiple genetic alterations, including the activation of oncogenes and inactivation of tumor suppressor genes, are required for malignancy in human cancers and are correlated with increased stages of carcinogenesis and further tumor progression with many characteristics, such as fast infiltrating growth, metastasis in early stage, high-grade malignancy, and poor therapeutic efficacy [9-11]. HCC prognoses are poor, and early detection is of the utmost importance [12, 13]. Most of HCC patients died quickly because of the rapid tumor progression, and hepatic resection or transplantation is the only potential curative treatment for HCC. Treatment options are severely limited by the frequent presence of metastases. Therefore, it is the 3rd leading cause of cancer-induced death worldwide with a very poor prognosis [14]. Growing understanding of the molecular mechanisms underlying the carcinogenesis of HCC is a multi-factor, multi-step, and complex process, involving chromosomal aberrations, gene mutations, epigenetic alterations, and activation of complex signaling pathways [15, 16].

Recently, studies have discovered changes in the insulin-like growth factor (IGF) axis that affect the molecular pathogenesis of HCC, and IGF-II is a polypeptide hormone secreted by many organs of the fetus [17, 18]. IGF axis (Figure.1) has emerged as an important pathway in the development and progression of HCC and as a potential therapeutic target. Human IGF-

II gene contains 9 exons (E_1~E_9) and 4 promoters (P_1~P_4, Figure1A). IGF system consists of the ligands, cell surface receptors, and the IGF binding proteins (IGFBPs) [19]. IGF receptors (IGF-1R and IGF-2R) are tyrosine kinase cell-surface receptor that binds either IGF-I or IGF-II. IGFBPs have key roles in regulating ligand bioavailability. IGF-II interacts with IGF-IR, IGF-IIR (lacks tyrosine kinase domain), and the exon 11-lacking (A) form of the insulin receptor (IR), and the IGFBPs. Hybrid receptors form from dimerization of IGF-IR and IR hemireceptors. These hybrid receptors retain high affinity for IGF-I, but have a significantly reduced affinity for insulin [20, 21].

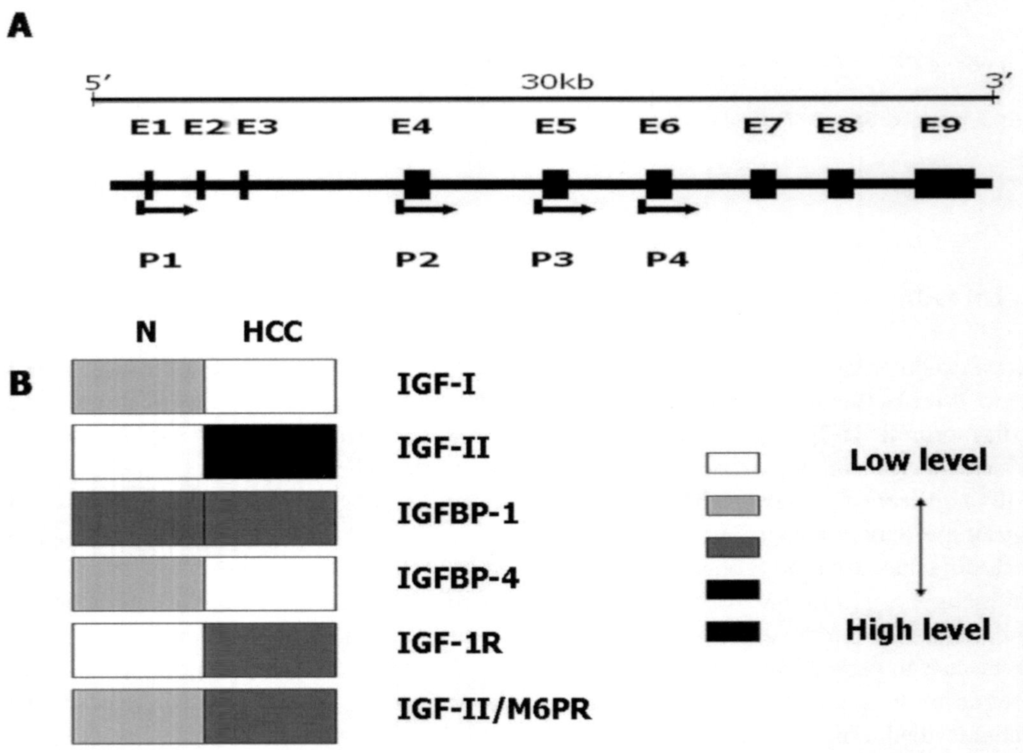

Figure 1. Schematic illustration demonstrating the structure of IGF-II gene (A) and the IGFs representative results (B) from immunohistochemical analysis or in situ hybridisation of antisense mRNA to normal liver (N) and HCC tissues. The intensity of gene expression is directly proportional to the darkness of the section. IGF, insulin-like growth factor; IGFBP, IGF binding protein; IGF-IR, IGF-I receptor; and IGF-II/M6PR, mannose 6-phosphate receptor.

IGFs, including IGF-I, IGF-II, IGF binding proteins, and their receptors (IGF-1R and IGF-2R) were well characterized in primary HCC tissue (Figure 1B) [22]. The IGFs system regulates many key aspects of cellular and whole- organism physiology and plays a crucial role in the regulation of cell growth, energy metabolism, differentiation, as well as key aspects of tumors such as transformation and anti-apoptotic signaling (Figure 2). Now, little is known of relationship between IGF-II gene's promoter methylation status and hepatocarcinogenesis.

http://dx.doi.org/10.5772/55418

IGF-II gene has complex regulation of transcription, resulting in multiple mRNA initiated by different promoters. Here, we review the complexity of IGF axis and focus on the expression of hepatic IGF-II and their gene during the malignant transformation of hepatocytes, the hepatic expression and circulating level of IGF-II in patients with liver diseases for prospectively elucidating the relationship between IGF-II level and the pathological features as well as the diagnosis and metastasis of HCC, and the effect of miRNA silencing IGF-II gene on inhibition of HepG2 cell proliferation with an urgent need to search for novel effective therapies for HCC. [23, 24]

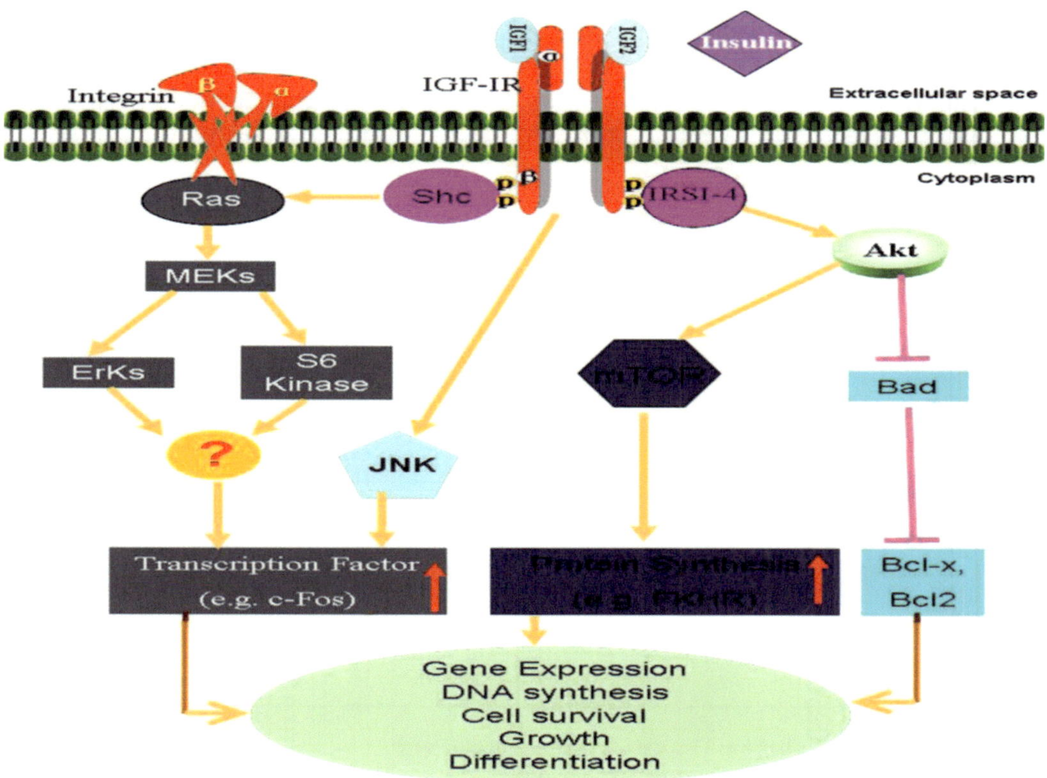

Figure 2. The IGF-II/IGF-1R intracellular pathway. Binding of the ligands IGF-I and IGF-II to IGF-IR activates its intrinsic tyrosine kinase activity resulting in signaling through cellular pathways that stimulates proliferation and inhibits apoptosis. The key downstream signaling pathways include PI3K-AKT-TOR and the RAF-MEK-ERK pathway. Therapeutic approaches that target the IGF-IR are being tested clinically and include antibodies directed at the extracellular portion of the receptor and small molecule tyrosine kinase inhibitors with specificity for IGF-IR. **ErK**, extracellular signal-related kinase; **IGF**, insulin-like growth factor; **IGF-IR**, IGF-I receptor; **mTOR**, mammalian TOR, target of rapamycin; **IRS**, insulin receptor substrate; **AKt**, Ak transforming; **Shc**, Src homology 2 domain-containing; **Ras**, rat sarcoma viral oncogene homolog.

2. Dynamic expression IGF-II during HCC development

IGF-II is a fetal growth peptide produced by the liver, which is over expressed in a wide variety of neoplasms including HCC and involved in experimental liver carcinogenesis [25-27]. 48 male Sprague-Dawley rats, 4~6 weeks old and weighing 120~160 g, were randomly divided into groups of 6 per cage, including control group and experimental groups. The control rats were given a standard diet, and the experimental rats were fed with 0.05 % 2-fluorenylacetamide (2-FAA, Sigma, USA) in an air-conditioned environment. One control rat and a group of experimental rats were sacrificed under mild ether anesthesia every 2 weeks(wk), blood was drawn from the heart and the serum was separated. The livers were washed free of blood, one part was used for pathological examination and immunohistochemical analysis, and the others were stored at -80 ℃. All procedures were conducted in accordance with the guidelines for experimental animals approved by the Animal Care and Use Committee of Nantong University. The morphological changes in rat liver cells were clearly seen during HCC development. The histological examination confirmed changes in hepatocytes from granule-like degeneration to atypical hyperplasia to HCC formation inducing with 2-FAA (Table 1).

Group		*n*	Histopathological change (HE staining)			
			Normal	Degeneration	Precancerous	HCC
Control		6	6	0	0	0
Experimental:	2nd wk	6	0	6	0	0
	4th wk	6	0	6	0	0
	6th wk	6	5	1	0	0
	8th wk	6	0	3	2	1
	10th wk	6	0	2	1	3
	12th wk	6	0	0	2	4
Total		42	6	22	6	8

Table 1. Histopathological Changes of Rat Liver during HCC Development

At the early stage during HCC induction process, the granular degeneration appeared in the cytoplasm and a large heterogeneous nucleus was seen (the degeneration group). At the intermediate stage, hepatic plate cell layers increased, focal cell layers surpassed three, the nuclear chromatin was denser, and the ratio of nucleus to cytoplasm increased (the precancerous group). At the later stage, the hepatic structure disappeared, the cells arranged into nido or funicular form, nuclei became middling large and the chromatin was denser, and the ratio of nucleus to cytoplasm increased. All of these were highly differentiated HCC (the HCC group).

http://dx.doi.org/10.5772/55418

At the same time, the expression levels of IGF-II in hepatic tissues and sera progressively increased (Table 2). *In vivo*, IGF-II is a growth factor that plays an important role during HCC development. It is synthesized and activated through tyrosine kinase and the IGF-I receptor. The process of IGF-II activation and expression has been confirmed in the liver tissues of HCC rats, transgenic rats and experimental animals infected with hepatitis virus. When the expression of IGF-II in the transgenic rat rise continuously, the risk of HCC increases. The reason for the high expression of IGF-II is the reactivation of the embryonic IGF-II gene. In the precancerous condition, IGF-II-mediated hepatocyte proliferation is mainly via IGF-IR by a paracrine mechanism. IGF-II was distributed in the cytoplasm of hepatocytes and over-expressed in the precancerous group, and the levels of IGF-II expression suggest that it may be secreted by hepatoma cells themselves and stimulate their proliferation via an autocrine mechanism. Although different levels of IGF-II expression were found in rat livers with different histopathological changes, the expression of IGF-II was detected in the hepatic cytoplasm of all rats fed with 2-FAA and none in the control group [28].

			IGF-II expression intensity			
Group	***n***	**Positive (%)**	**-**	**+**	**++**	**+++**
Control	6	0 (0.0)	6	0	0	0
Degeneration	22	8 (36.36)	4	6	1	1
Precancerous	6	6 (100)*	0	3	2	1
HCC	8	8 (100)*	0	1	2	5

*P<0.01 vs. the control group.

Table 2. Dynamic Alteration of IGF-II Expression during Rat HCC Development

IGFs are potent autocrine and paracrine mitogens for liver cancer cell proliferation, and their bioactivity is reduced by IGFBP-3 [29]. Human embryonic liver cell lines also express IGF-II, suggesting that hepatoma cells may regain some embryonic characteristics like AFP secretion. A smaller proportion of IGF-II is associated with other IGFBPs, while less than 5% of IGF-II exists in the unbound or free form that is believed to be the biologically active fraction, capable of binding to the IGF-2R. IGF-II present in the ternary complex is not easily dissociated. However, IGF-II contained in low molecular weight binding complexes has a rapid turnover and may be the source of much of the free IGF-II detected. The levels of serum IGF-II protein were significantly higher in the HCC group than in the precancerous, degeneration and control groups (Table 3). Its main mechanism possibly is that the abnormal activation and over-expression cause precancerous cells in a high multiplication condition which transforms and finally induces HCC. The levels of IGF-II expression reflect the degree of pathological change in rat liver. Hepatic IGF-II may participate in liver cancer induction, and detection of IGF-II expression during HCC development could be a useful molecular marker for early diagnosis and prognosis of HCC [28].

	Serum IGF-II (ng/L)			Liver IGF-II (ng/mg protein)		
Group	***n***					
	Mean ± SD	***t***	***P value****	**Mean ± SD**	***t***	***P value****
Normal	6	149.7±19.1	7.40 <0.01	52.3±4.5	8.85	<0.01
Degeneration	22	174.2±43.4	6.75 <0.01	54.9±12.8	6.79	<0.01
Precancerous	6	274.1±24.1	4.30 <0.01	70.3±8.4	2.42	<0.05
HCC	8	450.3±112.6		80.7±7.4		

*P<0.01, vs. the HCC group.

Table 3. Dynamic Quantitative Analysis of Liver and Serum IGF-II Expression during Rat HCC Development

IGF-II is a kind of fetal growth factor, a mitogenic polypeptide closely related to insulin, highly expressed in hepatocarcinogenesis, and causes mitosis in different cell types. IGF-II may promote hepatocyte proliferation via a paracrine mechanism in the pre-cancerous stage. When hepatocytes are transformed into malignant cells, they may secrete IGF-II and promote malignant cell proliferation by an autocrine mechanism [30]. Identification of molecular abnormalities associated with an increased risk of HCC is particularly important to improve knowledge of both the pathways of liver carcinogenesis and the outcomes. Its gene has complex regulation of transcription, resulting in multiple mRNAs initiated by different promoters, which contribute to cell proliferation, differentiation, anti-apoptosis, and invasive behavior.

3. Difference of IGF-II expression in human HCC tissues

3.1. Alteration of fetal IGF-II promoter methylation status

Carcinogenesis of hepatocytes is a multi-factor, multi-step, and complex process. Genetic and epigenetic changes are the core biological processes in HCC. DNA cytosine methylation is a central epigenetic modification that has essential roles in cellular processes including genome regulation, development and disease [31-33]. Epigenetic changes include DNA methylation, histone modification, and DNA methylation is performed by DNA methyltransferase. The methylation status is closely associated with the development and progression of carcinoma. Hepatic IGF-II gene contains 4 promoters (P_1~P_4, Figure1A), P_1 for adult liver and P_2~P_4 for fetal liver [34-36].

The methylation status of IGF-II promoter and IGF-II expression were analyzed in HCC-, their surrounding-, and noncancerous- tissues, and the patterns by MPS were shown in Figure 3. The incidences of IGF-II P_3 methylation was 0% (0 of 40) in human HCC, 47.5% (19 of 40) in their surrounding, and 100% (40 of 40) in normal tissues, respectively; and the incidence was increased gradually (Table 4) from cancerous to non-cancerous parts of liver tissues, with significant differences among them (Table 4, χ^2 = 37.623, P < 0.001). The methylation

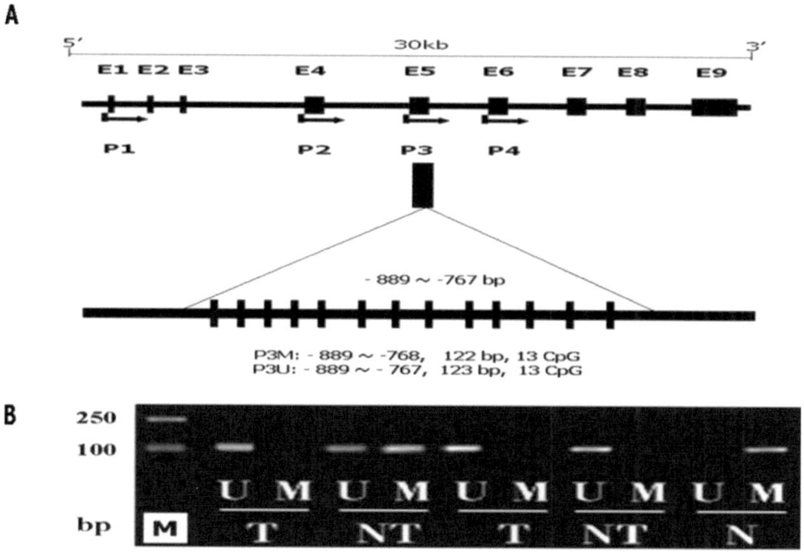

Figure 3. Methylation analysis of IGF-II promoter 3 region in human HCC tissues and IGF-II expression. A, Exon-intron and 4 promoter structure of human IGF-II gene. Exons are shown as numbered boxes (plain are coding). The 122 bp (P_3M) or 123 bp (P_3U) fragment of IGF-II promoter3 amplified for methylation analysis is enlarged below. Vertical lines indicate 13 CpG positions. **B,** The patterns of promoter methylation of hepatic IGF-II in different liver tissues. T-HCC; NT-Adjacent; N-Normal; U-Demethylation; M-Methylation; m, DNA marker.

rate of IGF-II P_3 in the adjacent tissues in poorly differentiated HCC were lower than well-differentiated ones (P<0.001), suggesting the positive correlation between demethylation status of IGF-II P_3 and hepatocarcinogenesis, suggesting aberrant methylation occurs before mutation and is an early event in the development of HCC. IGF-II is highly expressed in the fetal liver and early after birth, which is mainly based on activation of $P_2 \sim P_4$. But its expression is strongly reduced in adulthood, mainly based on activation of P_1. Several studies have shown elevated expression levels of IGF-II in preneoplastic lesions and very high levels in HCC, and so was the IGF-II P_2~P_4, suggesting the correlation between IGF-II gene expression and promoter.

Group	n	M (%)	PM (%)	UM (%)	Z	P
HCC	40	0(0)	0(0)	40(100)	6.708	0.000
Adjacent	40	0(0)	19(47.5)	21(52.5)	4.290	0.000
Non-HCC	40	40 (100)	0(0)	0(0)		

P<0.01, compared with non-cancerous group; M, methylation of liver IGF-II gene P3 promoter; PM, part methylation of liver IGF-II gene P3 promoter; UM, unmethylation of of liver IGF-II gene P3 promoter.

Table 4. The Status of IGF-II Promoter 3 Methylation in Different Liver Tissues

Tumor differentiation and gene methylation while gene displayed different methylation profiles at different levels of differentiation, only two showed statistically significant differences. However, there was no correspondence with tumor progression toward poor differentiation. Only the gene displayed lower methylation in the normal progression of a tumor from well to moderate to poor differentiation. These findings might underscore the role of these genes in the tumor differentiation process. Tumor stage and gene methylation profile gene showed different methylation profiles at different tumor stages, with the gene displaying statistically significant differences with higher methylation at lower methylation at higher methylation at advanced stages [37].

3.2. Alteration of GF-II expression in different liver tissues

The expression of hepatocyte IGF-II was analyzed in HCC, their surrounding, and nocancerous tissues by immunohistochemistry were shown in Figure 4. Positive staining of hepatic IGF-II showed brown particles, located in cytoplasm with only a few in cellular nuclei but none in cell membrane. Positive cells were mostly located in the margin of portal area or near the central vein. The expression level of IGF-II went up with the histological changes. It was significantly higher in the HCC or the surrounding group than in the nocancerous group, and its levels in HCC group were obviously higher than in the surrounding group (*P*<0.05). There were 11 samples showed positive staining of IGF-II in degeneration group and 54.5 % of them were staining moderately and above. Five samples in precancerous lesion group showed positive staining of IGF-II and 80 % of them were staining moderately and above. Eight samples in cancerization group were positive for IGF-II staining and 87.5 % of them showed moderate and above. Thus we concluded that the expression intensities of IGF-II were associated with the morphological changes of hepatocytes [38, 39].

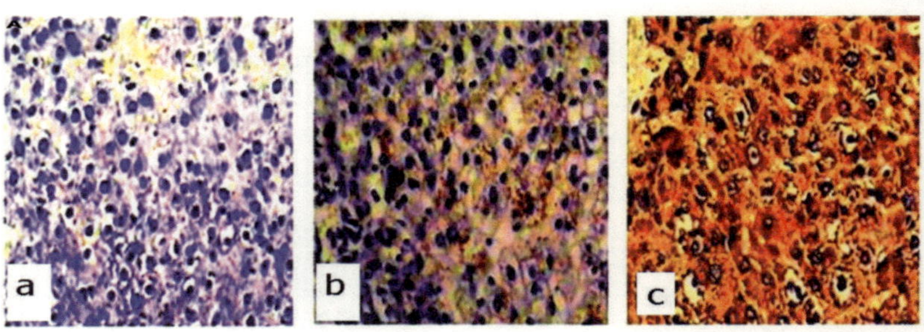

Figure 4. Immunohistochemical analysis with anti-human IGF-II in HCC tissues; a, the absence of cytoplamic staining for IGF-II (S-P, original magnification ×200) from non- cancerous tissues of human HCC; b, the IGF-II weakly positive staining in cytoplasm and cell membrane from the surrounding tissues; and c, the IGF-II strongly positive staining in cytoplasm and cell membrane (S-P, original magnification ×100) from human HCC tissues.

3.3. Expression of total RNA and IGF-II mRNA in HCC tissues

IGF-II may be a biological marker in the early diagnosis of HCC. The expression levels of IGF-II mRNA are different in different parts of HCC liver tissues. Different expression of hepatic total RNA (μg/mg wet liver tissue) was found in the different parts of 36 HCC tissues. The total RNA levels were significantly lower in HCC tissues (17.9 ± 27.7 μg/mg wet liver tissue) than in self-control surrounding- (32.9 ± 31.2 μg/mg wet liver tissue, $P<0.05$) or non-cancerous liver tissues (41.4 ± 50.3 μg/mg wet liver tissue, $P < 0.01$), respectively [38].

Studies found that the amplified fragments of IGF-II mRNA by RT-PCR were identical to original designed ones with size of 170 bp and confirmed by sequencing analysis (Figure 5). The dilution experiments revealed that the lowest sensitivity of our system was 2 ng/L of total RNA (Figure 5A), the size of IGF-II DNA was identical to the original designed one, and confirmed by DNA sequencing analysis (Figure 5B). The incidence of positive IGF-II mRNA fragments was 100 % in HCC tissues, and significantly higher ($P<0.01$) than that in their surrounding (53.3 %) or in their non-cancerous (0%) liver tissues, respectively. [38, 39]

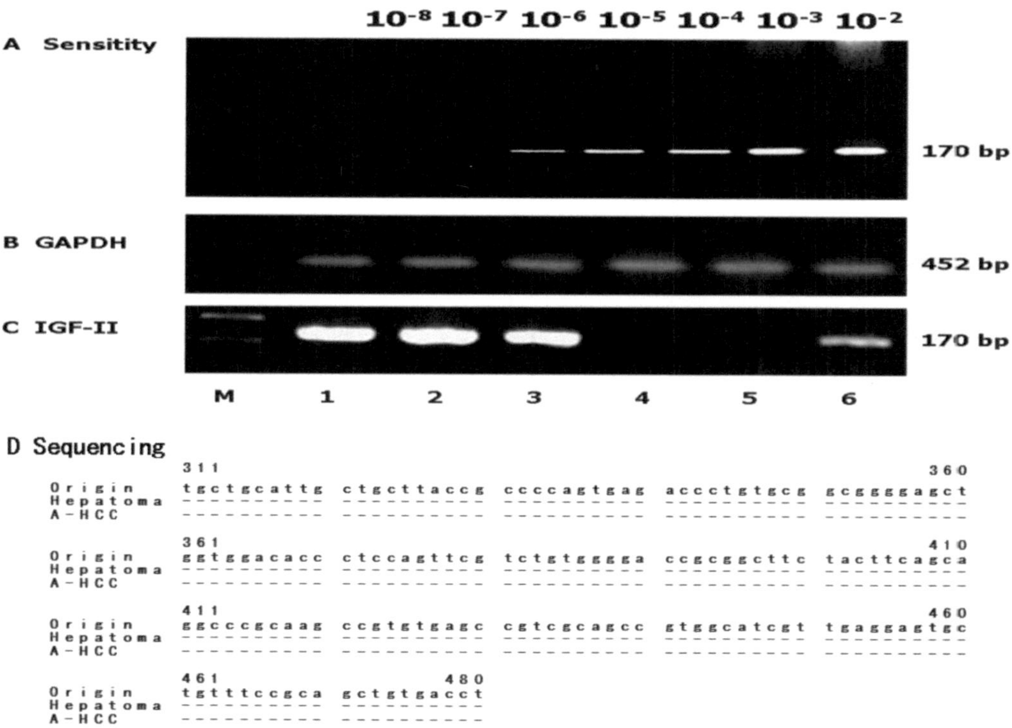

Figure 5. Amplification of IGF-II genomes from human liver tissues of HCC patients. IGF-II mRNAs were synthesized according to IGF-II cDNA with random hexamers and moloney murine leukemia virus reverse-transcriptase, and detected with different primer pairs by nested PCR (170 bp). The positive fragments of IGF-II genome were found distinctly in HCC or surrounding tissues. A, the sensitive limitation of the detection system (2 ng/L), using total RNA with 10^{-2} ~10^{-8} fold dilution and then amplified by nested PCR; B, the amplified fragments (452 bp) of glyceraldehyde-3-phosphate dehydrogenase genome from liver tissues; C, the amplification of IGF-II genomes in human liver tissues (No. 1~6). No. 1~3, the positively amplified fragments of IGF-II mRNA from cancerous tissues of HCC patients; No. 4~5, no positively amplified fragment from para-cancerous or non-cancerous tissue of HCC patients; No. 6, the positively

amplified fragments of IGF-II mRNA from para-cancerous tissue of HCC. GAPDH: glyceraldehyde-3 -phosphate dehydrogenase. M: DNA molecular weight marker. D, Alignment of nucleotide sequences of the amplified fragments of IGF-II genome from different liver tissues in patients with HCC by sequence analysis. Origin: the cited sequence (170 bp, nt 311-480) of human IGF-II genome; Hepatoma: the amplification fragment of IGF-II genome from human HCC tissue; A-HCC: the amplified fragment of IGF-II genome from the surrounding tissue in HCC patients. HCC, hepatocellular carcinoma.

4. Expression of IGF-II associated with HBV or HCV infection

HCC is mainly associated with HBV and HCV infection. Activation of cell growth stimulator IGF-II gene is observed in tumor formation especially in viral associated HCC [5, 6, 11, 13]. IGF-II signaling is mediated through IGF-1R, up-regulation of IGF-II in some hepatocytes may lead to high focal IGF-II levels sufficient to saturate local IGF-II binding capacities, and may result in an increased susceptibility to cellular dedifferentiation and, ultimately, liver cancer. Elevated focal IGF-II transcript levels may therefore indicate an increased risk for HCC. SNPs sites (frequency ≥5%) of 376 HCC patients (312/21/43; HBV/HCV/NBNC) was found in angiogenic genes including VEGF, HIF-1α, and IGF-II (TT genotype more common). T allele (TT+CT genotype) at -13021C in IGF-II were independent risk factors in HCC recurrence. The SNPs in IGF-II genes may be important risk factors for the recurrence of HCC [40].

4.1. Expression of IGF-II and HBV Infection

In HBV, HBx protein promotes cell cycle progression, inactivates negative growth regulators, and binds to and inhibits the expression of p53 tumor suppressor gene and other tumor suppressor genes and senescence-related factors. During recent years evidence has accumulated that HBx protein modulates transcription of methyl transferases, causing regional DNA hypermethylation that results in silencing of tumor suppressor genes, or global hypomethylation that results in chromosomal instability, thereby playing a role in hepatocarcinogenesis. Particularly important among the anti- apoptotic properties is inhibition of p53 [41].

Recent experimental observations suggest that HBx protein may increase the expression of TERT and telomerase activity, prolonging the life-span of hepatocytes and contributing to malignant transformation. Carboxy-terminal truncated HBx protein loses its inhibitory effects on cell proliferation and pro-apoptotic properties, and it may enhance the protein's ability to transform oncogenes. Dysregulation of IGF-II enhances proliferation and anti-apoptotic effects of oncogenes, resulting in uncontrolled cell growth. Significant increase in fetal transcripts is associated with the p53 mutation and poor prognosis of the HCC patients and might serve as one of identification parameters of poor HCC prognosis. HBx product become transcriptional transactivators of cellular and viral genes, are known to play causative roles in HCC development [42, 43]

Using 240 different combinations of three one-base anchored oligo-dT primers and 80 arbitrary 13 mers, 16 genes were differentially expressed in the HBx- positive HCC. Unexpectedly, upregulated genes in association with functional HBV proteins were different from those reportedly transactivated by HBV viral proteins in vitro. Ten genes were downregulated, including three novel genes. In contrast, 15 genes in HCC tissue negative for HBx-expression were preferentially expressed including IGF-II and 10 ribosomal proteins genes. Cellular genes involved in the viral protein-transactivation may generally differ from those not associated with transactivation in established HCC, and that the specific oncogenic coordination through the transactivation by viral proteins which works in experiments in vitro, may play only a potential role in hepatocarcinogenesis in vivo [43, 44].

HBV infection is one of the most important factors for HCC, especially HBV X gene (HBX) is closely related to hepatocarcinogenesis. And more than 80% of HCC cases are associated with HBV. Many studies showed HBV infection contributed to hypermethylation of tumour suppressor genes. The methylation rates of IGF-II P_3 in positive surface antigen HCC patients was significantly lower than those with negative surface antigen, suggesting DNA demethylation could related to HBV infection. DNA methylation may be the molecular-targeted therapies of HCC [41]. Further studies will allow us to investigate the changes of IGF-II gene promoter methylation status in patients' peripheral blood with HCC, and will elevate early diagnosis and monitor metastasis of HCC. These reference epigenomes provide a foundation for future studies exploring this key epigenetic modification in human disease and development. DNA cytosine methylation is a central epigenetic modification that has essential roles in cellular processes including genome regulation, development and disease [45, 46].

4.2. Expression IGF-II and HCV infection

In HCV, core protein is believed to transactivate host IGF-II receptor through PKC pathway and the inhibition of tumor cell growth can be achieved by blocking IGF-II pathway either at transcriptional level or increasing its binding with IGFBPs (IGF binding proteins) at C-terminal, so that it is not available in free form. IGFBP-6 is a specific inhibitor of IGF-II actions. Affinity of IGFBPs with IGFs is controlled by post- translational modifications. Phosphorylation of IGFBPs inhibits IGFs action on target cells while O-glycosylation prevents binding of IGFBP-6 to glycosamino- glycans and cell membranes and resulting in a 10-fold higher affinity for IGF-II. O-glycosylation and phosphorylation operate the functional expression of cellular proteins, this switching on and off the protein expression is difficult to monitor in vivo [44]. By using neural network based prediction methods, alternate O-β-GlcNAc modification and phosphorylation on Ser 204 control the binding of IGFBP-6 with IGF-II. This information may be used for developing new therapies by regulating IGFBP-6 assembly with IGF-II to minimize the risk of viral associated HCC [44].

During HCV/HBV infection, O-β-GlcNAc of IGFBP-6 at Ser 204 diminish their binding with IGF-II, increase IGF-II cellular expression and promote cancer progression which can lead to hepatocellular carcinoma. Furthermore, this site can be used for developing new therapies to control the IGF-II actions during viral infection to minimize the risk of hepatocellular carcinoma [46]. The possibility that HCV core gene product (HCV-core) acts as a transactivator in IGF-II gene transcription was tested. HCV-core protein increases endogenous IGF-II expression from promoter 4 (P_4) of the IGF-II gene through two cis-acting elements: Sp1 and Egr1 binding sites. Sp1 and Egr1 both bind to IGF-II P4 and functionally cooperate in mediating the maximal activity of IGF-II P4. HCV-core protein induced the binding of Sp1 and Egr1 on its binding sites on IGF-II P4. In addition, Sp1 and Egr1 were stimulated to phosphorylate by HCV-core, and its DNA binding activity was up-regulated upon HCV-core transfection [47].

Transfection with HCV-core in HepG2 cells stimulated the membrane translocation of protein kinase C (PKC) and the treatment of HCV-core transfected cells with calphostin C, a PKC inhibitor, blocked induction of Sp1 and Egr1 DNA binding activity, and eventually transcriptional transactivations of the IGF-II gene. Increasing the DNA binding activity of the phosphorylated form of Sp1 and Egr1 might be an important mechanism for regulating IGF-II gene expression and for promoting cell division during hepatic carcinogenesis. HCV-core functions as a positive regulator of IGF-II transcription through the PKC pathway and that Sp1 and Egr1 are direct targets of the transcriptional regulation of the IGF-II gene which plays an important role in HCV pathogenesis during the formation of HCC. [47]

5. Circulating IGF-II and clinicopathological features

There were 156 patients with HCC enrolled for this study at Affiliated Hospital of Nantong University, China. The patients' ages ranged from 26 to 74 years (median, 46 years). 134 patients (86 %) had a history of cirrhosis, and 22 (14%) had a history of chronic hepatitis [48]. All patients were diagnosed by blood biochemical tests, viral histology and B-ultrasonic examination. The incidence of hepatitis virus in these patients was 76 % (118 of 156) in HBsAg, and 10 % (16 of 156) in antibody to hepatitis C virus (ELISA, Beijing, China). The serum AFP level ranged from 33 to 2,500 ng/mL (median, 243 ng/mL). Serum AFP more than 50 ng/mL was taken as a positive result. Other cases included 39 patients with acute hepatitis, 72 patients with chronic hepatitis, 75 patients with decompensated cirrhosis, and 60 healthy subjects with negative-HBV markers (HBsAg, HBcAb, and HBV-DNA) and with normal serum ALT levels from the Nantong Central Blood Bank. All peripheral blood samples were collected in the morning, with anti-clot heparin, and peripheral blood mononuclear cells were separated immediately, according to the method as described previously. AFP-mRNA in peripheral blood was also detected in this study as described elsewhere. Ethics Statement, this study was approved by the Institutional Review Board, Affiliated Hospital of Nantong University, and written informed consent was obtained. The diagnosis of HCC and viral hepatitis was based on the criteria proposed by Chinese National Collaborative Cancer Research Group and the 2000 Prevention and Cure Scheme of Viral Hepatitis, respectively.

The levels of IGF-II expression in the serum of 224 patients with liver diseases was significantly higher (P< 0.001) in patients with HCC than in patients with liver cirrhosis or chronic hepatitis. Also, the level of serum IGF-II in patients with HCC was significantly higher (P < 0.001) than in patients with nonliver tumors or acute hepatitis. The evaluation of serum IGF-II and AFP levels for HCC diagnosis using the ROC curves is shown in Figure 6. The analysis of 2 markers for the whole range of sensitivities and specificities using the area (0.823 for AFP and 0.771 for IGF-II) under ROC curves indicated that the abnormality of serum IGF-II level could be a useful molecular marker for HCC diagnosis [48, 49].

http://dx.doi.org/10.5772/55418

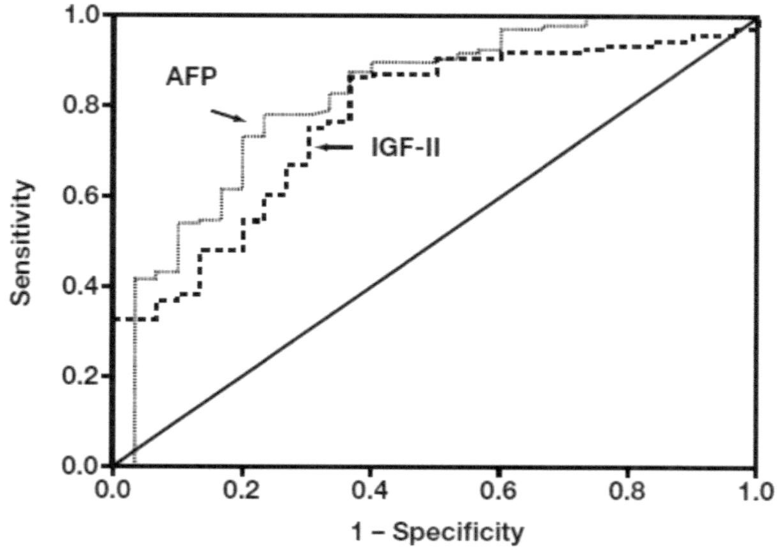

Figure 6. The diagnostic value of circulating IGF-II level for HCC. Receiver operating characteristic (ROC) curves for the serum insulin-like growth factor II (IGF-II) investigated marker for hepatocellular carcinoma. Sensitivity, true-positive rate; specificity, false-positive rate. The area under the ROC curves was 0.823 for α-fetoprotein (AFP) and 0.771 for IGF-II [50].

The positive frequency of circulating IGF-II mRNA was 34% in HCC, and no amplified fragment was found in other liver diseases, extrahepatic tumors, and normal controls. The circulating IGF-II mRNA was correlated with the stage of HCC, and its incidence was 100% in HCC with extrahepatic metastasis, and 35% in HCC with AFP-negative. No significant difference was found between tumor sizes and circulating IGF-II mRNA fragment and IGF-II mRNA can only be detected in the peripheral blood of HCC patients. The levels of circulating IGF-II mRNA and its diagnostic value increase with clinical stage of HCC and with distant metastases. Circulating IGF-II mRNA could be a useful molecular marker for HCC diagnosis, especially in monitoring extrahepatic metastases.

However, little is known about the diagnostic value of circulating IGF-II in the early stage of HCC. In the present study, we analyzed the localization and expression of IGF-II during the malignant transformation process in rat hepatic cells by immunohistochemistry, detected the dynamic changes of IGF-II expression in the liver and sera of HCC model rats, and discussed the possibility of circulating IGF-II becoming a marker for early diagnosis of HCC. Hence the abnormal expressions of IGF-II and IGF-II mRNA are useful tumor markers for HCC diagnosis, differentiation of extrahepatic metastasis, and monitoring postoperative recurrence. The pathologic characteristics of circulating IGF-II expression are shown in Table 5. The higher expression of hepatic IGF-II in patients with HCC was associated with HBV infection ($P<0.001$). However, no significant difference was found between IGF-II expression and patient sex, age, tumor size, extrahepatic metastasis, or AFP level ($P > 0.05$) [50, 51].

Group		No. of Cases	Mean ± SD IGF-II (ng/mL)	*t*	*P*
HCC		146	3.74 ± 0.67	—	—
Sex	Male	108	3.73 ± 0.65	0.224	0.823
	Female	38	3.77 ± 0.77		
Age (yr)	≥50	109	3.74 ± 0.64	0.117	0.907
	<50	37	3.75 ± 0.77		
Tumor size (cm)	≥5.0	66	3.77 ± 0.76	0.491	0.624
	<5.0	80	3.71 ± 0.59		
Extrahepatic metastasis	With	38	3.88 ± 0.69	2.013	0.058
	Without	108	3.62 ± 0.67		
α-Fetoprotein (ng/mL)	≥400.0	67	3.83 ± 0.67	1.564	0.120
	<400.0	79	3.66 ± 0.66		
Hepatitis B surface antigen	Positive	110	3.93 ± 0.50	5.390	0.000
	Negative	36	3.16 ± 0.80		

HCC, hepatocellular carcinoma; IGF-II, insulin-like growth factor II. *IGF-II values are given in conventional units; to convert to Système International (SI) units (nMol/L), multiply by 0.131. To convert the conventional units for alpha-fetoprotein to SI units (μg/L), multiply by 1.0.

Table 5. Pathologic Characteristics of Circulating IGF-II Expression in Patients with HCC*

6. Targeting IGF-1R

The IGF signaling axis is comprised of two receptors (IGF-1R and IGF-2R), the ligands IGF-1 and IGF-2, and a system of at least six binding proteins and attendant proteases that modulate ligand availability [52, 53]. Insulin also binds to the IGF-1R, but with 100- to 1000-fold lower affinity than that of the IGFs. The supporting preclinical and clinical data highlighting the significance of this pathway in HCC, and the early clinical trials of targeting this axis in advanced HCC. However, the underlying mechanisms that lead to malignant transformation of infected cells remain unclear. The efficacy profile seems to be promising [54, 55]. However, further studies are needed to define the exact role of IGF-1R inhibitors in clinical practice. IGF-1R with its ligands and intracellular pathway is involved in cell growth and survival control.

Many studies have shown how IGF-1R is over-expressed in HCC cell lines and histological samples [56, 57]. In recent years many trials have been conducted investigating IGF-1R as a possible cancer therapy, with major efforts focusing on the use of monoclonal antibodies and small molecules directed against the IGF-1R-driven pathway. Several drugs are currently under intense investigation and in different experimental phases. Available data suggest that this class of drugs is well tolerated with mild to moderate side effects, when used alone or in combination with other therapeutic agents [58, 59].

It is speculated to serve as an autocrine growth factor in various cancers because they often co-express IGF-II and IGF-IR in hepatocarcinogenesis, and re-expression of IGF-II gene has recently been described in HCC. To date, several therapeutic strategies have been developed in order to specifically inhibit IGF-1R while sparing IR, Phase I/II studies have shown that a monotherapy with this class of drug seems to give stability of disease rather than responses. More recent studies are, in fact, investigating combination of anti-IGF-1R therapy with chemotherapy or other targeted agents, in order to give a wider tumor response through multiple blocking of intracellular pathways or DNA damages. Anti-IGF-1R drugs seem to be a very promising class of targeted agents for cancer therapy, although the real potential of this class of drugs, whether alone or in combination, needs to be further investigated in randomized studies. Another key point on which research should focus is to find a biological marker of potential efficacy of this class of drugs, in order to select which patients should really benefit from this treatment approach [60].

7. Inhibition of IGF-II on effect of HCC cell proliferation

Abnormal expression of IGF-II is associated with the hepatocyte malignant transformation and HCC progress [61-63]. Specific IGF-II miRNA plasmids were constructed and transfected to HepG2 cells to knockdown IGF-II expression for observing effects on the cell proliferation, survival, apoptosis, angiogenesis, and anchorage-independent colony formation [64-66]. IGF-II mRNA was evaluated by quantitative real-time polymerase chain reaction, and the level of IGF-II or VEGF was quantitatively analyzed by ELISA. Our data shown that down-regulation of IGF-II expression resulted in the viability alteration, proliferation inhibition, and apoptosis occurrence of HepG2 cells [67]. The level of VEGF expression in the supernatant of HepG2 cells in the IGF-II-miRNA-transfected group was significantly decreasing ($P<0.01$) than those in the untransfected group or the miRNA-neg-transfected group, with the susceptibility to anoikis and decreasing of anchorage-independent colony formation of HepG2 cells. Thus, concluding that IGF-II is a potential molecular target for HCC gene therapy [68, 69].

HepG2 cells transfected with four recombinant targeting IGF-II plasmids: pCMV-IGF-II-miR-1, pCMV-IGF-II-miR-2, pCMV-IGF-II-miR-3, and pCMV- IGF-II-miR-4, containing green fluorescent protein, are shown in Figure 7. After the HepG2 cells transfected with a high efficiency at 24 h (Figure 7a, b), the alterations of IGF-II gene expression at transcriptional level showed the four different silencing efficiencies, and one of the best plasmids was the pCMVIGF-II-miR-2. After the HepG2 cells were transfected with the pCMV-IGF-II-miR-2, the expression of IGF-II gene at transcriptional level at 48 h was significantly inhibited (down to 15 %, $P < 0.001$, Figure 7c), and the same interference effects ($P < 0.001$) were observed at protein level (Figure 7d), with the IGF-II protein down to 25 % compared with the miR-neg group, indicating that the highly specific and efficient miRNA could suppress the activation of IGF-II expression in hepatoma cells at transcriptional or protein level.

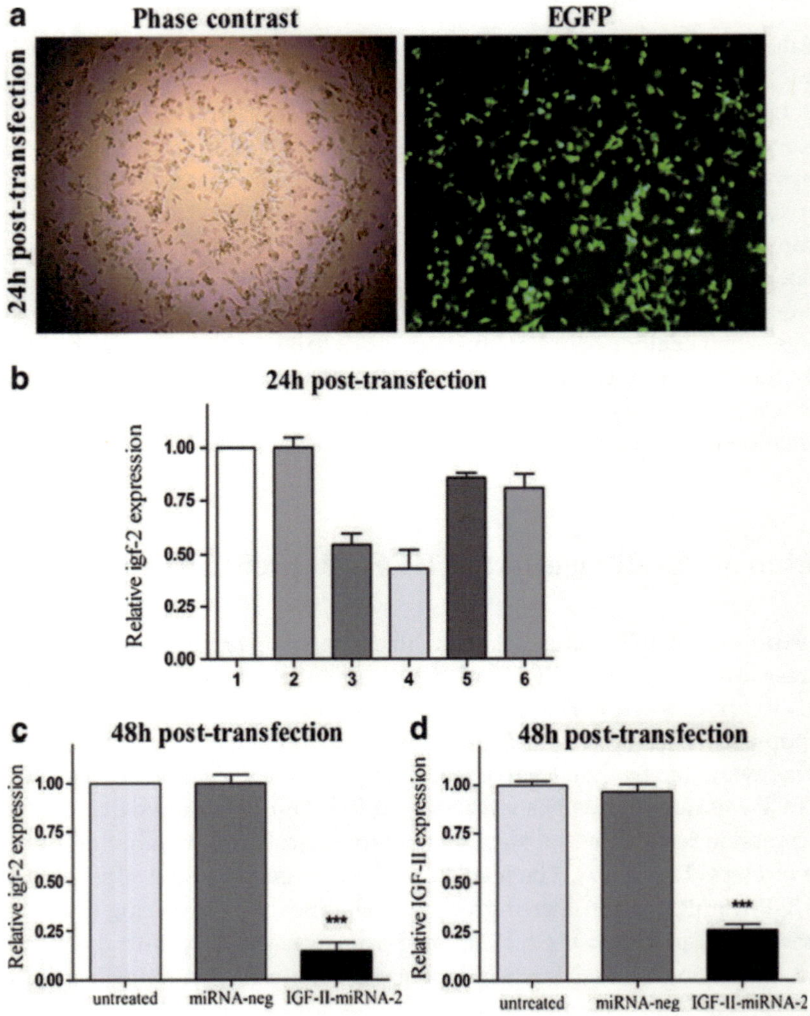

Figure 7. Suppression of IGF-II activation in HepG2 cells with different miRNAs. [67] HepG2 cells were transfected according to the preoptimized instructions. At 24 or 48 h after the HepG2 cells transfected with different IGF-II miRNAs, the cells were then harvested and checked. a The phase contrast and fluorescence photomicrographs (100× magnification) of the HepG2 cells transfected with different constructed pCMV-IGF-II-miR plasmid vectors containing green fluorescent protein at 24 h. b Analysis of IGF-II gene at transcriptional level in the HepG2 cells transfected with different pCMV-miR at 24 h. Lanes 1 the untreated HepG2 cells, 2 the HepG2 cells with IGF-II-miR-neg, 3 the HepG2 cells with IGF-II-miR-1, 4 the HepG2 cells with IGF-II-miR-2, 5 the HepG2 cells with IGF-II-miR-3, 6 the HepG2 cells with IGF-II-miR-4. c IGF-II gene transcriptional level at 48 h after the HepG2 cells were transfected with IGF-II-miR-2; d IGF-II protein level at 48 h after the HepG2 cells were transfected with IGF-II-miR-2 by ELISA. Data were expressed as mean ± SD from three independent experiments. ***$P<0.001$ vs. the IGF-II-miR-neg group.

The viability inhibition after the HepG2 cells transfected with miRNA determined by a trypan blue exclusion assay is shown in Figure 8. Compared with the control (miR-neg) group, the viability of the HepG2 cells transfected with IGF-II-miR-2 (Figure 8a) was notably inhibited at a time-dependent manner. The rapid growth of the HepG2 cells leads to insufficient blood supply, and solid cancer cells should evolve to tolerate nutrition starvation. The effect of IGF-II on the death of serum-deprived HepG2 cells was also evaluated by trypan blue staining. Compared with the miR-neg group, the IGF-II-miR-2-transfected group displayed higher death rates for both 48 h (31.3 % vs. 17.3 %, $P < 0.01$) and 72 h (68.7 % vs. 36.7 %, $P < 0.001$) after serum starvation (Figure 8b), whereas the miR-neg group showed a similar frequency of death as untreated group, indicating that highly IGF-II expression might increases the growth and survival of HepG2 cells *in vitro* [67]

The downregulation of IGF-II expression, which inhibited the proliferation of HepG2 cells by apoptosis mechanism, is shown in Figure 7c. The proliferation and apoptosis of the HepG2 cells were analyzed by EdU incorporation assay based on the measurement of DNA synthesis regarded as a gold standard for measuring the cell proliferation. Under common culture conditions (10 % FBS), the EdU incorporation assay displayed that DNA synthesis of the cells was significantly inhibited in the IGF-II-miR-2-transfected group as compared with the miR-neg-transfected group (P <0.01; Figure 7c, d). Furthermore, the analysis of apoptosis revealed that the amount of apoptosis in the IGF-II-miR-2-transfected HepG2 group is increased as compared with the control group ($P < 0.01$; Figure 8c, e), indicating that downregulation of IGF-II expression might inhibit HepG2 cell proliferation. [67]

IGF-II is involved in the process of HCC development and has exhibited numerous genetic abnormalities as well as epigenetic alterations including modulation of DNA methylation. Targeted therapy to the IGF system is being studied in combination with chemotherapy as demonstrated by the phase II study. Other combination strategies are also being employed in breast cancer, given the important links between the ER and the IGF-IR pathway that have been discovered in experimental models. Constitutive activation of the IGF-signaling axis is frequently observed in human HCC. Especially the overexpression of the fetal growth factor IGF-II, IGF-IR, and cytoplasmic downstream effectors such as IRS contribute to proliferation, anti-apoptosis, and invasive behavior [70, 71].

8. Perspectives

The IGF system is emerging as a promising new target in cancer therapy and promises to revolutionize the way we select therapies in combination with chemotherapy, endocrine therapy, and other biological agents. The relevant alterations in this signaling pathway and independent in vivo models that support the central role IGF-II signaling during HCC development and progression. Since this pathway has become the center of interest as a target for potential anti-cancer therapy in many types of malignancies, various experimental strategies have been developed, including neutralizing antibodies and selective receptor kinase inhibitors, with respect to the specific and efficient reduction of oncogenic IGF-II/IGF-

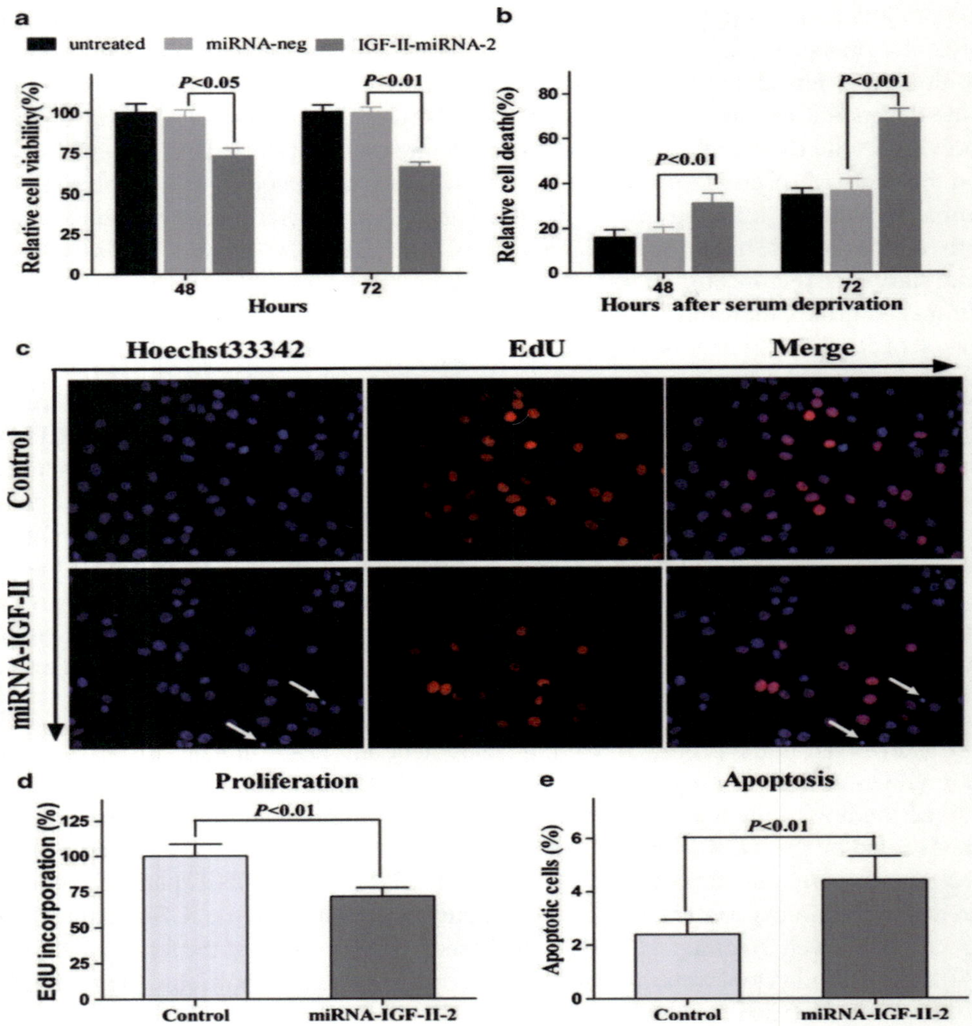

Figure 8. Silencing IGF-II expression on effect of HepG2 cell growth and survival. a The downregulation of IGF-II expression inhibition of HepG2 cell viability. At 48 h after transfection, the HepG2 cells were plated into 6-well plates (50×10^4 cells per plate). After 48 and 72 h, cell viability was assayed with a trypan blue assay; b Suppression of IGF-II inhibits HepG2 cells survival. After transfection at 48 h, HepG2 cells were plated into 6-well plates (50×10^4 cells per plate). After 4 h, the adherent cells were switched to serum-free medium and harvested for the trypan blue staining at different time points (48 or 72 h); then the trypan blue positive cells were counted and calculated as percent of total cell number. Data represented the mean ± SD from three independent experiments. c After the HepG2 cells (200×) transfected with miRNA were stained with the EdU incorporation and Hoechest 33342. At 48 h, the cells were plated in 96-well plates (2.0×103 cells per well) in triplicate for other 24 h, then exposed to EdU for 2 h, and visualized under a fluorescence microscopy. EdU (red), DNA synthesis; Hoechst 33342 (blue), nuclear staining; Apoptotic cells (white arrows) showed shrunken nuclei with a bright fluorescence appearance. d Quantitative analysis of the EdU incorporation assay. Data are represented from three independent experiments; e quantification of apoptotic events (white arrows) as determined in Figure 7c. The number of cells with nuclear morphological features of apoptosis was counted after staining with Hoechest 33342. Data are expressed as percentage of apoptotic cells based on counting 100 cells in randomly selected fields. Data are from three separate experiments, and mean values ± SD, from three independent experiments [67]

IR-signaling[72, 73]. Several laboratories have implicated constitutive activation of miRNA as one of the early key events involving in neoplastic progression of the liver. Further studies will permit us to analyze mechanism of human hepatocarcinogenesis and pay attention to these areas to be more practical up to present [74, 75].

Acknowledgements

This work was supported by the Projects of Jiangsu Medical Science (HK201102 and BL2012053), the Priority Academic Program Development of Jiangsu Higher Education Institution, the Program of Nantong Society Undertaking and Technological Innovation (HS2011012, HS2012039), and the Grant from International Science & Technology Cooperation Program (No.2013DFA32150), China.

Author details

Min Yao, Li Wang, Meijuan Yan, Xiaodi Yan and Dengfu Yao*

*Address all correspondence to: Yaodf@ahnmc.com

Research Center of Clinical Medicine, Affiliated Hospital, Departments of Immunology and Informatics, School of Medicine; Nantong University, Nantong, China

References

[1] Yang JD, Roberts LR. Hepatocellular carcinoma: a global view. Nat Rev Gastroenterol Hepatol, 2010; 7: 449-58 [PMID: 20628345]

[2] El-Serag HB, Marrero JA, Rudolph L, Reddy KR. Diagnosis and treatment of hepatocellular carcinoma. Gastroenterol, 2008; 134: 1752-63 [PMID: 18471552]

[3] Yao DF, Huang ZW, Chen SZ, Huang JF, Lu JX, Xiao MB, Meng XY. Diagnosis of hepatocellular carcinoma by quantitative detection of hepatoma-specific bands of serum gamma-glutamyltransferase. Am J Clin Pathol. 1998; 110: 743-9 [PMID: 9844586]

[4] Ito S, Yao DF, Nii C, Horie T, Kamamura M, Nishikado T, Honda H, Shibata H, Shimizu I, Meng XY. Incidence of hepatitis C virus (HCV) antibodies and HCV- RNA in blood donors and patients with liver diseases in the inshore area of the Yangtze River. J Gastroenterol Hepatol. 1994; 9: 245-9. [PMID: 7519896]

[5] Ito S, Yao DF, Nii C, Hibino S, Kamamura M, Nisikado T, Honda H, Shimizu I, Meng XY. Epidemiological characteristics of the incidence of hepatitis C virus (C100-3) anti-

bodies in patients with liver diseases in the inshore area of the Yangtze River. J Gastroenterol Hepatol. 1993; 8: 232-7. [PMID: 7686055]

[6] El-Serag HB. Epidemiology of viral hepatitis and hepatocellular carcinoma. Gastroenterology. 2012; 142: 1264-73 [PMID: 22537432]

[7] Aravalli RN, Steer CJ, Cressman EN. Molecular mechanisms of hepatocellular carcinoma. Hepatology 2008; 48: 2047-63 [PMID: 19003900]

[8] Ubagai T, Kikuchi T, Fukusato T, Ono Y. Aflatoxin B1 modulates the insulin-like growth factor-2 dependent signaling axis. Toxicol In Vitro. 2010; 24: 783-9. [PMID: 20036727]

[9] Jain S, Singhal S, Lee P, Xu R. Molecular genetics of hepatocellular neoplasia. Am J Transl Res, 2010; 2: 105-18 [PMID: 20182587]

[10] Morisawa T, Marusawa H, Ueda Y, Iwai A, Okazaki IM, Honjo T, Chiba T. Organ-specific profiles of genetic changes in cancers caused by activation-induced cytidine deaminase expression. Int J Cancer. 2008; 123: 2735-40 [PMID: 18781563]

[11] Couvert P, Carrié A, Pariès J, Vaysse J, Miroglio A, Kerjean A, Nahon P, Chelly J, Trinchet JC, Beaugrand M, Ganne-Carrié N. Liver insulin-like growth factor 2 methylation in hepatitis C virus cirrhosis and further occurrence of hepatocellular carcinoma. World J Gastroenterol. 2008; 14: 5419-27 [PMID: 18803353]

[12] Yao DF, Dong ZZ, Yao M. Specific molecular markers in hepatocellular carcinoma. Hepatobiliary Pancreat Dis Int. 2007; 6: 241-7 [PMID: 17548245]

[13] Kim DG. Differentially expressed genes associated with hepatitis B virus HBx and MHBs protein function in hepatocellular carcinoma. Methods Mol Biol. 2006; 317: 141-55[PMID: 16264227]

[14] Effendi K, Sakamoto M. Molecular pathology in early hepatocarcinogenesis. Oncology. 2010; 78: 157-60 [PMID: 20389138]

[15] Hoshida Y. Molecular signatures and prognosis of hepatocellular carcinoma. Minerva Gastroenterol Dietol. 2011; 57: 311-22 [PMID:21769080]

[16] Breuhahn K, Schirmacher P. Reactivation of the insulin-like growth factor- signaling pathway in human hepatocellular carcinoma. World J Gastroenterol, 2008, 14: 1690-8 [PMID: 21074736]

[17] Scharf JG, Dombrowski F, Ramadori G. The IGF axis and hepatocarcinogenesis. Mol Pathol 2001; 54: 138-44 [PMID: 11376124]

[18] Nussbaum T, Samarin J, Ehemann V, Bissinger M, Ryschich E, Khamidjanov A, Yu X, Gretz N, Schirmacher P, Breuhahn K. Autocrine insulin-like growth factor-II stimulation of tumor cell migration is a progression step in human hepato- carcinogenesis. Hepatology. 2008; 48: 146-56 [PMID: 18537183]

[19] Scharf JG, Braulke T. The role of the IGF axis in hepatocarcinogenesis. Horm Metab Res. 2003; 35: 685-93 [PMID: 14710347]

[20] Tovar V, Alsinet C, Villanueva A, Hoshida Y, Chiang DY, Solé M, Thung S, Moyano S, Toffanin S, Mínguez B, Cabellos L, Peix J, Schwartz M, Mazzaferro V, Bruix J, Llovet JM. IGF activation in a molecular subclass of hepatocellular carcinoma and preclinical efficacy of IGF-1R blockage. J Hepatol. 2010; 52: 550- 9 [PMID: 20206398]

[21] Chen YW, Boyartchuk V, Lewis BC. Differential roles of insulin-like growth factor receptor- and insulin receptor-mediated signaling in the phenotypes of hepato- cellular carcinoma cells. Neoplasia. 2009; 11: 835-45 [PMID: 19724677]

[22] Breuhahn K, Schirmacher P. Reactivation of the insulin-like growth factor-II signaling pathway in human hepatocellular carcinoma. World J Gastroenterol. 2008 21; 14: 1690-8 [PMID: 18350600]

[23] Jeng YM, Chang CC, Hu FC, Chou HY, Kao HL, Wang TH, Hsu HC. RNA- binding protein insulin-like growth factor II mRNA-binding protein 3 expression promotes tumor invasion and predicts early recurrence and poor prognosis in hepatocellular carcinoma. Hepatology. 2008; 48: 1118-27 [PMID: 18802962]

[24] Cantarini MC, de la Monte SM, Pang M, Tong M, D'Errico A, Trevisani F, Wands JR. Aspartyl-asparagyl beta hydroxylase over-expression in human hepatoma is linked to activation of insulin-like growth factor and notch signaling mechanisms. Hepatology. 2006; 44: 446-57 [PMID: 16871543]

[25] Mukherjee B, Ghosh S, Das T, Doloi M. Characterization of insulin-like- growth factor II (IGF II) mRNA positive hepatic altered foci and IGF II expression in hepatocellular carcinoma during diethylnitrosamine-induced hepatocarcinogenesis in rats. J Carcinog. 2005; 4: 12 [PMID: 16092956]

[26] Breuhahn K, Vreden S, Haddad R, Beckebaum S, Stippel D, Flemming P, Nussbaum T, Caselmann WH, Haab BB, Schirmacher P. Molecular profiling of human hepatocellular carcinoma defines mutually exclusive interferon regulation and insulin-like growth factor II overexpression. Cancer Res. 2004; 64: 6058-64 [PMID: 15342387]

[27] Alexia C, Fallot G, Lasfer M, Schweizer-Groyer G, Groyer A. An evaluation of the role of insulin-like growth factors (IGF) and of type-I IGF receptor signalling in hepatocarcinogenesis and in the resistance of hepatocarcinoma cells against drug- induced apoptosis. Biochem Pharmacol. 2004; 68: 1003-15 [PMID: 15313394]

[28] Qiu LW, Yao DF, Zong L, Lu YY, Huang H, Wu W, Wu XH. Abnormal expression of insulin-like growth factor-II and its dynamic quantitative analysis at different stages of hepatocellular carcinoma development. Hepatobiliary Pancreat Dis Int. 2008; 7: 406-11 [PMID: 18693177]

[29] Himoto T, Kuriyama S, Zhang JY, Chan EK, Nishioka M, Tan EM. Significance of autoantibodies against insulin-like growth factor II mRNA-binding proteins in patients with hepatocellular carcinoma. Int J Oncol. 2005; 26: 311-7 [PMID: 15645114]

[30] Wang Z, Ruan YB, Guan Y, Liu SH. Expression of IGF-II in early experimental hepatocellular carcinomas and its significance in early diagnosis. World J Gastroenterol 2003; 9: 267-70 [PMID: 12532445]

[31] Esteller M. Cancer epigenomics: DNA methylomes and histone-modification maps. Nat Rev Genet, 2007, 8: 286–98 [PMID:17339880]

[32] Wu J, Qin Y, Li B, He WZ, Sun ZL. Hypomethylated and hypermethylated profiles of H19DMR are associated with the aberrant imprinting of IGF2 and H19 in human hepatocellular carcinoma. Genomics. 2008; 91: 443-50 [PMID: 18358696]

[33] Tang SH, Yang DH, Huang W, Zhou HK, Lu XH, Ye G. Hypomethylated P4 promoter induces expression of the insulin-like growth factor-II gene in hepato- cellular carcinoma in a Chinese population. Clin Cancer Res. 2006; 12: 4171-7 [PMID: 16857788]

[34] Tang SH, Yang DH, Huang W, Zhou M, Zhou HK, Lu XH, Ye G. Differential promoter usage for insulin-like growth factor-II gene in Chinese hepatocellular carcinoma with hepatitis B virus infection. Cancer Detect Prev. 2006; 30: 192-203 [PMID: 16697535]

[35] Poirier K, Chalas C, Tissier F, Couvert P, Mallet V, Carrié A, Marchio A, Sarli D, Gicquel C, Chaussade S, Beljord C, Chelly J, Kerjean A, Terris B. Loss of parental-specific methylation at the IGF2 locus in human hepatocellular carcinoma. J Pathol. 2003; 201: 473-9 [PMID: 14595760]

[36] Couvert P, Carrié A, Pariès J, Vaysse J, Miroglio A, Kerjean A, Nahon P, Chelly J, Trinchet JC, Beaugrand M, Ganne-Carrié N. Liver insulin-like growth factor 2 methylation in hepatitis C virus cirrhosis and further occurrence of hepatocellular carcinoma. World J Gastroenterol. 2008; 14: 5419-27 [PMID: 18803353]

[37] Yao X, Hu JF, Daniels M, Shiran H, Zhou X, Yan H, Lu H, Zeng Z, Wang Q, Li T, Hoffman AR. A methylated oligonucleotide inhibits IGF2 expression and enhances survival in a model of hepatocellular carcinoma. J Clin Invest. 2003; 111: 265-73 [PMID: 12531883]

[38] Dong ZZ, Yao DF, Wu XH, Shi GS, Qiu LW, Wu W, Su XQ. Early diagnostic value of abnormal expression of insulin-like growth factor (IGF)-II and IGF-II- mRNA in hepatocellular carcinoma patients. Zhonghua Gan Zang Bing Za Zhi. 2005; 13: 866-8. Chinese[PMID: 16313745]

[39] Mukherjee B, Ghosh S, Das T, Doloi M. Characterization of insulin-like-growth factor II (IGF II) mRNA positive hepatic altered foci and IGF II expression in hepatocellular carcinoma during diethylnitrosamine-induced hepatocarcinogenesis in rats. J Carcinog. 2005; 4: 12 [PMID: 16092956], 4, 12.

[40] Lee SH, Chung YH, Kim JA, Lee D, Jin YJ, Shim JH, Jang MK, Cho EY, Shin ES, Lee JE, Park NH, Yu E, Lee YJ. Single nucleotide polymorphisms associated with metastatic tumour antigen 1 overexpression in patients with hepatocellular carcinoma. Liver Int. 2012; 32: 457-66. [PMID: 22098246]

[41] Tang SH, Yang DH, Huang W, Zhou M, Zhou HK, Lu XH, Ye G. Differential promoter usage for insulin-like growth factor-II gene in Chinese hepatocellular carcinoma with hepatitis B virus infection. Cancer Detect Prev. 2006; 30: 192-203. [PMID: 16697535]

[42] Kim DG.Differentially expressed genes associated with hepatitis B virus HBx and MHBs protein function in hepatocellular carcinoma. Methods Mol Biol. 2006; 317: 141-55. [PMID: 16264227]

[43] Kew MC. Hepatitis B virus x protein in the pathogenesis of hepatitis B virus- induced hepatocellular carcinoma. J Gastroenterol Hepatol. 2011; 26 Suppl 1: 144- 52. [PMID: 21199526]

[44] Ahmad W, Shabbiri K, Ijaz B, Asad S, Nazar N, Nazar S, Fouzia K, Kausar H, Gull S, Sarwar MT, Shahid I, Hassan S. Serine 204 phosphorylation and O-β-GlcNAC interplay of IGFBP-6 as therapeutic indicator to regulate IGF-II functions in viral mediated hepatocellular carcinoma.Virol J. 2011; 8: 208. [PMID: 21548981], 8, 208.

[45] Kim YJ, Yoon JH, Kim CY, Kim LH, Park BL, Shin HD, Lee HS. IGF2 polymorphisms are associated with hepatitis B virus clearance and hepatocellular carcinoma. Biochem Biophys Res Commun. 2006; 346: 38-44 [PMID: 16750516]

[46] Otsuka M, Aizaki H, Kato N, Suzuki T, Miyamura T, Omata M, Seki N. Differential cellular gene expression induced by hepatitis B and C viruses.Biochem Biophys Res Commun. 2003; 300: 443-7.[PMID:12504104]

[47] Lee S, Park U, Lee YI. Hepatitis C virus core protein transactivates insulin-like growth factor II gene transcription through acting concurrently on Egr1 and Sp1 sites. Virology. 2001; 283: 167-77. [PMID: 11336542]

[48] Yao DF, Dong ZZ, Liu YH, Zhao L, Huang JF, Meng XY. Amplification of peripheral blood insulin-like growth factor II-mRNA and its clinical significance in the diagnosis of hepatocellular carcinoma. Zhonghua Gan Zang Bing Za Zhi. 2003; 11: 695-6. Chinese [PMID: 14636457]

[49] Dong ZZ, Yao DF, Yao DB, Wu XH, Wu W, Qiu LW, Jiang DR, Zhu JH, Meng XY. Expression and alteration of insulin-like growth factor II-messenger RNA in hepatoma tissues and peripheral blood of patients with hepatocellular carcinoma. World J Gastroenterol. 2005; 11(30): 4655-60 [PMID: 16094705]

[50] Qian J, Yao D, Dong Z, Wu W, Qiu L, Yao N, Li S, Bian Y, Wang Z, Shi G. Characteristics of hepatic igf-ii expression and monitored levels of circulating igf-ii mRNA in

metastasis of hepatocellular carcinoma. Am J Clin Pathol. 2010; 134: 799-806 [PMID: 20959664]

[51] Wachter DL, Kristiansen G, Soll C, Hellerbrand C, Breuhahn K, Fritzsche F, Agaimy A, Hartmann A, Riener MO. Insulin-like growth factor II mRNA-binding protein 3 (IMP3) expression in hepatocellular carcinoma. A clinicopathological analysis with emphasis on diagnostic value. Histopathology. 2012; 60: 278-86 [PMID: 22211286]

[52] Zhao H, Desai V, Wang J, Epstein DM, Miglarese M, Buck E. Epithelial- mesenchymal transition predicts sensitivity to the dual IGF-1R/IR inhibitor OSI-906 in hepatocellular carcinoma cell lines. Mol Cancer Ther. 2012; 11: 503-13 [PMID: 22161861]

[53] Bodzin AS, Wei Z, Hurtt R, Gu T, Doria C. Gefitinib resistance in HCC mahlavu cells: upregulation of CD133 expression, activation of IGF-1R signaling pathway, and enhancement of IGF-1R nuclear translocation. J Cell Physiol. 2012; 227: 2947-52 [PMID: 21959795]

[54] Yao WF, Liu JW, Sheng GL, Huang DS. Blockade of IGF-IR exerts anticancer effects in hepatocellular carcinoma. Mol Med Report. 2011; 4: 719-22 [PMID: 21567089]

[55] Aleem E, Nehrbass D, Klimek F, Mayer D, Bannasch P. Upregulation of the insulin receptor and type I insulin-like growth factor receptor are early events in hepatocarcinogenesis. Toxicol Pathol. 2011; 39: 524-43 [PMID: 21411721]

[56] Zeng C, Wang R, Li D, Lin XJ, Wei QK, Yuan Y, Wang Q, Chen W, Zhuang SM. A novel GSK-3 beta-C/EBP alpha-miR-122-insulin-like growth factor 1 receptor regulatory circuitry in human hepatocellular carcinoma. Hepatology. 2010; 52: 1702-12 [PMID: 21038412]

[57] Weng CJ, Hsieh YH, Tsai CM, Chu YH, Ueng KC, Liu YF, Yeh YH, Su SC, Chen YC, Chen MK, Yang SF. Relationship of insulin-like growth factors system gene polymorphisms with the susceptibility and pathological development of hepatocellular carcinoma. Ann Surg Oncol. 2010; 17: 1808-15[PMID: 20119675]

[58] Huynh H, Ngo VC, Koong HN, Poon D, Choo SP, Toh HC, Thng CH, Chow P, Ong HS, Chung A, Goh BC, Smith PD, Soo KC. AZD6244 enhances the anti-tumor activity of sorafenib in ectopic and orthotopic models of human hepatocellular carcinoma (HCC). J Hepatol. 2010; 52: 79-87 [PMID: 19910069]

[59] Desbois-Mouthon C, Baron A, Blivet-Van Eggelpoël MJ, Fartoux L, Venot C, Bladt F, Housset C, Rosmorduc O. Insulin-like growth factor-1 receptor inhibition induces a resistance mechanism via the epidermal growth factor receptor/HER3/ AKT signaling pathway: rational basis for cotargeting insulin-like growth factor-1 receptor and epidermal growth factor receptor in hepatocellular carcinoma. Clin Cancer Res. 2009; 15: 5445-56 [PMID: 19706799]

[60] Freise C, Ruehl M, Erben U, Neumann U, Seehofer D, Kim KY, Trowitzsch- Kienast W, Stroh T, Zeitz M, Somasundaram R. A hepatoprotective Lindera obtusiloba extract suppresses growth and attenuates insulin like growth factor-1 receptor signal-

ing and NF-kappaB activity in human liver cancer cell lines. BMC Complement Altern Med. 2011; 11: 39 [PMID: 21569410], 11, 39.

[61] Ranke MB, Maier KP, Schweizer R, Stadler B, Schleicher S, Elmlinger MW, Flehmig B. Pilot study of elevated levels of insulin-like growth factor-binding protein-2 as indicators of hepatocellular carcinoma. Horm Res. 2003; 60: 174-80 [PMID: 14530605]

[62] Cheng W, Tseng CJ, Lin TT, Cheng I, Pan HW, Hsu HC, Lee YM. Glypican-3 -mediated oncogenesis involves the insulin-like growth factor- signaling pathway. Carcinogenesis. 2008; 29: 1319-26 [PMID: 18413366]

[63] Iizuka N, Oka M, Tamesa T, Hamamoto Y, Yamada-Okabe H. Imbalance in expression levels of insulin-like growth factor 2 and H19 transcripts linked to progression of hepatocellular carcinoma. Anticancer Res. 2004; 24: 4085-9 [PMID: 15736456]

[64] Nussbaum T, Samarin J, Ehemann V, Bissinger M, Ryschich E, Khamidjanov A, Yu X, Gretz N, Schirmacher P, Breuhahn K. Autocrine insulin-like growth factor-II stimulation of tumor cell migration is a progression step in human hepato- carcinogenesis. Hepatology. 2008; 48: 146-56 [PMID: 18537183]

[65] Lund P, Schubert D, Niketeghad F, Schirmacher P. Autocrine inhibition of chemotherapy response in human liver tumor cells by insulin-like growth factor-II. Cancer Lett. 2004; 206: 85-96 [PMID: 15019164]

[66] Alexia C, Lasfer M, Groyer A. Role of constitutively activated and insulin-like growth factor-stimulated ERK1/2 signaling in human hepatoma cell proliferation and apoptosis: evidence for heterogeneity of tumor cell lines. Ann N Y Acad Sci. 2004; 1030: 219-29 [PMID: 15659801]

[67] Yao N, Yao D, Wang L, Dong Z, Wu W, Qiu L, Yan X, Yu D, Chen J, Sai W, Zhang H, Yang J. Inhibition of autocrine IGF-II on effect of human HepG2 cell proliferation and angiogenesis factor expression.Tumour Biol. 2012; 33: 1767-76. [PMID: 22684773]

[68] Rehem RN, El-Shikh WM. Serum IGF-1, IGF-2 and IGFBP-3 as parameters in the assessment of liver dysfunction in patients with hepatic cirrhosis and in the diagnosis of hepatocellular carcinoma. Hepatogastroenterology 2011; 58: 949-54 [PMID: 21830422]

[69] Gish RG, Lencioni R, Di Bisceglie AM, Raoul JL, Mazzaferro V. Role of the multi-disciplinary team in the diagnosis and treatment of hepatocellular carcinoma. Expert Rev Gastroenterol Hepatol. 2012; 6: 173-85 [PMID: 22375523]

[70] Tanaka S, Arii S. Molecularly targeted therapy for hepatocellular carcinoma. Cancer Sci. 2009; 100: 1-8[PMID: 19038007]

[71] Faivre S, Bouattour M, Raymond E. Novel molecular therapies in hepatocellular carcinoma. Liver Int. 2011; 31: 151-60 [PMID: 21205154]

[72] Li D, Liu X, Lin L, Hou J, Li N, Wang C, Wang P, Zhang Q, Zhang P, Zhou W, Wang Z, Ding G, Zhuang SM, Zheng L, Tao W, Cao X. MicroRNA-99a inhibits hepatocellu-

lar carcinoma growth and correlates with prognosis of patients with hepatocellular carcinoma. J Biol Chem. 2011; 286: 36677-85 [PMID: 21878637]

[73] Augello C, Vaira V, Caruso L, Destro A, Maggioni M, Park YN, Montorsi M, Santambrogio R, Roncalli M, Bosari S. MicroRNA profiling of hepatocarcino- genesis identifies C19MC cluster as a novel prognostic biomarker in hepato- cellular carcinoma. Liver Int. 2012; 32: 772-82 [PMID: 22429613]

[74] Wu J, Zhu AX. Targeting insulin-like growth factor axis in hepatocellular carcinoma. J Hematol Oncol. 2011; 4: 30 [PMID: 21729319], 4, 30.

[75] Wong VW, Chan HL. Prevention of hepatocellular carcinoma: a concise review of contemporary issues. Ann Hepatol, 2012; 11: 284-93[PMID: 22481445]

Chapter 14

Simultaneous Changes in Expression of Bile Canalicular CD10 and Sinusoidal CD105 (Endoglin) in Chronic Hepatitis and Liver Cirrhosis

Toshitsugu Nakamura

Additional information is available at the end of the chapter

http://dx.doi.org/10.5772/56734

1. Introduction

Liver tissue contains hepatic sinusoids and bile canaliculi among hepatocyte plates. Dynamic changes of these components during a sequence of chronic hepatitis (CH) to liver cirrhosis (LC) have been an interesting subject from a standpoint of cellular injury and regeneration. It is known that proliferative activity of hepatocytes is significantly correlated with the severity of CH [1-3]. On the other hand, the dynamic changes of proliferative sinusoidal cells have been analyzed in experimental liver injury [4,5], but not enough in human cases of CH/LC in relation to inflammatory activity or fibrosis stage. Similarly, bile canalicular changes in CH/LC have not been analyzed until recently, because the bile canaliculi are difficult to recognize morphologically.

Recent identification of markers for bile canaliculi or hepatic sinusoids facilitated the analysis of phenotypic changes in these components in CH/LC. Some markers for bile canaliculi, such as CD10, CD13 and biliary glycoprotein I, are known at present [6,7]. CD10, also called common acute lymphoblastic lymphoma antigen (CALLA) or neprilysin, is a 100kD type II cell-surface metalloproteinase [8] and modulates the enkephalin-mediated inflammatory response [9]. It is expressed in various tissues, including brush border of enterocytes, renal tubules/glomeruli, endometrial stroma, hepatic bile canaliculi and lymphoid precursor cells [10]. It is also a useful marker for neoplastic counterpart of these tissues such as some lymphoma/leukemia [11], renal cell carcinoma, endometrial stromal sarcoma [12] and hepatocellular carcinoma (HCC) [6,7,13,14]. However, changes of expression pattern of CD10 in bile canaliculi (CD10(BC)) during a sequence of CH/LC have not been examined except for a report by Shousha *et al.* [15]

CD105, also known as endoglin, is an 180kD homodimeric transmembrane glycoprotein forming part of transforming growth factor-β (TGF-β) receptor complex [16,17]. It is expressed with marked tissue-specificity, predominantly in vascular endothelial cells of tissues undergoing active angiogenesis such as regenerating or inflamed tissue and tumoral stroma [18,19]. In particular, its expression in the stromal vessels of various carcinomas is associated with unfavorable prognosis [19-22]. Thus, CD105 has been attracted considerable attention, not only as a biological marker of tumor growth but also as a target molecule for diagnostic and therapeutic application against cancer [23,24]. On the other hand, CD105 expression has also been examined in the active/proliferative vessels of stromal tissues other than carcinomas, such as hemorrhoids [25], inflammation and wound healing [26,27], endometrial tissue throughout the menstrual cycle [28], or CH/LC [29-32]. Although expression of CD105 along hepatic sinusoids (CD105(HS)) in CH/LC has been reported [29-32], a correlation between CD10 and CD105 expression has not been examined so far. We previously reported changes in expression of CD10 and CD105 in the hepatic tissue around tumors including HCC and metastatic carcinoma [33]. In the present study, we analyzed CH/LC in the same way as in the previous report.

2. Materials and methods

2.1. Tissue samples

Fifty-two cases of surgically resected liver specimens were retrieved from a pathological database file at Suwa Red Cross Hospital (Suwa, Japan). The cases showing fatty metamorphosis or treated before operation by trans-arterial embolization or radiofrequency ablation for tumors were excluded. The resected livers had HCC with CH or LC (40 cases, consisted of 26 cases of type C, 4 of type B and 10 of non-B/non-C type), metastatic carcinoma (11 cases; 8 for colorectal origin and 1 for breast, stomach and Vater's papilla origin in each) and biliary cystadenoma (1 case). None of the cases of metastatic carcinoma and cystadenoma showed features of CH/LC clinically or histopathologically. All specimens had been fixed in 10% phosphate-buffered formalin immediately after resection and embedded in paraffin. In each case, representative paraffin blocks of the background hepatic tissue of tumors were selected and serial tissue sections were subjected to Azan-Mallory and immunohistochemical stainings. The sections contained part of the tumor nodule in 46 cases.

2.2. Evaluation of chronic hepatitis/cirrhosis

The inflammatory activity (A) and fibrosis stage (F) of CH/LC were evaluated by histological observation of sections with hematoxylin-eosin and Azan-Mallory stainings according to the new Inuyama Classification of Japan [34], which well corresponds to the International Classification of chronic hepatitis [35]. The inflammatory activity was classified as A0 (no inflammation or necrosis), A1 (mild), A2 (moderate) and A3 (severe), and the fibrosis stage as F0 (no fibrosis), F1 (fibrous extension of Glisson's sheathes), F2 (bridging fibrosis), F3 (distorted bridging fibrosis or pre-cirrhotic state) and F4 (LC). The background hepatic tissues apart enough from the tumor nodule in the cases of metastatic carcinoma or cystadenoma were used as controls.

2.3. Immunohistochemistry and evaluation of staining

The tissue sections were stained immunohistochemically using the streptavidin-biotin-peroxidase method. Endogenous peroxidase activity in the sections was eliminated in 0.3% hydrogen peroxide in methanol for 30 min. Thereafter, the sections were treated with 0.2% trypsin for 40min. at 37 degrees C (for CD105) or were submerged in 0.01mol/l citrate buffer (pH6.0) and boiled for 15 minutes in a microwave oven (for CD10) to retrieve the antigenecity [36]. After cooling to room temperature, these sections were incubated with monoclonal antibodies against CD10 (clone 56C6, Medical & Biological Laboratories, Nagoya, Japan, 1:50 dilution) and CD105 (clone SN6h, Dako, Glostrup, Denmark, 1:5 dilution), followed by biotinylated antibody against mouse immunoglobulin (Dako, 1:50 dilution), and finally reacted with peroxidase-conjugated streptavidin (Dako). The labeled peroxidase was visualized by 3,3′-diaminobenzidine-hydrogen peroxide method and counterstained by hematoxylin. Negative control sections for immunostaining were treated with phosphate-buffered saline instead of the primary antibodies and were confirmed to be unstained.

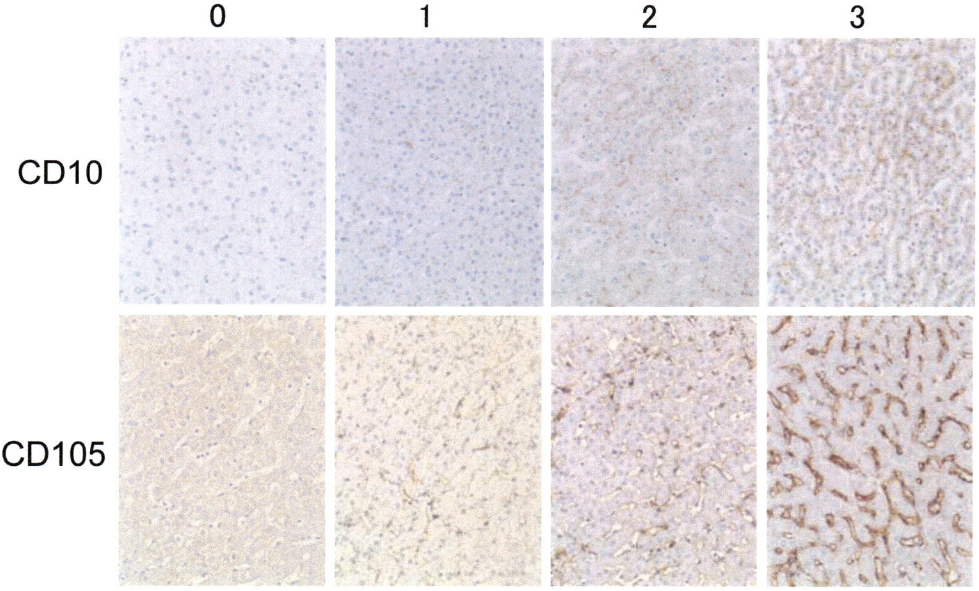

Figure 1. Representative features of CD10 score in bile canaliculi and CD105 score along hepativ sinusoids in lobular areas.

A scoring system was introduced for evaluation of expression of CD10 or CD105 in the background hepatic tissue, apart more than 5mm. from the tumor nodule. The intensity of CD10- or CD105-reactivity in the peri-portal and lobular areas were evaluated separately as 0 (no staining), 1 (weak), 2 (moderate) and 3 (intense) (Figure 1), and the sum of peri-portal and lobular scores was defined as CD10 score or CD105 score respectively. The immunoreactivity for CD10 in HCC was also evaluated as 0, 1, 2 and 3, and was defined as CD10-T. Statistical analyses of the scores were performed mutually or in relation to the severity of CH/LC by Mann-Whitney's test using Statmate III software (Atoms, Tokyo, Japan). Spearman's rank correlation coefficient between CD10 score and CD105 score was calculated by Statmate III.

3. Results

3.1. Control hepatic tissues

Out of 12 cases of metastatic carcinoma or biliary cystadenoma, the background hepatic tissues in 10 cases were evaluated as A0/F0 and those in the remaining 2 as A1/F0 and A0/F1 respectively. CD10(BC) expression was not uniform, while a difference of immunoreactivity was not conspicuous between peri-portal and lobular areas. CD10 score was more than 4 (moderate to intense staining) in 7 out of these 12 cases (Figure 2A, Table 1), including a case of A0/F1.

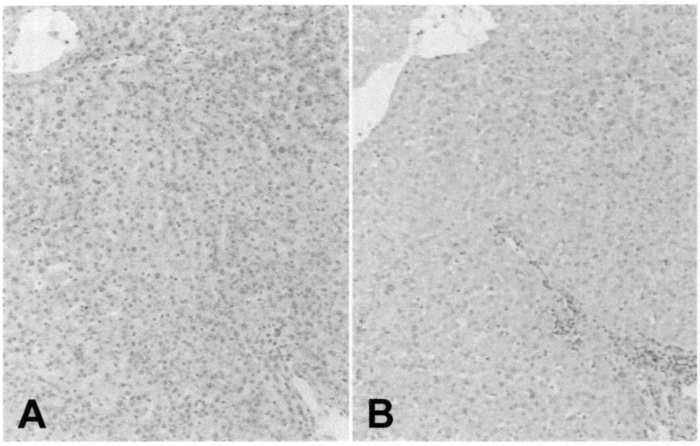

Figure 2. Expression of CD10 (A) and CD 105 (B) in the control hepatic tissue (serial sections). Bile canaliculi are moderately to intensely immunoreactive for CD10, whereas CD105 is not expressed in any regions.

As for CD105, 5 cases (including a case of A0/F1) showed no expression in any region of the background hepatic tissues (Figure 2B, Table 2). The other 7 cases did not reveal CD105(HS)-immunoreactivity in peri-portal areas but showed focal/weak expression in the lobular areas.

3.2. Chronic hepatitis/cirrhosis

CD10(BC) expression in the cases with CH/LC was not uniform, as in the control hepatic tissue, while CD10 scores were, in general, significantly lower than those in the control hepatic tissue (Figure 3A, Table 1). However, CD10(BC)-immunoreactivity was well preserved in the areas that the hepatocyte plates were regularly arranged with distinct trabecular pattern in some

http://dx.doi.org/10.5772/56734

cases (Figure 3B). In relation to inflammatory activity or fibrosis, a significant difference of CD10 score was demonstrated between the cases of A0 and A1-3 or between those of F0 and F1-4, but, among each group, only between A0 and A1 or F1-2 and F3 (Figures 4 B and 4E, Table 1).

CD105-positive hepatic sinusoids also revealed uneven distribution in the hepatic lobules. Although CD105 score was variable from case to case (Figures 4 C and 4F), the scores in CH/LC were significantly higher than those in the control hepatic tissue (Table 2). They also showed a tendency to be high in the cases of prominent inflammatory activity but not in those of advanced fibrosis stage (Table 2).

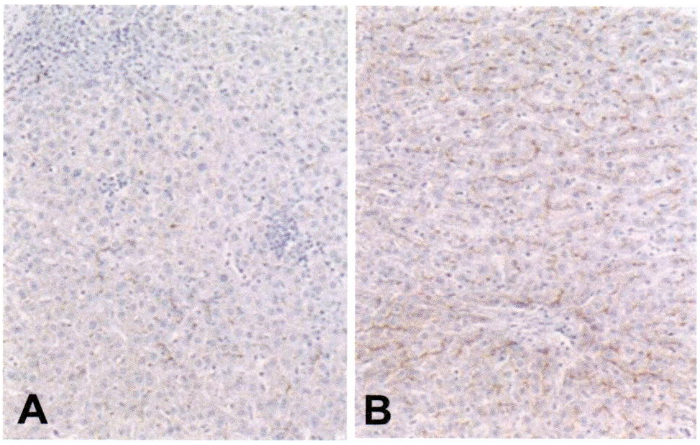

Figure 3. CD10 expression in a case of chronic hepatitis (A2/F2). (A) Decreased expression in the area of moderate inflammatory acitivity. (B) Intense expression in the area of mild inflammatory activity and well-preserved trabecular arrangement of hepatocyte plates.

CD10 score	0	1	2	3	4	5	6	
Control (12)		1	1	3	2	2	3	control vs. CH/LC: $p<0.05$
CH/LC (40)	12	6	8	7	4	3		
A0 (11)		1		3	2	2	3	A0 vs. A1-3: $p<0.001$
A1 (20)	6	1	6	4	1	2		A0 vs. A1: $p<0.01$
A2 (18)	5	4	2	3	3	1		A1 vs. A2: NS
A3 (3)	1	1	1					
F0 (13)		1	2	4	2	2	2	F0 vs. F1-4: $p<0.005$
F1 (4)				2		1	1	F1 vs. F1-2: NS
F2 (5)			2		2	1		F1-2 vs. F3: $p<0.001$
F3 (11)	5	2	3	1				F3 vs. F4: NS
F4 (19)	7	4	2	3	2	1		NS: not significant

( ): number of cases

Table 1. CD10 score in bile canaliculi in control liver and CH/LC in relation to inflammatory acitivity and degree of fibrosis

CD105 score	0	1	2	3	4	5
control (12)	5	5	2			
CH/LC (40)	4	9	11	10	4	2
A0 (11)	5	4	2			
A1 (20)	3	8	5	3	1	
A2 (18)	1	2	6	5	3	1
A3 (3)				2		1
F0 (13)	4	6	3			
F1 (4)	2	1			1	
F2 (5)	2		1	1		1
F3 (11)	1	4	4		1	1
F4 (19)		3	5	9	2	

( ): number of cases

control vs. CH/LC: p<0.001

A0 vs. A1-3: p<0.01
A0 vs. A1: p<0.05
A1 vs. A2: p<0.05

F0 vs. F1-4: p<0.005
F0 vs. F1-2: NS
F1-2 vs. F3: NS
F3 vs. F4: NS

NS: not significant

Table 2. CD105 score along hepatic sinusoid in control liver and CH/LC in relation to inflammatory activity and degree of fibrosis

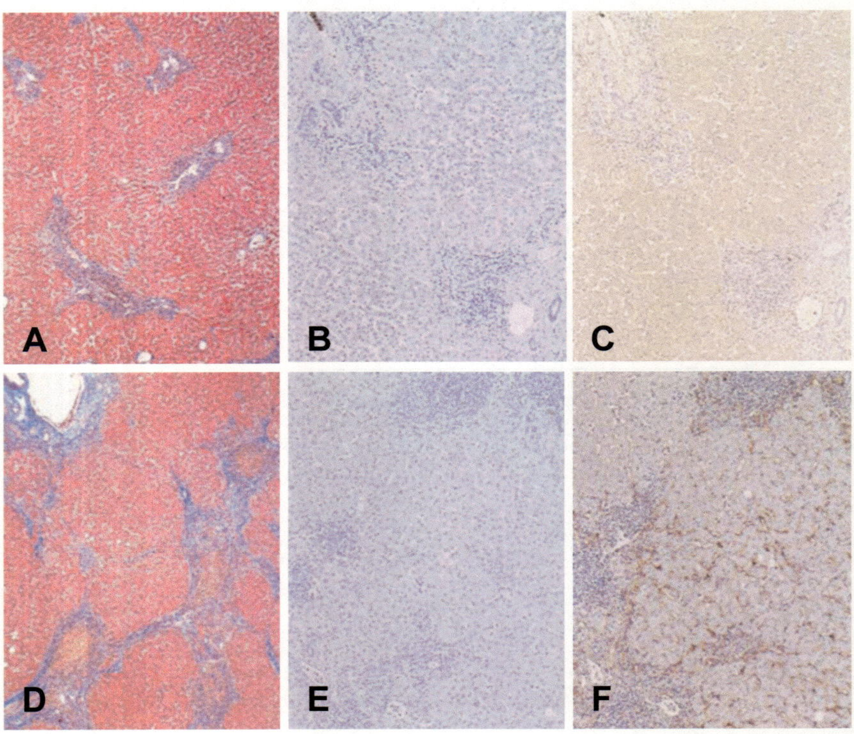

Figure 4. Representative cases of chronic hepatitis (CH): (A)-(C) CH (A1/F1), (D)-(F) CH (A2/F3). (A)(D) Azan-Mallory staining, (B) CD10 score 3, (C) CD105 score 0 (serial section of (B)), (E) CD10 score 0, (F) CD105 score 4 (serial section of (E)).

Figure 5 shows a correlation between CD10 score and CD105 score in all cases examined (including CL/LC and control hepatic tissues). There was a significant inverse correlation and Spearman's rank correlation coefficient was -0.533.

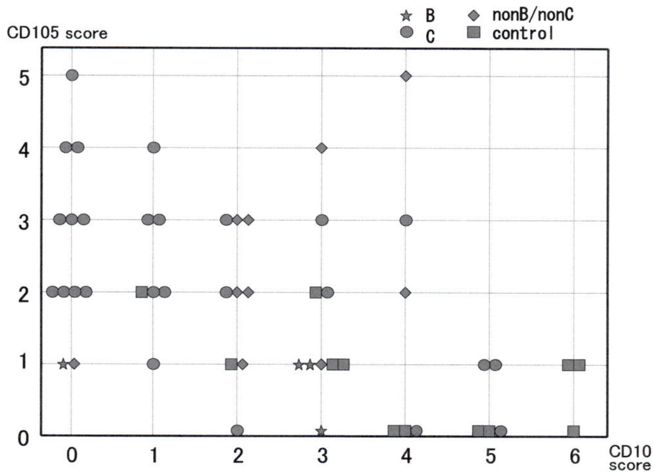

Figure 5. Inverse correlation of CD10 score and CD105 score (r_s=-0.533).

3.3. CD10 expression in HCC and background hepatic tissue

CD10 expression was observed, at least in part of HCC tissue, in 20 (58.8%) out of 34 cases examined (Figure 6). Although the immunoreactivity was variable, the cases with CD10-positive tumor tissues showed significantly higher CD10 score in the background hepatic tissue than those with no intra-tumoral CD10 expression (Table 3).

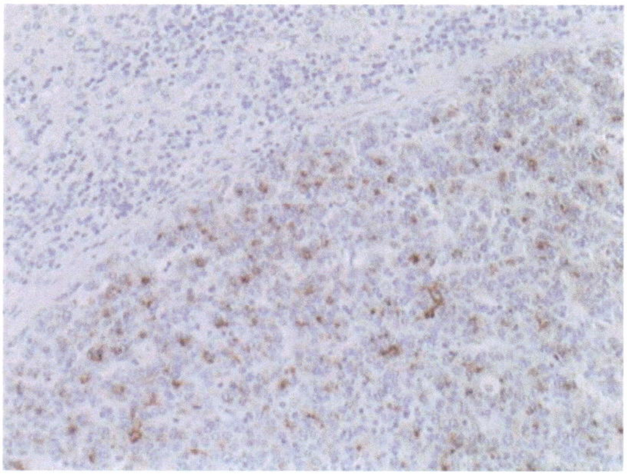

Figure 6. Expression of CD10 in hepatocellular carcinoma.

CD10 score in background liver tissue		0	1	2	3	4	5	
CD10 in HCC	(−)	6	2	2	2	1	1	$p<0.05$
	(+)	4	1	6	5	2	2	

Table 3. CD10 expression in hepatocellular carcinoma and CD10 score in background liver tissue

4. Discussion

In normal human liver, CD10 is detected in the bile canaliculi and interlobular bile ducts [6,7]. The present study indicated a decrease of CD10(BC) expression in CH/LC, a similar finding to what has been recently reported [15]. The distribution of CD10-immunoreactivity was not uniform, while the regularly arranged hepatocyte plates with distinct sinusoids maintained CD10-positive bile canaliculi. These observations may indicate, in CH/LC, a loss of differentiation and/or a functional impairment of bile canaliculi due to persistent hepatocyte injury. According to Shousha *et al.* [15], the loss of CD10(BC) reactivity was significantly correlated with fibrosis stage, but not with necro-inflammatory grade. In our study, however, a significant difference of CD10(BC) expression was demonstrated according to the presence or absence of inflammatory activity or fibrosis, but not necessarily between the groups of different grades of them. These results suggest that a decrease of CD10(BC) expression does not simply depend on the grade of inflammatory activity or fibrosis. Concerning other factors in relation to the severity of CH/LC, Shousha *et al.* reported a correlation of decreased CD10(BC) expression with abnormalities in liver function tests in CH/LC [15]. Meanwhile, our preliminary examination on alanine aminotransferase (ALT), aspartate aminotransferase (AST), lactic dehydrogenase (LDH), alkaline phosphatase (ALP) and gamma-glutamyl transpeptidase (gamma-GTP) showed that there was no distinct correlation between CD10 score and any data described above (data not shown). Further investigation on the mechanism of change in expression of CD10(BC) is warranted.

CD10 has also been used as a reliable marker for pathological diagnosis of HCC. The positive rate (58.8%) of CD10 expression in HCC in the present study was consistent with the previous reports (about 52-68%) [6,7,13,14]. In addition, CD10 in HCC was significantly correlated with the CD10 score of background hepatic tissue, although there was no significant correlation between CD10-T in HCC and CD score *in the lobular areas* in the previous report [33]. The present study suggests a phenotypic similarity of neoplastic and non-neoplastic hepatic tissue and also indicates the importance of evaluation of CD10 score in the all (peri-portal and lobular) areas.

The current study disclosed a significant inverse correlation between CD10 score and CD105 score in CH/LC. It has been reported that CD105 is not or minimally expressed in sinusoidal endothelial cells in normal human liver and is up-regulated in various types of chronic diseases, such as viral CH [29-32], autoimmune hepatitis [37], primary biliary cirrhosis [37,38],

http://dx.doi.org/10.5772/56734

alcoholic liver disease [39,40] and various benign nodular lesions [27]. Recently, it has been reported that increased CD105(HS) expression is significantly associated with progressive hepatic fibrosis in chronic hepatitis C virus infection [31]. The present study also showed up-regulation of CD105(HS)-immunoreactivity in CH/LC, indicating neoangiogenesis of hepatic sinusoids [30], and it was significantly correlated with the degree of inflammatory activity but not with the degree of fibrosis. The discrepancy between the two reports may reflect differences of methods of grading and scoring system. As for the type of hepatitis virus, CD105 score in CH/LC caused by hepatitis B virus was 0 or 1 in all cases in the present study. A correlation between CD105 score and type of hepatitis virus, however, could not be clarified because the number of cases of type B CH/LC was too small. Further cases of hepatitis B virus-positive CH/LC should be analyzed, although its infectious rate has been recently decreased due to vaccination [41].

In conclusion, the present study indicates simultaneous down-regulation of CD10(BC) and up-regulation of CD105(HS) in CH/LC. Although the phenotypic changes of bile canaliculi and hepatic sinusoids may be caused by separate mechanisms, they seem to represent different aspects induced by a common event, i.e., persistent hepatic injury.

5. Summary

The present study was undertaken in order to examine expression of CD10 in bile canaliculi (CD10(BC)) in relation to that of CD105 (endoglin) along hepatic sinusoids (CD105(HS)) in chronic hepatitis and liver cirrhosis (CH/LC). Fifty-two cases of resected liver, bearing hepatocellular carcinoma (HCC), metastatic carcinoma or biliary cystadenoma, were immunostained for CD10 and CD105. The immunoreactivity for CD10(BC) and CD105(HS) in the background hepatic tissue of tumors was scored separately. In the background hepatic tissue of metastatic carcinoma or cystadenoma (as controls), CD10(BC) was moderately or markedly expressed in more than half of the cases, whereas CD105(HS) was not or minimally positive. Compared with the controls, CH/LC cases significantly showed a decrease of CD10 score and an increase of CD105 score, the latter indicating neoangiogenesis, with inverse correlation (r_s = -0.533). The down-regulation of CD10 was not necessarily correlated with inflammatory activity or degree of fibrosis, whereas the up-regulation of CD105 was significantly correlated with inflammatory activity. These results indicate that the expression pattern of CD10(BC) and CD105(HS) changed simultaneously in CH/LC by persistent hepatic injury, although the mechanism of change of these markers may be different.

Acknowledgements

The author thanks Dr. S. Kajikawa for providing surgical specimens, and Ms. M. Morozumi, Mr. S. Hokibara, Mr. M. Shimomura and Mr. M. Yajima for their excellent technical assistance.

This work was approved by Institutional Review Board on ethical aspects at Suwa Red Cross Hospital (Suwa, Japan).

Author details

Toshitsugu Nakamura*

Address all correspondence to: pathology@suwa.jrc.or.jp

Department of Pathology, Suwa Red Cross Hospital, Suwa, Japan

References

[1] Nakamura T, Hayama M, Sakai T, Hotchi M, Tanaka E. Proliferative activity of hepatocytes in chronic viral hepatitis as revealed by immunohistochemistry for proliferating nuclear cell antigen. Human Pathology 1993; 24: 750-753.

[2] Farinati F, Cardin R, D'Errico A, De Maria N, Naccarato R, Cecchetto A, Grigioni W. Hepatocyte proliferative activity in chronic liver damage as assessed by the monoclonal antibody MIB1 Ki67 in archival material: the role of etiology, disease activity, iron, and lipid peroxidation. Hepatology 1996; 23: 1468-1475.

[3] Kaita KD, Pettigrew N, Minuk GY. Hepatic regeneration in humans with various liver disease as assessed by Ki-67 staining of formalin-fixed paraffin-embedded liver tissue. Liver 1997; 17: 13-16.

[4] Nakamura T, Hotch M. Changes in DNA strand breakd in non-parenchymal cells following heptocyte regeneration in CCl4-induced rat liver injury. Virchows Archiv B: Cell Pathology including Molecular Pathology 1992; 63: 11-16.

[5] Taniguchi E, Sakisaka S, Matsuo K, Tanikawa K, Sata M. Expression and role of vascular endothelial growth factor in liver regeneration after partial hepatectomy in rats. Journal of Histochemistry and Cytochemistry 2001; 49: 121-130.

[6] Borscheri N, Roessner A, Rocken C. Canalicular staining of neprilysin (CD10) as a diagnostic marker of hepatocellular carcinoma. American Journal of Surgical Pathology 2001; 25: 1297-1303.

[7] Rocken C, Licht J, Roessner A, Carl-McGrath S. Canalicular immunostaining of aminopeptidase N (CD13) as a diagnostic marker for hepatocellular carcinoma. Journal of Clinical Pathology 2005; 58: 1069-1075.

[8] McIntosh GG, Lodge AJ, Watson P, Hall AG, Wood K, Anderson JJ, Angus B, Horne CH, Milton ID. NCL-CD10-270: A new monoclonal antibody recognizing CD10 in paraffin-embedded tissue. American Journal of Pathology 1999; 154: 77-82.

[9] Shipp MA, Stefano GB, Switzer SN, Griffin JD, Reinherz EL. CD10 (CALLA) neutral endopeptidase 24.11 modulates inflammatory peptide-induced changes in neutrophil morphology, migration, and adhesion proteins and is itselt regulated by neutrophil activation. Blood 1991; 78: 1834-1841.

[10] Lebien TW, McCormack RT. The common acute lymphoblastic leukemia antigen (CD10): emancipation from a functional enigma. Blood 1989; 73: 625-635.

[11] Borella L, Sen L, Casper JT. Acute lymphoblastic leukemia (ALL) antigens detected with antisera to E rosette-forming and non-E rosette forming ALL blasts. Journal of Immunology 1977; 118: 309-315.

[12] Chu P, Arber DA. Paraffin-section detection of CD10 in 505 nonhematopoietic neoplasms. Frequent expression in renal cell carcinoma and endometrial stromal sarcoma. American Journal of Clinical Pathology 2000; 113: 374-382.

[13] Chu PG, Ishizawa S, Wu E, Weiss LM. Hepatocyte antigen as a marker of hepatocellular carcinoma: an immunohistochemical comparison to carcinoembryonic antigen, CD10, and alpha-fetoprotein. American Journal of Surgical Pathology 2002: 26: 978-988.

[14] Morrison C, Marsh W Jr, Frankel WL. A comparison of CD10 to pCEA, MOC-31, and hepatoyte for the distinction of malignant tumors in the liver. Modern Pathology 2002; 15: 1279-1287.

[15] Shousha S, Gadir F, Peston D, Bansi D, Thillainaygam AV, Murray-Lyon IM. CD10 immunostaining of bile canaliculi in liver biopsies: change of staining pattern with the development of cirrhosis. Histopathology 2004; 45: 335-342.

[16] Duff SE, Li C, Garland JM, Kumar S. CD105 is important for angiogenesis: evidence and potential applications. The FASEB Journal 2003; 17: 984-992.

[17] Fonsatti E, Maio M. Highlights on endoglin (CD105): from basic findings towards clinical applications in human cancer. Journal of Translational Medicine 2004; 2: 18 (http://www.translational-medicine.com/content/ 2/1/18) (accessed 5 October 2012)

[18] Ho JW, Poon RT, Sun CK, Xue W-C, Fan S-T. Clinicopathological and prognostic implications of endoglin (CD105) expression in hepatocellular carcinoma and its adjacent non-tumorous liver. World Journal of Gastroenterology 2005; 11: 176-181.

[19] Yu J-X, Zhang X-T, Liao Y-Q, Zhang Q-Y, Chen H, Lin M, Kumar S. Relationship between expression of CD105 and growth factors in malignant tumors of gastrointestinal tract and its significance. World Journal of Gastroenterology 2003; 9: 2866-2869.

[20] Salvesen HB, Gulluoglu MG, Stefansson I, Akslen LA. Significance of CD105 expression for tumor angiogenesis and prognosis in endometrial carcinoma. Acta Pathologica Microbiologica et Immunologica Scandinavica 2003; 111: 1011-1018.

[21] Saad RS, Liu YL, Nathan G, Celebrezze J, Medich D, Silverman JF. Endoglin (CD105) and vascular endothelial growth factor as prognostic markers in colorectal cancer. Modern Pathology 2004; 17: 197-203.

[22] Kyzas PA, Agnantis NJ, Stefanou D. Endoglin (CD105) as a prognostic factor in head and neck squamous cell carcinoma. Virchows Archiv 2006; 448: 768-775.

[23] Fonsatti E, Sigalotti L, Arslan P, Altomonte M, Maio M. Emerging role of endoglin (CD105) as a marker of angiogenesis with clinical potential in human malignancies. Current Cancer Drug Targets 2003; 3: 427-432.

[24] Fonsatti E, ALtomonte M, Nicotra MR, Natali PG, Maio M. Endoglin (CD105): a powerful therapeutic target on tumor-associated angiogenetic blood vessels. Oncogene 2003; 22: 6557-6563.

[25] Chung YC, Hou YC, Pan AC. Endoglin (CD105) expression in the development of hemorrhoids. European Journal of Clinical Investigation 2004; 34: 107-112.

[26] Tasman F, Dagdeviren A, Kendir B, Er N, Atac A. Endothelial cell and stromal antigens in human periapical granulation tissue. Journal of Endodontics 2000; 26: 81-84.

[27] Torsney E, Charlton R, Parums D, Collis M, Arthur HM. Inducible expression of human endoglin during inflammation and wound healing in vivo. Inflammation Research 2002; 51: 464-470.

[28] Zhang EG, Smith SK, Charnock-Jones DS. Expression of CD105 (endoglin) in arteriolar endothelial cells of human endometrium throughout the menstrual cycle. Reproduction 2002; 124: 703-711.

[29] Garcia-Monzon C, Sanchez-Madrid F, Garcia-Buey L, Garcia-Arroyo A, Garcia-Sanchez A, Moreno-Otero R. Vascular adhesion molecule expression in viral chronic hepatitis: evidence of neoangiogenesis in portal tracts. Gastroenterology 1995; 108: 231-241.

[30] Asanza CG, Garcia-Monzon C, Clemente G, Salcedo M, Garcia-Buey L, Garcia-Iglesias C, Banares R, Alvarez E, Moreno-Otero R. Immunohistochemical evidence of immunopathogenetic mechanisms in chronic hepatitis C recurrence after liver transplantation. Hepatology 1997; 26: 755-763.

[31] Clemente M, Nunez O, Lorente R, Rincon D, Matilla A, Salcedo M, Catalina MV, Ripoll C, Iacono OL, Banares R, Clemente G, Garacia-Monzon C. Increased intrahepatic and circulating levels of endoglin, a TGF-α co-receptor, in patients with chronic hepatitis C virus infection: relationship to histological and serum markers of hepatic fibrosis. Journal of Viral Hepatitis 2006; 13: 625-632.

[32] Yu D, Zhuang L, Sun X, Chen J, Yao Y, Meng K, Ding Y. Particular distribution and expression pattern of endoglin (CD105) in the liver of patients with hepatocellular carcinoma. BMC Cancer 2007; 7: 122.

[33] Nakamura T. Changes in expression of bile canalicular CD10 and sinusoidal CD105 (endoglin) in peritumoral hepatic tissue. Tumori 2009; 95: 495-500.

[34] Ichida F, Tsuji T, Omata M, Ichida T, Kamimura T, Yamada G et al. New Inuyama Classification: new criteria for histological assessment of chronic hepatitis. International Hepatology Communications 1996; 6: 112-119.

[35] Desmet VJ, Gerber M, Hoofnagle JH, Manns M, Scheuer PJ. Classification of chronic hepatitis: diagnosis, grading and staging. Hepatology 1994; 19: 1513-1520.

[36] Shi SR, Cote RJ, Taylor CR. Antigen retrieval techniques: current perspectives. Journal of Histochemistry and Cytochemistry 2001; 49: 931-937.

[37] Medina J, Sanz-Cameno P, Garcia-Buey L, Martin-Vilchez S, Lopez-Cabrera M, Moreno-Otero R. Evidence of angiogenesis in primary biliary cirrhosis: an immunohistochemical descriptive study. Journal of Hepatology 2005; 42: 124-131.

[38] Xu B, Broome U, Uzunel M, Nava S, Kumagai-Braesch M, Hultenby K et al. Capillarization of hepatic sinusoid by liver endothelial cell-reactive autoantibodies in patients with cirrhosis and chronic hepatitis. American Journal of Pathology 2003; 163: 1275-1289.

[39] Urashima S, Tsutsumi M, Nakase K, Wang JS, Takada A. Studies on capillarization of the hepatic sinusoids in alcoholic liver disease. Alcohol and Alcoholism, Supplement 1B 1993; 77-84.

[40] Xu GF, Wang XY, Ge GL, Li PT, Jia X, Tian DL et al. Dynamic changes of capillarization and peri-sinusoid fibrosis in alcoholic liver diseases. World Journal of Gastroenterology 2004; 10: 238-243.

[41] Yoshizawa A, Suzuki K, Abe A, Tanaka T, Yamaguchi K, Tanaka T, Ishikawa Y, Minegishi K, Gotanda Y, Yugi H, Uchida S, Satake M, Mizoguchi H, Tadokoro K. Effect of selective vaccination on a decrease in the rate of hepatitis B virus-positive Japanese first-time blood donors. Transfusion Medicine 2009; 19: 172-179.

Chapter 15

Hepatocellular Carcinoma, Steroid Hormones and Metalloproteases

Noemí Eiró, Belen Fernandez-Garcia, Antonio Altadill, Luis O. González and Francisco J. Vizoso

Additional information is available at the end of the chapter

http://dx.doi.org/10.5772/56877

1. Introduction

Liver cancer is the fifth and seventh most frequently diagnosed cancer worldwide in men and women, respectively, but the second most frequent cause of cancer death in men [1]. In addition, hepatocellular carcinoma (HCC) represents the major histological subtype of primary liver cancers, accounting up to 90% of the total liver cancer burden worldwide [2]. The incidence of HCC has increased significantly over the past 10 years and is expected to increase because of the actual high prevalence of viral hepatitis C-seropositive individuals and also because of the known long latency period to HCC development from the initial hepatitis C virus (HCV) infection, which may take 2-3 decades [3]. Despite of the varied treatment options, the prognosis of HCC remains poor. Thus, estimated 5-year survival rates are in the range of 26% to 50%, and disease-free survival is 13% to 29% [4]. At present, systemic chemotherapy is quite ineffective in HCC treatment, and is also known to express the multidrug-resistance gene MDR-1 [5]. Therefore, is necessary to identify and characterize molecular abnormalities of clinical significance in HCC. Besides the heterogeneity of different HCC subtypes, these tumors may use different cellular pathways and oncogenic mechanisms at different development stages, and this is of essential importance to develop biologically-based clinical trials.

2. Steroid hormone receptors and hepatocellular carcinoma

Although sex differences in liver cancer may be attributed to differences in lifestyle [6-8], there are several epidemiological and experimental studies suggesting that HCC might be, in part, hormone-related. Liver cancer is predominantly a male disease, with approximately three times higher incidence and mortality among men than women [9]. This male predominance is further supported by the fact that chronic liver disease progresses more rapidly to cirrhosis in males than in females, and therefore cirrhosis-derived HCC is largely seen in men and postmenopausal women disease [10].

The role of estrogens in modulating morphological and physiological features of liver became evident in early 1970s when a possible correlation between occurrence of hepatic neoplasms and use of oral contraceptives was suggested [11-12]. On the basis of these data, several *in vitro* and *in vivo* studies have explored the importance of sex hormones in HCC. Animal model-based studies indicate that sex hormones play a key role in tumor progression, showing that ovarian estrogens protect against tumor progression, whereas androgens promote tumorigenesis [13-15]. It has been reported that the protective effect of estrogens against chemically induced liver tumors is mediated by prolactin (PRL) through liver prolactin receptors (PRLR) [16-18]. Nevertheless, the precise role of male and female sex hormones and their receptors in HCC remains still poorly understood. There is not enough information regarding the mechanism of estrogen and androgen in HCC.

Estrogen and androgen mediate their biological functions through binding to their specific receptors, the estrogen receptor (ER) and the androgen receptor (AR). Both ER and AR belong to the nuclear receptors family that, as transcription factors, regulate the expression level of several genes such as those involved in triggering immune responses, cell proliferation and apoptosis [19-21]. Therefore, sex hormones play a key role in normal physiology of organs other than these of the reproductive system.

Variable expressions of ER and AR has been found in normal liver and HCC using different methods, such as immunohistochemistry, enzyme-immuno assays, or determining mRNA levels (Table 1 and Table 2 give the details of these studies for ER and AR, respectively), which indicate a relationship between sex hormones and pathogenesis of HCC. The percentage of positivity for these receptors varied between the different studies [22]. These differences may be due to several methodological aspects, such as differences in the origin of the studied patients populations, sample types or technologies determining the receptor expression. In a recent study, we determined the expression of sex hormones receptors in 31 HCC patients by immunohistochemistry using tissue micro-arrays technology [23]. Our results demonstrate a wide variability in the immunohistochemical values for steroid receptors among HCCs: 67.7% of tumors stained positively for AR, 51.6% for ER and 83.8% for progesterone receptor (PgR), but, among the positive cases, immunostaining score values for each protein were largely variable.

Reference	Protein /mRNA	Type of liver tissue	Method	Localization	n	% positive cases	Country	Year
[122]	ER protein	Normal	BA	cytosolic	4	100	United Kingdom	1978
[123]	ER protein	Normal	BA	-	3	100	Germany	1978
[124]	ER protein	Normal	BA	-	2	100	United States	1982

Reference	Protein /mRNA	Type of liver tissue	Method	Localization	n	% positive cases	Country	Year
[125]	ER protein	Normal	BA	-	6	100	Germany	1982
[126]	ER protein	Normal	BA	-	6	100	United States	1983
[127]	ER protein	Normal	BA	cytosolic and nuclear	4	100	United Kingdom	1983
[128]	ER protein	Surrounding	BA	cytosolic	30	43	Japan	1986
[129]	ER protein	Non-cancerous	BA	cytosolic and nuclear	7	43	Japan	1986
[130]	ER protein	Non-cirrhotic	EIA	cytosolic	12	12	Japan	1987
[131]	ER protein	Normal		-	2	2	Japan	1988
[132]	ER protein	Surrounding	BA	cytosolic	17	65	Japan	1989
[133]	ER protein	Surrounding			22	64	Japan	1989
[134]	ER protein	Surrounding	BA	cytosolic	5	100	Japan	1990
[135]	ER protein	Normal	BA		9	9	United States, Italy	1991
[52]	ER protein	Non-cancerous	BA	cytosolic	26	42	Spain	1993
[136]	ER mRNA	Non-cancerous	ISH		13	54	Italy	1993
[137]	ER mRNA	Peritumoral	RT-PCR	-	32	88	Korea	2006
[124]	ER protein	HCC	BA	cytosolic	5	100	United States	1982
[127]	ER protein	HCC	BA	cytosolic and nuclear	5	100	United Kingdom	1983
[138]	ER protein	HCC	IHC	cytosolic	10	10	Singapore	1984
[128]	ER protein	HCC	BA	cytosolic	30	40	Japan	1986
[139]	ER protein	HCC	BA	cytosolic and nuclear	8	13	Japan	1986
[130]	ER protein	HCC	EIA	cytosolic	13	38	Japan	1987
[132]	ER protein	HCC	BA	cytosolic	19	37	Japan	1989
[24]	ER protein	HCC	BA	cytosolic	66	39	Japan	1990
[134]	ER protein	HCC	BA	cytosolic	6	17	Japan	1990
[140]	ER protein	HCC	BA	cytosolic	21	48	Japan	1991
[141]	ER protein	HCC	BA	cytosolic and nuclear	9	89	United States, Italy	1991
[135]	ER protein	HCC	BA	cytosolic and nuclear	9	89	United States, Italy	1991

Reference	Protein /mRNA	Type of liver tissue	Method	Localization	n	% positive cases	Country	Year
[52]	ER protein	HCC	EIA	cytosolic	26	15	Spain	1993
[136]	ER protein	HCC	IHC	-	15	0	Italy	1993
[136]	ER mRNA	HCC	ISH	-	15	73	Italy	1993
[142]	ER mRNA	HCC	RT-PCR	-	14	57	Italy	1995
[25]	ER protein	HCC	EIA	cytosolic	33	39	Germany	1997
[143]	ER protein	HCC	IHC	cytosolic	71	24	China	1997
[144]	ER mRNA	HCC	RT-PCR	-	40	70	Italy	1998
[145]	ER mRNA	HCC	RT-PCR	-	42	60	Italy	2003
[146]	ER protein	HCC	IHC	cytosolic and nuclear	45	71	United States/ Koreans	2004
[147]	ER protein	HCC	IHC	-	28	39	China	2004
[147]	ER mRNA	HCC	RT-PCR	-	28	89	China	2004
[137]	ER mRNA	HCC	RT-PCR	-	32	100	Korea	2006
[148]	ER protein	HCC	IHC	-	66	5	Mexico	2007
[23]	ER protein	HCC	IHC	Nuclear	31	52	Spain	2007

ER: Estrogen receptor; HCC: Hepatocellular carcinoma; BA: Binding assay; EIA: Enzyme immunoassay; ISH: *In situ* hybridization; RT-PCR: Reverse transcriptase-polymerase Chain reaction for ERα wild type; IHC: Immunohistochemistry.

Table 1. Estrogen expression in normal liver and hepatocellular carcinoma tissue samples.

Reference	Protein /mRNA	Type of liver tissue	Method	Localization	n	% positive cases	Country	Year
[127]	AR protein	Normal	BA	cytosolic and nuclear	4	0	United Kingdom	1983
[139]	AR protein	Non-cancerous	BA	cytosolic and nuclear	6	17	Japan	1986
[132]	AR protein	Non-cancerous	BA	cytosolic	17	65	Japan	1989
[133]	AR protein	Surrounding			21	33	Japan	1989
[134]	AR protein	Surrounding	BA	cytosolic	10	80	Japan	1990
[135]	AR protein	Normal	-	-	9	100	United States, Italy	1991
[137]	AR mRNA	Peritumoral	RT-PCR		32	100	Korea	2006

Reference	Protein /mRNA	Type of liver tissue	Method	Localization	n	% positive cases	Country	Year
[127]	AR protein	HCC	BA	cytosolic and nuclear	5	100	United Kingdom	1983
[138]	AR protein	HCC	IHC	cytosolic	10	50	Singapore	1984
[149]	AR protein	HCC	BA	cytosolic	19	74	Japan	1985
[150]	AR protein	HCC	BA	cytosolic and nuclear	5	100	United Kingdom	1985
[139]	AR protein	HCC	BA	cytosolic and nuclear	8	50	Japan	1986
[151]	AR protein	HCC	BA	cytosolic	13	100	United Kingdom	1988
[132]	AR protein	HCC	BA	cytosolic	19	37	Japan	1989
[27]	AR protein	HCC	BA	cytosolic	45	69	Japan	1989
[134]	AR protein	HCC	BA	cytosolic	11	64	Japan	1990
[140]	AR protein	HCC	BA	cytosolic	21	86	Japan	1991
[135]	AR protein	HCC	BA	cytosolic and nuclear	9	100	United States, Italy	1991
[152]	AR protein	HCC	BA	cytosolic	5	100	Japan	1992
[52]	AR protein	HCC	BA	cytosolic	26	54	Spain	1993
[28]	AR protein	HCC	BA	cytosolic	43	65	Spain	1995
[23]	AR protein	HCC	IHC	nuclear	31	68	Spain	2007
[129]	AR mRNA	HCC	ISH	-	22	73	Italy	1994
[153]	AR mRNA	HCC	RT-PCR	-	38	89	Italy	2002
[137]	AR mRNA	HCC	RT-PCR	-	32	100	Korea	2006

AR: Androgen receptor; HCC: Hepatocellular carcinoma; BA: Binding assay; ISH: *In situ* hybridization; RT-PCR: Reverse transcriptase-polymerase Chain reaction; IHC: Immunohistochemistry.

Table 2. Androgen receptor expression in normal liver and hepatocellular carcinoma tissue samples.

Several studies have analyzed the relationship between ER or AR and clinicopathological parameters from HCCs patients and their clinical outcome (Table 3). In general, ER expression was associated with higher tumor aggressiveness and/or worse prognosis in HCC patients [24-26], whereas AR expression was negatively associated with recurrence [27-29]. It is remarkable the finding that the presence of the ERα variant has been associated with shortened overall survival in patients with resectable HCC [30,26].

3. Steroid receptors and hepatitis virus

It is of special interest the interaction between sex estrogen receptors and viral proteins in hepatitis B virus (HBV) and hepatitis C virus (HCV)-induced HCC. It has been reported that a HBV protein (HBx) interacts with ERα. HBx is a multifunctional protein involved in neoplastic transformation in cultured cells and in HCC induction in transgenic mice. Both HBx and vERα (Delta 5 deletion variant of ERα) have additive effects on suppressing ERα transactivation [31]. In addition, it was reported that tamoxifen inhibits ERα actions and suppresses HCV genome replication [32], which may be of potential interest to develop new anti-HCV strategies based on anti-ER drugs. On the other hand, higher serum androgen concentrations or a specific AR gene, which leads to higher AR activities, have also been associated to higher risk in HBV-mediated HCC [33-34]. Likewise, it has been reported that the combination of male gender and HBV infection had a significant synergistic effect on HCC progression [35]. Most recently, Ming-Heng *et al.* found that hepatic AR increases the HBV viral titer by enhancing HBV RNA transcription through direct binding to the androgen response element near the viral core promoter. This activity forms a positive feedback mechanism with the cooperation of its downstream target, the HBx protein, to promote hepatocarcinogenesis. In addition in these same study administration of a chemical compound that selectively degrades AR, ASC-J9, was able to suppress HCC tumor size in a transgenic HBV mouse model that developed HCC upon exposure to a low dose of N'-N'-diethylnitrosamine (DEN). These results demonstrate that targeting the AR, rather than the androgen, could be developed as a new therapy to battle HBV-induced HCC [36].

Reference	Protein / mRNA	clinicopathological parameters	Correlation	n	year	country
[128]	ER protein	Serum alpha-fetoprotein, HBV profile, tumor histology, carcinoembryonic antigen	-	30	1986	Japan
[132]	ER and AR protein	Serum alpha-fetoprotein, Histopathology, HBV markers	-	19	1989	Japan
[24]	ER protein	Sex, age, alcohol consumption, hepatic function, other liver disease, tumor size, hepatic resection, tumor recurrence, long-term survival rate	ER- patients showed higher rate of resection and larger tumor size	66	1990	Japan
[49]	ER and AR protein	Local recurrence	AR expression was associated with intrahepatic recurrence	78	1995	Japan
[25]	ER protein	Survival after curative resection	ER+ tumor have a negative effect on patient survival after curative resection	28	1997	Germany

Reference	Protein / mRNA	clinicopathological parameters	Correlation	n	year	country
[26]	ER mRNA	Survival	Wild type ERs tumors showed long survival in patients	96	2000	Italy
[132]	AR protein	Recurrence and survival rate	AR+ patients showed higher recurrence rates. AR- patients showed better survival rates.	45	1989	Japan
[28]	AR protein	Tumor size and tumor recurrence	AR expression correlated with smaller tumor size. Higher tumor recurrence in AR+ surrounding tissues.	43	1995	Spain
[29]	AR protein	Tumor size and survival time	AR+ tumor correlated with higher tumor size and lower survival rates.	32	1998	China

ER: Estrogen receptor; AR: Androgen receptor

Table 3. Relationship between estrogen or androgen receptors with clinicopathological parameters and clinical outcome of patients with HCC.

4. Endocrine therapy in hepatocellular carcinoma

Considering both the epidemiologic and the experimental data supporting the sex steroids influence in growth and progression from HCCs, different clinical studies analyzed if endocrine therapy could be interesting in advanced disease. Table 4 gives details of some of these studies. Trials using several agents, such as the anti-estrogen tamoxifen, megestrol acetate, progestin, the gonadotropin releasing hormone (GnRH) agonist leuprorelin and the anti-androgen flutamide have been uniformly disappointing [37-40]. At present, experts have concluded that hormonal manipulation should not be a part of the current management of patients with HCC [41-42]. However, it is possible that the rational design of an endocrine therapy requires a more complete understanding of the role of sex hormones in the tumorigenic process and how hormones and organ systems interact during this process [18], in addition to careful selection of the new studies patient populations, since patient stratification based on gender may uncover signals of activity of hormonal therapy in these settings. Notably, it has been shown that the anti-estrogens tamoxifen and raloxifene, behave differently in different tissues, producing estrogen-agonist activity in one tissue while behaving as an antagonist in another [43-44]. In addition, *in vitro* studies in the liver cell line Hep3B, indicate that raloxifene induces the insulin-like growth factor (IGF-I) gene transcription, whereas estradiol or tamoxifen inhibits it [45]. On the other hand, the lack of hormone efficacy in these clinical studies, in terms of tumor growth and survival, could be due to either a low expression of ER or AR in HCC or to mutated receptors expression. Therefore, further studies will be necessary to improve patient selection on the basis of gender, ER tumor expression and their functional status. With regard to this latter aspect, considering that PgR is an estrogen inducible protein, it led us to consider that this steroid receptor could be a possible marker of ER functional status in HCC, to select candidate patients to an anti-estrogenic therapy. In addition, we demonstrated that PgR expression have a prognostic implication in patients with resected HCCs, being a factor associated with better prognostic [23], which is a clinical finding previously demonstrated in breast cancer [46-47]. This finding is very important considering also our reported positive association between PgR expression and HCV infection [23], which represents an increasing aetiology of HCC in our patient's population [3].

Several data suggest that blocking AR may be interesting in HCC therapy. Studies in animal models suggest that increased hepatic AR expression correlated with accelerated tumor development [48], or even AR expression was associated with intrahepatic recurrence in HCC [49]. However, AR expression has also been reported to be associated to small tumor size, but not with a higher rate of recurrence [28]. More recent data indicate that suppression of androgen or AR signals also led to an increase in the number of infiltrating cells, such as macrophages as well as B or T-cells [50], which shows diverse and important roles in the promotion of HCC tumorigenicity [51]. Although there is few data on the effect of anti-androgens in HCC patients, it has been suggested that anti-androgen therapy may have some benefit in patients with androgen-positive tumors [52]. Likewise, recently it has been reported that a multicenter trial with anti-androgens in HCC male patients, has been interrupted because of digestive side effects [39]. Nevertheless, further studies will be necessary to assess whether AR status may be a useful marker to select more accurately candidate patients to further anti-androgenic therapies. Notably, it has been reported that expression of androgen-induced proteins, such as apolipoprotein D or Zinc-alpha2-glycoprotein, is associated with poor prognosis in HCC.

Apolipoprotein D (ApoD) is an androgen-induced protein increased in both prostate and breast cancer cells [53-55]. A report of Utsunomiya *et al.* showed that low ApoD expression correlated significantly with less-differentiated HCCs and therefore with a worse prognosis of patients [56]. However, we did not found any relationship between ApoD expression and the hormonal receptor status in HCC [23]. Nevertheless, further studies will be also necessary in order to assess the possible value of ApoD as a biological marker of androgen response and/or other hormonal pathways in HCC. Thus, with regard to this latter aspect, although ApoD is an androgen-regulated protein, it can also been induced by other hormonal steroids or substances such as glucocorticoids, retinoic acid or 1,25-dihydroxyvitamin D_3, that might be involved in the regulation of this ApoD in human tumors [54,57-58]. This is relevant since it has been described that both retinoid and glucocorticoid receptors have been also detected in HCC [59-60], and that preliminary data show that retinoids are considered of clinical interest as cancer chemotherapeutic agents in advanced HCC [61].

Zinc-alpha2-glycoprotein (ZA2G) is also an androgen-induced protein increased in breast cancer [58,62]. Recently, ZA2G expression was found to be decreased in HCC tissues at both mRNA and protein levels. Moreover, low expression of ZA2G was notably more prevalent in

http://dx.doi.org/10.5772/56877

Hormone Receptor/ mRNA	Valuation parameters	Treatment	n	Clinical outcomes	Year	Reference
ER (previous patient group)	Tumor growth	Progestin	5	Tumor regression in 2	1982	[124]
NA	Anti-tumoral effect. Survival.	Tamoxifen 20 mg twice daily.	33	No effect on the tumor, in 8 remained stable between 5 and 13 months. Prolonged survival in 4 patients (over 18 months).	1990	[154]
NA	Anti-tumoral effect. Survival.	Tamoxifen 20 mg daily.	120 (placebo = 62)	No effect on the tumor. No effect on survival.	1995	[155]
Wild type and variant ER RNA m	Tumor growth.	Tamoxifen 80 mg daily in patients with wild-ERs or megestrol 160 mg daily in patients with variant ERs.	8 patients, 4 with wild ERs and 4 with variant ERs.	Tumor regression to half size in patients with wild type ERs following tamoxifen treatment. Megestrol slowed down tumor growth in tumors with variant ERs.	1996	[30]
ER y PR	Survival.	Tamoxifen.	119 (placebo = 58)	No effects on survival, regardless of the type of receptor expressed.	2000	[156]
Variant ER mRNA.	Tumor growth. Survival.	Megestrol 160 mg daily.	45 (placebo = 24).	Significantly slowed down tumor growth and improved survival in treated patients than placebo group.	2001	[157]
NA	Survival. Quality of life.	Tamoxifen 120 mg or 60 mg daily.	329	No effect on survival or on quality of life. Deleterious effects with the higher dose.	2002	[158]

ER= Estrogen receptor. NA=information not available. PR= Progesterone Receptor.

Table 4. Results of hormonal treatment in hepatocellular carcinoma

patients with poor tumor differentiation, advanced liver cirrhosis, high serum alpha fetoprotein (AFP) level and shorter survival time. These results suggest that ZA2G may be a promising novel prognostic biomarker for HCC [63], and advocate for the need for validation studies.

Recent data indicates that estrogens attenuate tumor progression in HCC *in vivo* by reducing tumor cell invasion, arresting cell cycle progression, and promoting apoptosis, which is characterized by an increased expression of cleaved caspase-3, and by a decrease in the expression of Proliferating Cell Nuclear Antigen (PCNA), cyclin A, cyclin D1, Bcl-2, and matrix metalloproteases (MMP) 2 and 9 [64]. It is relevant the data indicating that steroid hormones, such as estrogens, may inhibit MMPs in several experimental models [65-67]. This may be of great importance due to MMPs are proteolytic enzymes which participate in the degradation of the stromal connective tissue and basement membrane component, therefore facilitating tumor invasion and metastasis. Here, we show a negative relationship between ER expression and MMP2, MMP-9 or MMP-11 expression in HCC (Figure 1).

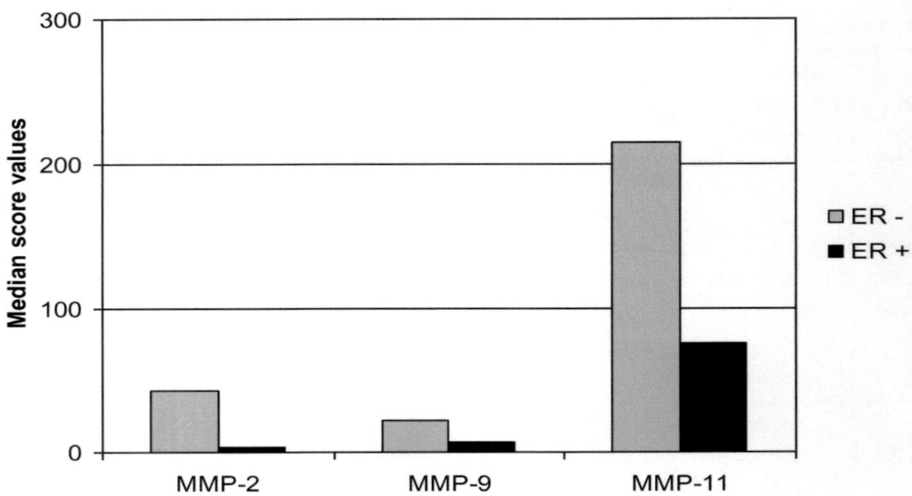

Figure 1. Relationship between ER expression and median score values of MMP2, MMP-9 or MMP-11 expression in HCC.

5. Metalloproteases and their inhibitors

Degradation of the stromal connective tissue and basement membrane components are key elements in tumor invasion and metastasis. Some components of the extracelluar matrix, particularly interstitial collagens, are very resistant to proteolytic attacks, being degraded only by matrix metalloproteases (MMPs) [68].

The human MMP family currently consists of 28 members of homologous zinc-dependent endopeptidases, which can be divided into eight structural classes or, based on their substrate specificity and primary structure, into the more familiar subgroups of collagenases (MMP-1, -8 and -13), gelatinases (MMP-2 and -9), stromelysins (MMP-3, -10, -11), membrane-associated MMPs (MMP-14, -15, -16, -17, -23, -24, -25) and other novel MMPs [69-71]. MMPs are synthesized as inactive zymogens, which are then activated predominantly pericellularly by other MMPs or by serine-proteases. MMPs' activity is specifically inhibited by the so-called tissue inhibitors of metalloproteases (TIMPs). Currently, four different TIMPs are known to exist: TIMP-1, -2, -3 and -4. In addition, there are other two additional aspects conferring relevance to this enzymatic system in cancer biology. First, MMPs are able to impact on tumor cell behavior *in vivo* as a consequence of their ability to cleave growth factors, cell surface receptors, cell adhesion molecules, or chemokines/cytoquines [72-77]. Furthermore, by cleaving proa-poptotic factors, MMPs may induce a more aggressive phenotype via generation of apoptotic resistant cells [78]. MMPs may also regulate angiogenesis in cancer, both positively through their ability to mobilize or activate proangiogenic factors [79-80], and negatively via generation of angiogenesis inhibitors, such as angiostatin and endostatin, cleaved from large protein precursors [81-83]. Second, it is now assumed that TIMPs are multifactorial proteins also involved in the induction of proliferation and the inhibition of apoptosis [84-85].

Previous studies have shown the expression of several MMPs in HCC [86-100]. These findings have a great interest because HCC is characterized by a disposition for vascular invasion and high metastatic potential, thus leading to high incidence of early postoperative recurrence and poor survival [101-102]. Although there is no basal membrane in the liver, HCC cancer cells grow surrounded by extracellular matrix proteins secreted as a consequence of cirrhosis, and therefore proteolytic activity is required to allow HCC cells to penetrate and cross over such tissue boundaries [103]. In fact, several studies have suggested the significance of some MMPs in the malignant behavior of HCC, such as MMP-2 [86-93], MMP-7 [88,94], MMP-9 [95-97,91,93,104], MMP-12 [105] or MMP-14 (MT1-MMP) [98,91,99-100]. In these studies, MMPs were associated with several parameters indicative of tumor aggressiveness and poor prognosis, although the cellular type expressing each factor (tumor cell and/or peritumor stromal cell) was not specifically considered.

There are few available data referring to the integrated expression of these factors in relation with HCC. In this context, we have described new findings about MMPs and TIMPs expressions in HCC, together with an important expression by tumor stromal cells, as well as their clinical relevance. It is known that MMPs expression in neoplastic tissues is high due to regulation, in a paracrine manner, by growth factors and cytokines secreted by either tumor or stromal cells [106]. Nevertheless, high MMPs and TIMPs expression by HCCs tissues may be also due to the interplay between transformed cells and their microenviron-ment, particularly the surrounding extracellular matrix. In human livers, fibrogenesis underlies the development of HCCs in at least 90% of cases [107], and HCC is typically surrounded by a fibrous capsule at an early stage [108]. In addition, several studies have shown that some MMPs (MMP-1, -2, -9 and -13) and TIMPs (TIMP-1 and -2) are in-volved in the liver fibrosis processes [90,109-112]. It has been demonstrated that extracellu-lar matrix deposition induces overexpression of MMPs and TIMPs, such as MMP-2, secreted by human mesenchymal cells but also by hepatoma cells [87].

Recently we reported that immunostaining for MMPs and TIMPs was localized predominantly in tumor cells, but also in peritumor stromal cells in a significant percentage of cases. However, we found no stromal expression of MMPs or TIMPs in normal liver samples [113]. We also found a positive and noteworthy association between MMP-1 expression by fibroblasts or by mononuclear inflammatory cells (MICs) and a larger tumor size. In addition, our data showed that MMP-1 expression by stromal fibroblasts, as well as the expression of MMP-13, TIMP-1 and 2, by MICs, were significantly associated with a shorter overall survival (Figure 2) [113].

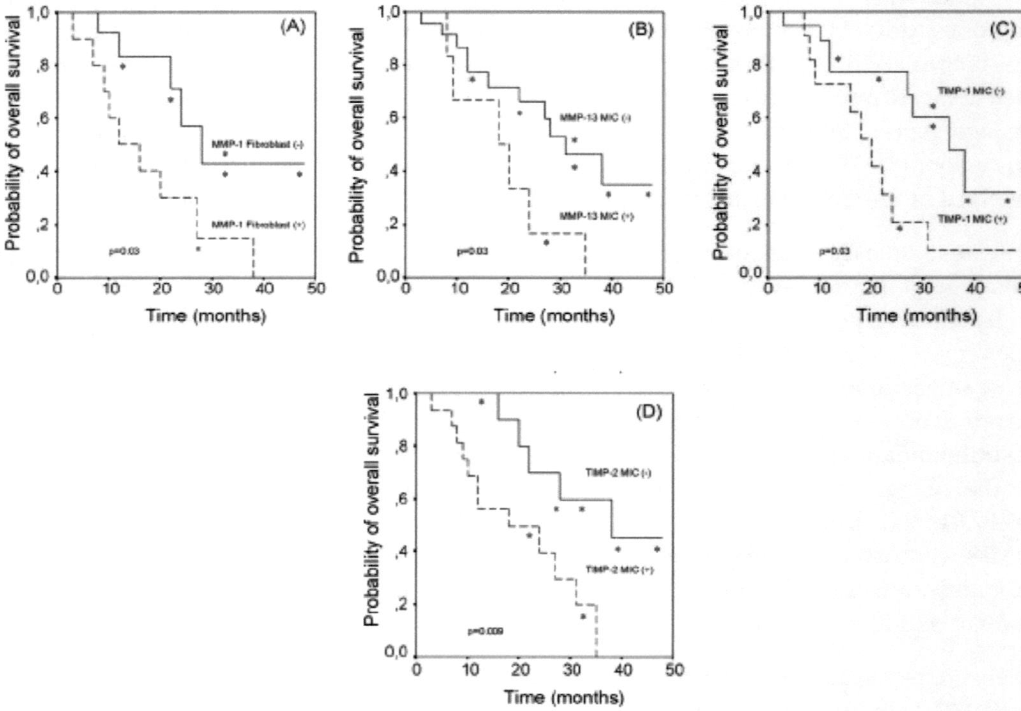

Figure 2. Kaplan-Meier survival curves as function of the expression by fibroblasts cells of MMP-1 (A); expression by MIC of MMP-13 (B), TIMP-1 (C) and TIMP-2 (D).

There are discrepancies between different studies regarding the prognostic significance of several of these factors in HCC, such as MMP-9 and MMP-2 expression in stromal compartments [113,93]. Nevertheless, it is worth considering the existence of possible differences in MMPs or TIMPs expression between different patient's populations. Thus, for example, in Asian countries HCC originates more frequently in healthy liver tissues, with less incidence of cirrhosis, than in Europe, whereas in the Mediterranean area as well as in the North American countries liver HCC only develops in chronically injured livers, where altered turn-over and increased deposition of ECM proteins has been described. In a such environment, upregulation of MMPs and TIMPs has been reported and it is possible for them to play an important role in the rearrangement of the liver tissue architecture an aspect that could influence the different expression pattern of MMPs and TIMPs in stromal HCC cells [110,114].

http://dx.doi.org/10.5772/56877

On the other hand, a decrease on TIMP-2 and -3 expression has been reported to be associated with invasion and metastases in HCC [115-116]. Certainly, if TIMPs inhibit MMPs *in vivo*, it should be expected that high levels of these inhibitors would prevent tumor progression and thus to be related with good outcome in cancer patients. However, TIMPs are multifunctional proteins that in addition to its MMP-inhibitory effect also shown distinct tumor-stimulatory functions, such as the induction of proliferation and the inhibition of apoptosis [84]. Thus, it is of note that TIMP-1 and -2 expressions by stromal cells were associated with shortened overall survival[113]. Accordingly, it has been reported that TIMP-1 overexpression leads to an increase of hepatoma cells migration [117], and also that it is associated with invasion and metastases in HCC [115,117].

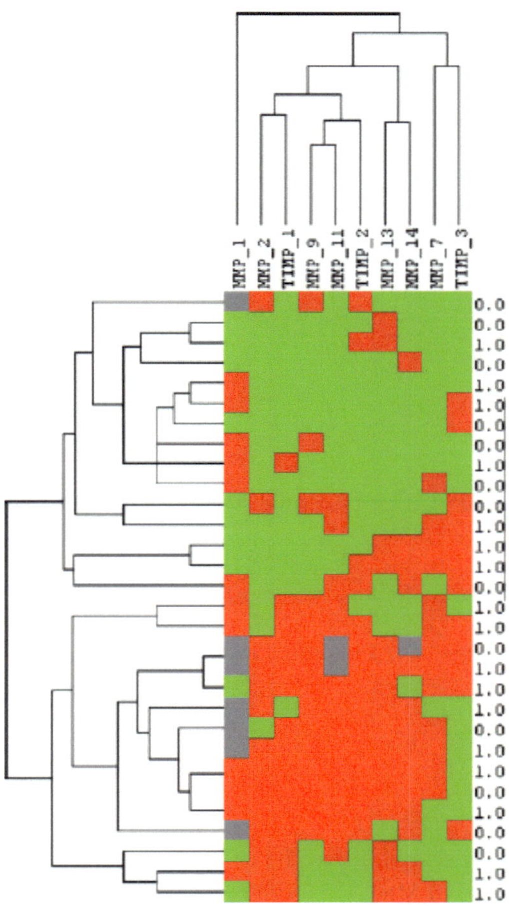

Figure 3. Graphical representation of two-dimensional unsupervised hierarchical clustering results on immunohistochemistry expression (score values) profile in 10 proteins (MMPs and TIMPs) in 30 samples of HCC tissue. Rows: tumor samples; columns: MMPs and TIMPs. Protein expressions are depicted according to a color scale: red: positive staining; green: negative staining; gray: missing data. At right bank of the figure is represented the overall survival status for each patient (0, alive; 1, death due tumor progression).

The unsupervised hierarchical cluster analysis of MMPs/TIMPs expressions in HCCs led us to identify 2 well-defined clusters of cases (Figure 3): one with low expression of MMPs and TIMPs (Group 1), and another with high expression of these factors (Group 2). This classification could have biological interest in order to identify patient candidates to new therapies based on enzymatic MMP inhibition. With regard to this, although there are no published data about use of MMP inhibitors in HCC, recently it has been reported that decreased MMP activity mediated by statins reduced progression and limits metastatic diffusion of established HCC [118]. Likewise, it was demonstrated that blocking the tumor-related glycoprotein HAb18G/CD147 by gene silence in HCC cells or with HA18 monoclonal antibody, resulted in a suppressive effect on MMP secretion and cell invasion [119]. More recent studies have shown an antimetastatic effect of Norcantharidin on HCC by transcriptional inhibition of MMP-9 [120], as well as a metastasis inhibition of HCC cells due to down-regulation of Osteopontin via a mechanism involving MMP-2 and urinary plasminogen activator (uPA) [121].

6. Conclusion

In summary, we consider that expression analysis of steroid hormone receptors, MMPs and TIMPs, contributes to a better knowledge in the biological characterization of HCC and highlights the need for further studies exploring new therapeutic targets for this common tumor.

Author details

Noemí Eiró, Belen Fernandez-Garcia, Antonio Altadill, Luis O. González and Francisco J. Vizoso*

*Address all correspondence to: fjvizoso@terra.es

Unidad de Investigación. Fundación Hospital de Jove. Gijón, Asturias, Spain

References

[1] Parkin DM, Bray F, Ferlay J, Pisani P (2005) Global cancer statistics, 2002. CA Cancer J Clin 55 (2):74-108. [PubMed: 15761078]

[2] Nordenstedt H, White DL, El-Serag HB (2010) The changing pattern of epidemiology in hepatocellular carcinoma. Dig Liver Dis 42 Suppl 3:S206-214. [PubMed: 20547305]

[3] El-Serag HB, Mason AC (1999) Rising incidence of hepatocellular carcinoma in the United States. N Engl J Med 340 (10):745-750. [PubMed: 10072408]

[4] Poon RT, Ng IO, Fan ST, Lai EC, Lo CM, Liu CL, Wong J (2001) Clinicopathologic features of long-term survivors and disease-free survivors after resection of hepatocellular carcinoma: a study of a prospective cohort. J Clin Oncol 19 (12):3037-3044. [PubMed: 11408499]

[5] Kato A, Miyazaki M, Ambiru S, Yoshitomi H, Ito H, Nakagawa K, Shimizu H, Yokosuka O, Nakajima N (2001) Multidrug resistance gene (MDR-1) expression as a useful prognostic factor in patients with human hepatocellular carcinoma after surgical resection. J Surg Oncol 78 (2):110-115. [PubMed: 11579388]

[6] Yu MC, Yuan JM (2004) Environmental factors and risk for hepatocellular carcinoma. Gastroenterology 127 (5 Suppl 1):S72-78. [PubMed: 15508106]

[7] Marrero JA, Fontana RJ, Fu S, Conjeevaram HS, Su GL, Lok AS (2005) Alcohol, tobacco and obesity are synergistic risk factors for hepatocellular carcinoma. J Hepatol 42 (2):218-224. [PubMed: 15664247]

[8] Ohishi W, Fujiwara S, Cologne JB, Suzuki G, Akahoshi M, Nishi N, Takahashi I, Chayama K (2008) Risk factors for hepatocellular carcinoma in a Japanese population: a nested case-control study. Cancer Epidemiol Biomarkers Prev 17 (4):846-854. [PubMed: 18398026]

[9] Shimizu I, Kohno N, Tamaki K, Shono M, Huang HW, He JH, Yao DF (2007) Female hepatology: favorable role of estrogen in chronic liver disease with hepatitis B virus infection. World J Gastroenterol 13 (32):4295-4305. [PubMed: 17708600]

[10] Shimizu I (2003) Impact of oestrogens on the progression of liver disease. Liver Int 23 (1):63-69. [PubMed: 12640729]

[11] Fechner RE (1977) Benign hepatic lesions and orally administered contraceptives. A report of seven cases and a critical analysis of the literature. Hum Pathol 8 (3): 255-268. [PubMed: 192659]

[12] Vana J, Murphy GP, Aronoff BL, Baker HW (1977) Primary liver tumors and oral contraceptives. Results of a survey. JAMA 238 (20):2154-2158. [PubMed: 199752]

[13] Kemp CJ, Leary CN, Drinkwater NR (1989) Promotion of murine hepatocarcinogenesis by testosterone is androgen receptor-dependent but not cell autonomous. Proc Natl Acad Sci U S A 86 (19):7505-7509. [PubMed: 2798421]

[14] Poole TM, Drinkwater NR (1995) Hormonal and genetic interactions in murine hepatocarcinogenesis. Prog Clin Biol Res 391:187-194. [PubMed: 8532716]

[15] Nakatani T, Roy G, Fujimoto N, Asahara T, Ito A (2001) Sex hormone dependency of diethylnitrosamine-induced liver tumors in mice and chemoprevention by leuprorelin. Jpn J Cancer Res 92 (3):249-256. [PubMed: 11267934]

[16] Yamamoto R, Iishi H, Tatsuta M, Yamamoto T, Koike K, Kanda Y, Miyake A, Tsuji M, Terada N (1995) Correlation between serum prolactin levels and hepatocellular

tumorigenesis induced by 3'-methyl-4-dimethylaminoazobenzene in mice. Br J Cancer 72 (1):17-21. [PubMed: 7599048]

[17] Ormandy CJ, Binart N, Helloco C, Kelly PA (1998) Mouse prolactin receptor gene: genomic organization reveals alternative promoter usage and generation of isoforms via alternative 3'-exon splicing. DNA Cell Biol 17 (9):761-770. [PubMed: 9778035]

[18] Bigsby RM, Caperell-Grant A (2011) The role for estrogen receptor-alpha and prolactin receptor in sex-dependent DEN-induced liver tumorigenesis. Carcinogenesis 32 (8):1162-1166. [PubMed: 21606321]

[19] Pettersson K, Gustafsson JA (2001) Role of estrogen receptor beta in estrogen action. Annu Rev Physiol 63:165-192. [PubMed: 11181953]

[20] Gavrilova-Jordan LP, Price TM (2007) Actions of steroids in mitochondria. Semin Reprod Med 25 (3):154-164. [PubMed: 17447205]

[21] Boonyaratanakornkit V, Edwards DP (2007) Receptor mechanisms mediating nongenomic actions of sex steroids. Semin Reprod Med 25 (3):139-153. [PubMed: 17447204]

[22] Kalra M, Mayes J, Assefa S, Kaul AK, Kaul R (2008) Role of sex steroid receptors in pathobiology of hepatocellular carcinoma. World J Gastroenterol 14 (39):5945-5961. [PubMed: 18932272]

[23] Vizoso FJ, Rodriguez M, Altadill A, Gonzalez-Dieguez ML, Linares A, Gonzalez LO, Junquera S, Fresno-Forcelledo F, Corte MD, Rodrigo L (2007) Liver expression of steroid hormones and Apolipoprotein D receptors in hepatocellular carcinoma. World J Gastroenterol 13 (23):3221-3227. [PubMed: 17589901]

[24] Nagasue N, Kohno H, Chang YC, Yamanoi A, Nakamura T, Yukaya H, Hayashi T (1990) Clinicopathologic comparisons between estrogen receptor-positive and -negative hepatocellular carcinomas. Ann Surg 212 (2):150-154. [PubMed: 2165386]

[25] Jonas S, Bechstein WO, Heinze T, Kling N, Lobeck H, Tullius SG, Steinmueller T, Neuhaus P (1997) Female sex hormone receptor status in advanced hepatocellular carcinoma and outcome after surgical resection. Surgery 121 (4):456-461. [PubMed: 9122877]

[26] Villa E, Moles A, Ferretti I, Buttafoco P, Grottola A, Del Buono M, De Santis M, Manenti F (2000) Natural history of inoperable hepatocellular carcinoma: estrogen receptors' status in the tumor is the strongest prognostic factor for survival. Hepatology 32 (2):233-238. [PubMed: 10915729]

[27] Nagasue N, Chang YC, Hayashi T, Galizia G, Kohno H, Nakamura T, Yukaya H (1989) Androgen receptor in hepatocellular carcinoma as a prognostic factor after hepatic resection. Ann Surg 209 (4):424-427. [PubMed: 2539062]

[28] Boix L, Castells A, Bruix J, Sole M, Bru C, Fuster J, Rivera F, Rodes J (1995) Androgen receptors in hepatocellular carcinoma and surrounding liver: relationship with tu-

mor size and recurrence rate after surgical resection. J Hepatol 22 (6):616-622. [PubMed: 7560855]

[29] Zhang X, He L, Lu Y, Liu M, Huang X (1998) Androgen receptor in primary hepatocellular carcinoma and its clinical significance. Chin Med J (Engl) 111 (12):1083-1086. [PubMed: 11263369]

[30] Villa E, Dugani A, Fantoni E, Camellini L, Buttafoco P, Grottola A, Pompei G, De Santis M, Ferrari A, Manenti F (1996) Type of estrogen receptor determines response to antiestrogen therapy. Cancer Res 56 (17):3883-3885. [PubMed: 8752151]

[31] Han J, Ding L, Yuan B, Yang X, Wang X, Li J, Lu Q, Huang C, Ye Q (2006) Hepatitis B virus X protein and the estrogen receptor variant lacking exon 5 inhibit estrogen receptor signaling in hepatoma cells. Nucleic Acids Res 34 (10):3095-3106. [PubMed: 16757575]

[32] Watashi K, Inoue D, Hijikata M, Goto K, Aly HH, Shimotohno K (2007) Anti-hepatitis C virus activity of tamoxifen reveals the functional association of estrogen receptor with viral RNA polymerase NS5B. J Biol Chem 282 (45):32765-32772. [PubMed: 17704057]

[33] Yu MW, Yang YC, Yang SY, Cheng SW, Liaw YF, Lin SM, Chen CJ (2001) Hormonal markers and hepatitis B virus-related hepatocellular carcinoma risk: a nested case-control study among men. J Natl Cancer Inst 93 (21):1644-1651. [PubMed: 11698569]

[34] Yu MW, Cheng SW, Lin MW, Yang SY, Liaw YF, Chang HC, Hsiao TJ, Lin SM, Lee SD, Chen PJ, Liu CJ, Chen CJ (2000) Androgen-receptor gene CAG repeats, plasma testosterone levels, and risk of hepatitis B-related hepatocellular carcinoma. J Natl Cancer Inst 92 (24):2023-2028. [PubMed: 11121465]

[35] Wang N, Zheng Y, Yu X, Lin W, Chen Y, Jiang Q (2009) Sex-modified effect of hepatitis B virus infection on mortality from primary liver cancer. Am J Epidemiol 169 (8): 990-995. [PubMed: 19224979]

[36] Wu MH, Ma WL, Hsu CL, Chen YL, Ou JH, Ryan CK, Hung YC, Yeh S, Chang C (2010) Androgen receptor promotes hepatitis B virus-induced hepatocarcinogenesis through modulation of hepatitis B virus RNA transcription. Sci Transl Med 2 (32): 32ra35. [PubMed: 20484730]

[37] Colleoni M, Nelli P, Vicario G, Mastropasqua G, Manente P (1995) Megestrol acetate in unresectable hepatocellular carcinoma. Tumori 81 (5):351-353. [PubMed: 8804452]

[38] Chao Y, Chan WK, Huang YS, Teng HC, Wang SS, Lui WY, Whang-Peng J, Lee SD (1996) Phase II study of flutamide in the treatment of hepatocellular carcinoma. Cancer 77 (4):635-639. [PubMed: 8616754]

[39] Randomized trial of leuprorelin and flutamide in male patients with hepatocellular carcinoma treated with tamoxifen (2004). Hepatology 40 (6):1361-1369. [PubMed: 15565568]

[40] Ruden DM, Xiao L, Garfinkel MD, Lu X (2005) Hsp90 and environmental impacts on epigenetic states: a model for the trans-generational effects of diethylstibesterol on uterine development and cancer. Hum Mol Genet 14 Spec No 1:R149-155. [PubMed: 15809267]

[41] Di Maio M, De Maio E, Morabito A, D'Aniello R, De Feo G, Gallo C, Perrone F (2006) Hormonal treatment of human hepatocellular carcinoma. Ann N Y Acad Sci 1089:252-261. [PubMed: 17261772]

[42] Di Maio M, Daniele B, Pignata S, Gallo C, De Maio E, Morabito A, Piccirillo MC, Perrone F (2008) Is human hepatocellular carcinoma a hormone-responsive tumor? World J Gastroenterol 14 (11):1682-1689. [PubMed: 18350599]

[43] Bryant HU, Dere WH (1998) Selective estrogen receptor modulators: an alternative to hormone replacement therapy. Proc Soc Exp Biol Med 217 (1):45-52. [PubMed: 9421206]

[44] Grese TA, Dodge JA (1998) Selective estrogen receptor modulators (SERMs). Curr Pharm Des 4 (1):71-92. [PubMed: 10197034]

[45] Fournier B, Gutzwiller S, Dittmar T, Matthias G, Steenbergh P, Matthias P (2001) Estrogen receptor (ER)-alpha, but not ER-beta, mediates regulation of the insulin-like growth factor I gene by antiestrogens. J Biol Chem 276 (38):35444-35449. [PubMed: 11457856]

[46] Stendahl M, Ryden L, Nordenskjold B, Jonsson PE, Landberg G, Jirstrom K (2006) High progesterone receptor expression correlates to the effect of adjuvant tamoxifen in premenopausal breast cancer patients. Clin Cancer Res 12 (15):4614-4618. [PubMed: 16899609]

[47] Punglia RS, Kuntz KM, Winer EP, Weeks JC, Burstein HJ (2006) The impact of tumor progesterone receptor status on optimal adjuvant endocrine therapy for postmenopausal patients with early-stage breast cancer: a decision analysis. Cancer 106 (12): 2576-2582. [PubMed: 16703595]

[48] Eagon PK, Elm MS, Epley MJ, Shinozuka H, Rao KN (1996) Sex steroid metabolism and receptor status in hepatic hyperplasia and cancer in rats. Gastroenterology 110 (4):1199-1207. [PubMed: 8613010]

[49] Nagasue N, Yu L, Yukaya H, Kohno H, Nakamura T (1995) Androgen and oestrogen receptors in hepatocellular carcinoma and surrounding liver parenchyma: impact on intrahepatic recurrence after hepatic resection. Br J Surg 82 (4):542-547. [PubMed: 7613907]

[50] Mercader M, Bodner BK, Moser MT, Kwon PS, Park ES, Manecke RG, Ellis TM, Wojcik EM, Yang D, Flanigan RC, Waters WB, Kast WM, Kwon ED (2001) T cell infiltration of the prostate induced by androgen withdrawal in patients with prostate cancer. Proc Natl Acad Sci U S A 98 (25):14565-14570. [PubMed: 11734652]

[51] Berasain C, Castillo J, Perugorria MJ, Latasa MU, Prieto J, Avila MA (2009) Inflammation and liver cancer: new molecular links. Ann N Y Acad Sci 1155:206-221. [PubMed: 19250206]

[52] Boix L, Bruix J, Castells A, Fuster J, Bru C, Visa J, Rivera F, Rodes J (1993) Sex hormone receptors in hepatocellular carcinoma. Is there a rationale for hormonal treatment? J Hepatol 17 (2):187-191. [PubMed: 8383159]

[53] Simard J, Dauvois S, Haagensen DE, Levesque C, Merand Y, Labrie F (1990) Regulation of progesterone-binding breast cyst protein GCDFP-24 secretion by estrogens and androgens in human breast cancer cells: a new marker of steroid action in breast cancer. Endocrinology 126 (6):3223-3231. [PubMed: 2351114]

[54] Simard J, de Launoit Y, Haagensen DE, Labrie F (1992) Additive stimulatory action of glucocorticoids and androgens on basal and estrogen-repressed apolipoprotein-D messenger ribonucleic acid levels and secretion in human breast cancer cells. Endocrinology 130 (3):1115-1121. [PubMed: 1537279]

[55] Sugimoto K, Simard J, Haagensen DE, Labrie F (1994) Inverse relationships between cell proliferation and basal or androgen-stimulated apolipoprotein D secretion in LNCaP human prostate cancer cells. J Steroid Biochem Mol Biol 51 (3-4):167-174. [PubMed: 7526888]

[56] Utsunomiya T, Ogawa K, Yoshinaga K, Ohta M, Yamashita K, Mimori K, Inoue H, Ezaki T, Yoshikawa Y, Mori M (2005) Clinicopathologic and prognostic values of apolipoprotein D alterations in hepatocellular carcinoma. Int J Cancer 116 (1): 105-109. [PubMed: 15756681]

[57] Lopez-Boado YS, Tolivia J, Lopez-Otin C (1994) Apolipoprotein D gene induction by retinoic acid is concomitant with growth arrest and cell differentiation in human breast cancer cells. J Biol Chem 269 (43):26871-26878. [PubMed: 7929425]

[58] Lopez-Boado YS, Diez-Itza I, Tolivia J, Lopez-Otin C (1994) Glucocorticoids and androgens up-regulate the Zn-alpha 2-glycoprotein messenger RNA in human breast cancer cells. Breast Cancer Res Treat 29 (3):247-258. [PubMed: 8049458]

[59] P'Eng F K, Lui WY, Chang TJ, Kao HL, Wu LH, Liu TY, Chi CW (1988) Glucocorticoid receptors in hepatocellular carcinoma and adjacent liver tissue. Cancer 62 (10): 2134-2138. [PubMed: 2460210]

[60] Sano K, Takayama T, Murakami K, Saiki I, Makuuchi M (2003) Overexpression of retinoic acid receptor alpha in hepatocellular carcinoma. Clin Cancer Res 9 (10 Pt 1): 3679-3683. [PubMed: 14506158]

[61] Clerici C, Castellani D, Russo G, Fiorucci S, Sabatino G, Giuliano V, Gentili G, Morelli O, Raffo P, Baldoni M, Morelli A, Toma S (2004) Treatment with all-trans retinoic acid plus tamoxifen and vitamin E in advanced hepatocellular carcinoma. Anticancer Res 24 (2C):1255-1260. [PubMed: 15154656]

[62] Diez-Itza I, Sanchez LM, Allende MT, Vizoso F, Ruibal A, Lopez-Otin C (1993) Zn-alpha 2-glycoprotein levels in breast cancer cytosols and correlation with clinical, histological and biochemical parameters. Eur J Cancer 29A (9):1256-1260. [PubMed: 8343263]

[63] Huang Y, Li LZ, Zhang CZ, Yi C, Liu LL, Zhou X, Xie GB, Cai MY, Li Y, Yun JP (2012) Decreased expression of zinc-alpha2-glycoprotein in hepatocellular carcinoma associates with poor prognosis. J Transl Med 10 (1):106. [PubMed: 22625427]

[64] Xu H, Wei Y, Zhang Y, Xu Y, Li F, Liu J, Zhang W, Han X, Tan R, Shen P (2012) Oestrogen attenuates tumour progression in hepatocellular carcinoma. J Pathol 228 (2): 216-229. [PubMed: 22374713]

[65] Gold SM, Sasidhar MV, Morales LB, Du S, Sicotte NL, Tiwari-Woodruff SK, Voskuhl RR (2009) Estrogen treatment decreases matrix metalloproteinase (MMP)-9 in autoimmune demyelinating disease through estrogen receptor alpha (ERalpha). Lab Invest 89 (10):1076-1083. [PubMed: 19668239]

[66] Claassen H, Steffen R, Hassenpflug J, Varoga D, Wruck CJ, Brandenburg LO, Pufe T (2010) 17beta-estradiol reduces expression of MMP-1, -3, and -13 in human primary articular chondrocytes from female patients cultured in a three dimensional alginate system. Cell Tissue Res 342 (2):283-293. [PubMed: 20941509]

[67] Zhou H, Kimura K, Orita T, Nishida T, Sonoda KH (2011) Inhibition by female sex hormones of collagen degradation by corneal fibroblasts. Mol Vis 17:3415-3422. [PubMed: 22219637]

[68] Nelson AR, Fingleton B, Rothenberg ML, Matrisian LM (2000) Matrix metalloproteinases: biologic activity and clinical implications. J Clin Oncol 18 (5):1135-1149. [PubMed: 10694567]

[69] McCawley LJ, Matrisian LM (2001) Matrix metalloproteinases: they're not just for matrix anymore! Curr Opin Cell Biol 13 (5):534-540. [PubMed: 11544020]

[70] Demers M, Couillard J, Belanger S, St-Pierre Y (2005) New roles for matrix metalloproteinases in metastasis. Crit Rev Immunol 25 (6):493-523. [PubMed: 16390324]

[71] Brinckerhoff CE, Rutter JL, Benbow U (2000) Interstitial collagenases as markers of tumor progression. Clin Cancer Res 6 (12):4823-4830. [PubMed: 11156241]

[72] Sternlicht MD, Werb Z (2001) How matrix metalloproteinases regulate cell behavior. Annu Rev Cell Dev Biol 17:463-516. [PubMed: 11687497]

[73] Egeblad M, Werb Z (2002) New functions for the matrix metalloproteinases in cancer progression. Nat Rev Cancer 2 (3):161-174. [PubMed: 11990853]

[74] Turk V, Kos J, Turk B (2004) Cysteine cathepsins (proteases)--on the main stage of cancer? Cancer Cell 5 (5):409-410. [PubMed: 15144947]

[75] Rifkin DB, Mazzieri R, Munger JS, Noguera I, Sung J (1999) Proteolytic control of growth factor availability. APMIS 107 (1):80-85. [PubMed: 10190283]

[76] Manes S, Llorente M, Lacalle RA, Gomez-Mouton C, Kremer L, Mira E, Martinez AC (1999) The matrix metalloproteinase-9 regulates the insulin-like growth factor-triggered autocrine response in DU-145 carcinoma cells. J Biol Chem 274 (11):6935-6945. [PubMed: 10066747]

[77] Noe V, Fingleton B, Jacobs K, Crawford HC, Vermeulen S, Steelant W, Bruyneel E, Matrisian LM, Mareel M (2001) Release of an invasion promoter E-cadherin fragment by matrilysin and stromelysin-1. J Cell Sci 114 (Pt 1):111-118. [PubMed: 11112695]

[78] Fingleton B, Vargo-Gogola T, Crawford HC, Matrisian LM (2001) Matrilysin [MMP-7] expression selects for cells with reduced sensitivity to apoptosis. Neoplasia 3 (6):459-468. [PubMed: 11774028]

[79] Yu Q, Stamenkovic I (2000) Cell surface-localized matrix metalloproteinase-9 proteolytically activates TGF-beta and promotes tumor invasion and angiogenesis. Genes Dev 14 (2):163-176. [PubMed: 10652271]

[80] Stetler-Stevenson WG (1999) Matrix metalloproteinases in angiogenesis: a moving target for therapeutic intervention. J Clin Invest 103 (9):1237-1241. [PubMed: 10225966]

[81] Dong Z, Kumar R, Yang X, Fidler IJ (1997) Macrophage-derived metalloelastase is responsible for the generation of angiostatin in Lewis lung carcinoma. Cell 88 (6): 801-810. [PubMed: 9118223]

[82] Cornelius LA, Nehring LC, Harding E, Bolanowski M, Welgus HG, Kobayashi DK, Pierce RA, Shapiro SD (1998) Matrix metalloproteinases generate angiostatin: effects on neovascularization. J Immunol 161 (12):6845-6852. [PubMed: 9862716]

[83] Ferreras M, Felbor U, Lenhard T, Olsen BR, Delaisse J (2000) Generation and degradation of human endostatin proteins by various proteinases. FEBS Lett 486 (3): 247-251. [PubMed: 11119712]

[84] Jiang Y, Goldberg ID, Shi YE (2002) Complex roles of tissue inhibitors of metalloproteinases in cancer. Oncogene 21 (14):2245-2252. [PubMed: 11948407]

[85] Baker AH, George SJ, Zaltsman AB, Murphy G, Newby AC (1999) Inhibition of invasion and induction of apoptotic cell death of cancer cell lines by overexpression of TIMP-3. Br J Cancer 79 (9-10):1347-1355. [PubMed: 10188875]

[86] Yamamoto H, Itoh F, Adachi Y, Sakamoto H, Adachi M, Hinoda Y, Imai K (1997) Relation of enhanced secretion of active matrix metalloproteinases with tumor spread in human hepatocellular carcinoma. Gastroenterology 112 (4):1290-1296. [PubMed: 9098015]

[87] Theret N, Musso O, Turlin B, Lotrian D, Bioulac-Sage P, Campion JP, Boudjema K, Clement B (2001) Increased extracellular matrix remodeling is associated with tumor

progression in human hepatocellular carcinomas. Hepatology 34 (1):82-88. [PubMed: 11431737]

[88] Ishii Y, Nakasato Y, Kobayashi S, Yamazaki Y, Aoki T (2003) A study on angiogenesis-related matrix metalloproteinase networks in primary hepatocellular carcinoma. J Exp Clin Cancer Res 22 (3):461-470. [PubMed: 14582707]

[89] McKenna GJ, Chen Y, Smith RM, Meneghetti A, Ong C, McMaster R, Scudamore CH, Chung SW (2002) A role for matrix metalloproteinases and tumor host interaction in hepatocellular carcinomas. Am J Surg 183 (5):588-594. [PubMed: 12034400]

[90] Sawada S, Murakami K, Murata J, Tsukada K, Saiki I (2001) Accumulation of extracellular matrix in the liver induces high metastatic potential of hepatocellular carcinoma to the lung. Int J Oncol 19 (1):65-70. [PubMed: 11408924]

[91] Maatta M, Soini Y, Liakka A, Autio-Harmainen H (2000) Differential expression of matrix metalloproteinase (MMP)-2, MMP-9, and membrane type 1-MMP in hepatocellular and pancreatic adenocarcinoma: implications for tumor progression and clinical prognosis. Clin Cancer Res 6 (7):2726-2734. [PubMed: 10914717]

[92] Cui J, Dong BW, Liang P, Yu XL, Yu DJ (2004) Effect of c-myc, Ki-67, MMP-2 and VEGF expression on prognosis of hepatocellular carcinoma patients undergoing tumor resection. World J Gastroenterol 10 (10):1533-1536. [PubMed: 15133868]

[93] Zhang Q, Chen X, Zhou J, Zhang L, Zhao Q, Chen G, Xu J, Qian F, Chen Z (2006) CD147, MMP-2, MMP-9 and MVD-CD34 are significant predictors of recurrence after liver transplantation in hepatocellular carcinoma patients. Cancer Biol Ther 5 (7): 808-814. [PubMed: 16775432]

[94] Gao ZH, Tretiakova MS, Liu WH, Gong C, Farris PD, Hart J (2006) Association of E-cadherin, matrix metalloproteinases, and tissue inhibitors of metalloproteinases with the progression and metastasis of hepatocellular carcinoma. Mod Pathol 19 (4): 533-540. [PubMed: 16474379]

[95] Arii S, Mise M, Harada T, Furutani M, Ishigami S, Niwano M, Mizumoto M, Fukumoto M, Imamura M (1996) Overexpression of matrix metalloproteinase 9 gene in hepatocellular carcinoma with invasive potential. Hepatology 24 (2):316-322. [PubMed: 8690399]

[96] Hayasaka A, Suzuki N, Fujimoto N, Iwama S, Fukuyama E, Kanda Y, Saisho H (1996) Elevated plasma levels of matrix metalloproteinase-9 (92-kd type IV collagenase/gelatinase B) in hepatocellular carcinoma. Hepatology 24 (5):1058-1062. [PubMed: 8903375]

[97] Sakamoto Y, Mafune K, Mori M, Shiraishi T, Imamura H, Takayama T, Makuuchi M (2000) Overexpression of MMP-9 correlates with growth of small hepatocellular carcinoma. Int J Oncol 17 (2):237-243. [PubMed: 10891530]

[98] Harada T, Arii S, Mise M, Imamura T, Higashitsuji H, Furutani M, Niwano M, Ishigami S, Fukumoto M, Seiki M, Sato H, Imamura M (1998) Membrane-type matrix

metalloproteinase-1(MT1-MTP) gene is overexpressed in highly invasive hepatocellular carcinomas. J Hepatol 28 (2):231-239. [PubMed: 9514536]

[99] Chen X, Cheung ST, So S, Fan ST, Barry C, Higgins J, Lai KM, Ji J, Dudoit S, Ng IO, Van De Rijn M, Botstein D, Brown PO (2002) Gene expression patterns in human liver cancers. Mol Biol Cell 13 (6):1929-1939. [PubMed: 12058060]

[100] Ip YC, Cheung ST, Leung KL, Fan ST (2005) Mechanism of metastasis by membrane type 1-matrix metalloproteinase in hepatocellular carcinoma. World J Gastroenterol 11 (40):6269-6276. [PubMed: 16419154]

[101] Bosch FX, Ribes J, Borras J (1999) Epidemiology of primary liver cancer. Semin Liver Dis 19 (3):271-285. [PubMed: 10518307]

[102] Poon RT, Fan ST, Lo CM, Liu CL, Ng IO, Wong J (2000) Long-term prognosis after resection of hepatocellular carcinoma associated with hepatitis B-related cirrhosis. J Clin Oncol 18 (5):1094-1101. [PubMed: 10694562]

[103] Giannelli G, Bergamini C, Fransvea E, Marinosci F, Quaranta V, Antonaci S (2001) Human hepatocellular carcinoma (HCC) cells require both alpha3beta1 integrin and matrix metalloproteinases activity for migration and invasion. Lab Invest 81 (4): 613-627. [PubMed: 11304581]

[104] Chen R, Cui J, Xu C, Xue T, Guo K, Gao D, Liu Y, Ye S, Ren Z (2012) The Significance of MMP-9 Over MMP-2 in HCC Invasiveness and Recurrence of Hepatocellular Carcinoma After Curative Resection. Ann Surg Oncol 19 Suppl 3:375-384. [PubMed: 21681378]

[105] Ng KT, Qi X, Kong KL, Cheung BY, Lo CM, Poon RT, Fan ST, Man K (2011) Overexpression of matrix metalloproteinase-12 (MMP-12) correlates with poor prognosis of hepatocellular carcinoma. Eur J Cancer 47 (15):2299-2305. [PubMed: 21683576]

[106] Stamenkovic I (2000) Matrix metalloproteinases in tumor invasion and metastasis. Semin Cancer Biol 10 (6):415-433. [PubMed: 11170864]

[107] Akriviadis EA, Llovet JM, Efremidis SC, Shouval D, Canelo R, Ringe B, Meyers WC (1998) Hepatocellular carcinoma. Br J Surg 85 (10):1319-1331. [PubMed: 9782009]

[108] Ozaki T, Mochizuki H, Ichikawa Y, Fukuzawa Y, Yoshida S, Morimoto M (2000) Persistence of hepatitis B surface antibody levels after vaccination with a recombinant hepatitis B vaccine: a 3-year follow-up study. J Oral Sci 42 (3):147-150. [PubMed: 11111325]

[109] Milani S, Herbst H, Schuppan D, Grappone C, Pellegrini G, Pinzani M, Casini A, Calabro A, Ciancio G, Stefanini F, et al. (1994) Differential expression of matrix-metalloproteinase-1 and -2 genes in normal and fibrotic human liver. Am J Pathol 144 (3): 528-537. [PubMed: 8129038]

[110] Benyon RC, Iredale JP, Goddard S, Winwood PJ, Arthur MJ (1996) Expression of tissue inhibitor of metalloproteinases 1 and 2 is increased in fibrotic human liver. Gastroenterology 110 (3):821-831. [PubMed: 8608892]

[111] Kapranos N, Karaiossifidi H, Kouri E, Vasilaros S (1996) Nm23 expression in breast ductal carcinomas: a ten year follow-up study in a uniform group of node-negative breast cancer patients. Anticancer Res 16 (6C):3987-3990. [PubMed: 9042324]

[112] Takahara T, Furui K, Yata Y, Jin B, Zhang LP, Nambu S, Sato H, Seiki M, Watanabe A (1997) Dual expression of matrix metalloproteinase-2 and membrane-type 1-matrix metalloproteinase in fibrotic human livers. Hepatology 26 (6):1521-1529. [PubMed: 9397993]

[113] Altadill A, Rodriguez M, Gonzalez LO, Junquera S, Corte MD, Gonzalez-Dieguez ML, Linares A, Barbon E, Fresno-Forcelledo M, Rodrigo L, Vizoso FJ (2009) Liver expression of matrix metalloproteases and their inhibitors in hepatocellular carcinoma. Dig Liver Dis 41 (10):740-748. [PubMed: 19372066]

[114] Preaux AM, Mallat A, Nhieu JT, D'Ortho MP, Hembry RM, Mavier P (1999) Matrix metalloproteinase-2 activation in human hepatic fibrosis regulation by cell-matrix interactions. Hepatology 30 (4):944-950. [PubMed: 10498646]

[115] Nakatsukasa H, Ashida K, Higashi T, Ohguchi S, Tsuboi S, Hino N, Nouso K, Urabe Y, Kinugasa N, Yoshida K, Uematsu S, Ishizaki M, Kobayashi Y, Tsuji T (1996) Cellular distribution of transcripts for tissue inhibitor of metalloproteinases 1 and 2 in human hepatocellular carcinomas. Hepatology 24 (1):82-88. [PubMed: 8707287]

[116] Zhang H, Wang YS, Han G, Shi Y (2007) TIMP-3 gene transfection suppresses invasive and metastatic capacity of human hepatocarcinoma cell line HCC-7721. Hepatobiliary Pancreat Dis Int 6 (5):487-491. [PubMed: 17897911]

[117] Roeb E, Bosserhoff AK, Hamacher S, Jansen B, Dahmen J, Wagner S, Matern S (2005) Enhanced migration of tissue inhibitor of metalloproteinase overexpressing hepatoma cells is attributed to gelatinases: relevance to intracellular signaling pathways. World J Gastroenterol 11 (8):1096-1104. [PubMed: 15754388]

[118] Taras D, Blanc JF, Rullier A, Dugot-Senant N, Laurendeau I, Vidaud M, Rosenbaum J (2007) Pravastatin reduces lung metastasis of rat hepatocellular carcinoma via a coordinated decrease of MMP expression and activity. J Hepatol 46 (1):69-76. [PubMed: 16935385]

[119] Xu J, Xu HY, Zhang Q, Song F, Jiang JL, Yang XM, Mi L, Wen N, Tian R, Wang L, Yao H, Feng Q, Zhang Y, Xing JL, Zhu P, Chen ZN (2007) HAb18G/CD147 functions in invasion and metastasis of hepatocellular carcinoma. Mol Cancer Res 5 (6):605-614. [PubMed: 17579119]

[120] Yeh CB, Hsieh MJ, Hsieh YH, Chien MH, Chiou HL, Yang SF (2012) Antimetastatic effects of norcantharidin on hepatocellular carcinoma by transcriptional inhibition of

MMP-9 through modulation of NF-kB activity. PLoS One 7 (2):e31055. [PubMed: 22363545]

[121] Chen RX, Xia YH, Xue TC, Zhang H, Ye SL (2011) Down-regulation of osteopontin inhibits metastasis of hepatocellular carcinoma cells via a mechanism involving MMP-2 and uPA. Oncol Rep 25 (3):803-808. [PubMed: 21174062]

[122] Duffy MJ, Duffy GJ (1978) Estradiol receptors in human liver. J Steroid Biochem 9 (3): 233-235. [PubMed: 651349]

[123] Macdonald JS, Lippman ME, Woolley PV, Petrucci PP, Schein PS (1978) Hepatic estrogen and progesterone receptors in an estrogen-associated hepatic neoplasm. Cancer Chemother Pharmacol 1 (3):135-138. [PubMed: 373914]

[124] Friedman MA, Demanes DJ, Hoffman PG, Jr. (1982) Hepatomas: hormone receptors and therapy. Am J Med 73 (3):362-366. [PubMed: 6289660]

[125] Bojar H, Schutte J, Staib W, Broelsch C (1982) Does human liver contain estrogen receptors? A comparative study of estrogen binding in human and rodent liver. Klin Wochenschr 60 (8):417-425. [PubMed: 7098385]

[126] Porter LE, Elm MS, Van Thiel DH, Dugas MC, Eagon PK (1983) Characterization and quantitation of human hepatic estrogen receptor. Gastroenterology 84 (4):704-712. [PubMed: 6825981]

[127] Iqbal MJ, Wilkinson ML, Johnson PJ, Williams R (1983) Sex steroid receptor proteins in foetal, adult and malignant human liver tissue. Br J Cancer 48 (6):791-796. [PubMed: 6317004]

[128] Nagasue N, Ito A, Yukaya H, Ogawa Y (1986) Estrogen receptors in hepatocellular carcinoma. Cancer 57 (1):87-91. [PubMed: 3000573]

[129] Negro F, Papotti M, Pacchioni D, Galimi F, Bonino F, Bussolati G (1994) Detection of human androgen receptor mRNA in hepatocellular carcinoma by in situ hybridisation. Liver 14 (4):213-219. [PubMed: 7968281]

[130] Kohigashi K, Fukuda Y, Imura H (1987) Estrogen receptors in hepatocellular carcinoma: is endocrine therapy for hepatocellular carcinoma likely to be effective? Gastroenterol Jpn 22 (3):322-330. [PubMed: 3040510]

[131] Ohnami S, Nakata H, Nagafuchi Y, Zeze F, Eto S (1988) [Estrogen receptors in human gastric, hepatocellular, and gallbladder carcinomas and normal liver tissues]. Gan To Kagaku Ryoho 15 (10):2923-2928. [PubMed: 2845868]

[132] Nagasue N, Kohno H, Chang YC, Hayashi T, Utsumi Y, Nakamura T, Yukaya H (1989) Androgen and estrogen receptors in hepatocellular carcinoma and the surrounding liver in women. Cancer 63 (1):112-116. [PubMed: 2535950]

[133] Hamazaki K, Miura H, Sakai H, Sato S, Yunoki M, Miichi N, Noda T, Mori M, Orita K (1989) [Estrogen and androgen receptors in hepatocellular carcinoma and in non-cancerous liver tissue]. Gan No Rinsho 35 (10):1109-1113. [PubMed: 2550681]

[134] Nagasue N, Kohno H, Chang Y, Hayashi T, Nakamura T (1990) Specificity of androgen receptors of hepatocellular carcinoma and liver in humans. Hepatogastroenterology 37 (5):474-479. [PubMed: 2174826]

[135] Eagon PK, Francavilla A, DiLeo A, Elm MS, Gennari L, Mazzaferro V, Colella G, Van Thiel DH, Strazl TE (1991) Quantitation of estrogen and androgen receptors in hepatocellular carcinoma and adjacent normal human liver. Dig Dis Sci 36 (9):1303-1308. [PubMed: 1654243]

[136] Pacchioni D, Papotti M, Andorno E, Bonino F, Mondardini A, Oliveri F, Brunetto M, Bussolati G, Negro F (1993) Expression of estrogen receptor mRNA in tumorous and non-tumorous liver tissue as detected by in situ hybridization. J Surg Oncol Suppl 3:14-17. [PubMed: 8389161]

[137] Wang AG, Lee KY, Kim SY, Choi JY, Lee KH, Kim WH, Wang HJ, Kim JM, Park MG, Yeom YI, Kim NS, Yu DY, Lee DS (2006) The expression of estrogen receptors in hepatocellular carcinoma in Korean patients. Yonsei Med J 47 (6):811-816. [PubMed: 17191310]

[138] Wong LY, Chan SH, Oon CJ, Rauff A (1984) Immunocytochemical localization of testosterone in human hepatocellular carcinoma. Histochem J 16 (6):687-692. [PubMed: 6330003]

[139] Ohnishi S, Murakami T, Moriyama T, Mitamura K, Imawari M (1986) Androgen and estrogen receptors in hepatocellular carcinoma and in the surrounding noncancerous liver tissue. Hepatology 6 (3):440-443. [PubMed: 3011631]

[140] Nagasue N, Kohno H, Yamanoi A, Kimoto T, Chang YC, Nakamura T (1991) Progesterone receptor in hepatocellular carcinoma. Correlation with androgen and estrogen receptors. Cancer 67 (10):2501-2505. [PubMed: 1849788]

[141] Francavilla A, Panella C, Amoruso A, Giangaspero A, Gennari L, Mazzaferro V, Colella G, Van Thiel DH, Starzl TE (1991) Role of estrogens and epidermal growth factor in hepatocellular carcinoma (HCC). Dig Dis Sci 36 (9):1299-1302. [PubMed: 1654242]

[142] Villa E, Camellini L, Dugani A, Zucchi F, Grottola A, Merighi A, Buttafoco P, Losi L, Manenti F (1995) Variant estrogen receptor messenger RNA species detected in human primary hepatocellular carcinoma. Cancer Res 55 (3):498-500. [PubMed: 7834616]

[143] Ng IO, Ng M, Fan ST (1997) Better survival in women with resected hepatocellular carcinoma is not related to tumor proliferation or expression of hormone receptors. Am J Gastroenterol 92 (8):1355-1358. [PubMed: 9260806]

[144] Villa E, Dugani A, Moles A, Camellini L, Grottola A, Buttafoco P, Merighi A, Ferretti I, Esposito P, Miglioli L, Bagni A, Troisi R, De Hemptinne B, Praet M, Callea F, Manenti F (1998) Variant liver estrogen receptor transcripts already occur at an early stage of chronic liver disease. Hepatology 27 (4):983-988. [PubMed: 9537437]

[145] Iavarone M, Lampertico P, Seletti C, Francesca Donato M, Ronchi G, del Ninno E, Colombo M (2003) The clinical and pathogenetic significance of estrogen receptor-beta expression in chronic liver diseases and liver carcinoma. Cancer 98 (3):529-534. [PubMed: 12879470]

[146] Moon WS, Chang K, Tarnawski AS (2004) Overexpression of metastatic tumor antigen 1 in hepatocellular carcinoma: Relationship to vascular invasion and estrogen receptor-alpha. Hum Pathol 35 (4):424-429. [PubMed: 15116322]

[147] Xing BC, Wang JH, Wang Y, Hao CY, Huang XF (2004) [Expression of wild type and variant estrogen receptors in human hepatocellular carcinoma]. Beijing Da Xue Xue Bao 36 (6):620-622. [PubMed: 15605095]

[148] Meza-Junco J, Montano-Loza AJ, Gamboa-Dominguez A, Green-Renner D (2007) Expression of oestrogen and growth factor receptors in hepatocellular carcinoma. Clin Oncol (R Coll Radiol) 19 (10):801-802. [PubMed: 17822888]

[149] Nagasue N, Ito A, Yukaya H, Ogawa Y (1985) Androgen receptors in hepatocellular carcinoma and surrounding parenchyma. Gastroenterology 89 (3):643-647. [PubMed: 2991072]

[150] Wilkinson ML, Iqbal MJ, Williams R (1985) Characterisation of high affinity binding sites of androgens in primary hepatocellular carcinoma. Clin Chim Acta 152 (1-2): 105-113. [PubMed: 2414040]

[151] Bannister P, Meystre CM, Losowsky MS (1988) Androgen receptor concentrations in needle biopsy specimens of human liver. Liver 8 (1):28-31. [PubMed: 3367706]

[152] Nagasue N, Yamanoi A, Kohno H, Kimoto T, Chang Y, Taniura H, Uchida M, Nakamura T (1992) Androgen receptor in cirrhotic liver, adenomatous hyperplastic nodule and hepatocellular carcinoma in the human. Hepatogastroenterology 39 (5): 455-460. [PubMed: 1334038]

[153] Tavian D, De Petro G, Pitozzi A, Portolani N, Giulini SM, Barlati S (2002) Androgen receptor mRNA under-expression in poorly differentiated human hepatocellular carcinoma. Histol Histopathol 17 (4):1113-1119. [PubMed: 12371139]

[154] Engstrom PF, Levin B, Moertel CG, Schutt A (1990) A phase II trial of tamoxifen in hepatocellular carcinoma. Cancer 65 (12):2641-2643. [PubMed: 2160313]

[155] Castells A, Bruix J, Bru C, Ayuso C, Roca M, Boix L, Vilana R, Rodes J (1995) Treatment of hepatocellular carcinoma with tamoxifen: a double-blind placebo-controlled trial in 120 patients. Gastroenterology 109 (3):917-922. [PubMed: 7657122]

[156] Liu CL, Fan ST, Ng IO, Lo CM, Poon RT, Wong J (2000) Treatment of advanced hepatocellular carcinoma with tamoxifen and the correlation with expression of hormone receptors: a prospective randomized study. Am J Gastroenterol 95 (1):218-222. [PubMed: 10638587]

[157] Villa E, Ferretti I, Grottola A, Buttafoco P, Buono MG, Giannini F, Manno M, Bertani H, Dugani A, Manenti F (2001) Hormonal therapy with megestrol in inoperable hepatocellular carcinoma characterized by variant oestrogen receptors. Br J Cancer 84 (7):881-885. [PubMed: 11286465]

[158] Chow PK, Tai BC, Tan CK, Machin D, Win KM, Johnson PJ, Soo KC (2002) High-dose tamoxifen in the treatment of inoperable hepatocellular carcinoma: A multicenter randomized controlled trial. Hepatology 36 (5):1221-1226. [PubMed: 12395333]